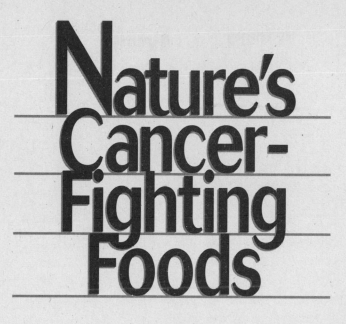

Nature's Cancer-Fighting Foods

Nature's Cancer-Fighting Foods

Prevent and Reverse
the Most Common Forms of Cancer
Using the Proven Power
of Great Food and Easy Recipes

Verne Varona

REWARD BOOKS

a member of
Penguin Putnam Inc.
New York

The information presented in this book is by no means intended to replace the advice of your personal medical professional. The author does not directly, or indirectly, dispense medical advice or prescribe the use of diet as a means of treating disease without prior medical approval. If you are seriously ill or undergoing medical treatment, please consult with a physician before making any dietary changes, taking supplements or begin any type of exercise program without first consulting the appropriate medical professinal. The author and publisher make no claims as to being able to prevent, treat, or cure any form of cancer or other disease and assume no responsibility for the health of the reader. We urge you to seek the best medical resources available to help you make informed decisions.

✦ Reward Books
a member of Penguin Putnam Inc.
375 Hudson Street
New York, NY 10014

Library of Congress Cataloging-in-Publication Data

Varona, Verne.
  Nature's cancer-fighting foods / Verne Varona.
    p. cm.
  Includes index.
  ISBN 0-7352-0176-5 (paperback)—ISBN 0-13-017087-9 (preprinted case)
  1. Cancer—Diet therapy.   2. Cancer—Prevention.   I. Title.

  RC271.D52 V37 2001
  616.99'40654—dc21

Printed in the United States of America

10 9 8 7 6 5 4 3 2 1   10 9 8 7 6 5 4

Most Reward Books are available at special quantity discounts for bulk purchases for sales promotions, premiums, fund-raising, or educational use. Special books, or book excerpts, can also be created to fit specific needs.

For details, write: Special Markets, Penguin Putnam Inc., 375 Hudson Street, New York, New York 10014.

In loving memory of my Mother and Father

Sara Irene Hertzovitz
and
Carlos Enrique Varona

CONTENTS

Preface   ix

Introduction   xv

CHAPTER 1

Eating Habits, Food Quality, and Cancer Prevention   1

CHAPTER 2

Carbohydrates, Fats, and Proteins: Myths, Truths,
and Healthy Advice   13

CHAPTER 3

Phytochemical Super Heroes and Amazing Antioxidants   43

CHAPTER 4

The Healing Power of Acid and Alkaline   59

CHAPTER 5

The Meat and Dairy Issue   85

CHAPTER 6

No-Guilt Craving Strategies for Eliminating Sugar,
Fat, and Overeating   103

CHAPTER 7

The Best Kept Secret of the Orient: The Soup
That Heals   137

CHAPTER 8

Harvesting the Good Earth—Medicinal Herbs
and Mushrooms   147

CHAPTER 9

Health Supportive Supplement Strategies   177

CHAPTER 10

Nature's Cancer-Fighting Food Plan   201

CHAPTER 11

Food Preparation and Cooking for Lifetime
Health Benefits   227

CHAPTER 12

Salud! Nutritious, Delicious, and Easy-to-Make
Recipes   263

Afterword   311

Acknowledgments   317

Resource Guide   325

Endnotes   337

Index   359

PREFACE

"He that conceals his grief finds no remedy for it."
—Turkish Proverb

Brooklyn, New York, 1965. Late October. The colors of autumn fell from the trees as the chilly morning air, tinged with frost, conspired to shorten the season. An anxious early winter was announcing its arrival.

A boy of thirteen, unconcerned about being marked truant, hid his schoolbooks behind a neighbor's shrubbery and hurried to a nearby subway that would take him from sleepy suburban Brooklyn into the pedestrian jungle of New York City. His concern, far from the typical concerns of most thirteen-year-olds rejoicing in long awaited teen-hood, were far more serious; his mother, at the age of thirty-five years, lay on her deathbed at a central Manhattan hospital, a passive host to a rapid breeding of cancer cells in the shape of multiple tumors. He'd convinced himself she would recover. It was just a matter of time, he thought. And these five words became his repetitive mantra; "just a matter of time . . . just a matter of time . . ."

Only two weeks earlier, while watching television in the living room of their two-story town home, he heard a loud thud echo from the second floor. It jarred the entire house and prompted him to race up the stairs. At the top landing, on the new tweed, blue-green carpet, his mother had fallen into a fetal posture. She lay unconscious, her body convulsing rhythmically as the white foam of saliva spilled from her lips. He stood for an instant, benumbed by the living picture that would be imprinted in his mind and heart forever.

Pushing aside anguish and helplessness, instinct rapidly took command and he managed to drag her limp body from the hallway into the bedroom and onto her bed. He mumbled words of comfort while desperately fighting his own demons of dread and confusion. Grabbing for the telephone he dialed an operator to send for an ambulance immediately. Then, he returned to her bedside and embraced her limp body, pleading with her through his tears not to die, telling her he loved her and that he would always take care of her when she got better.

Quick-moving ambulance attendants wheeled a stretcher into the house and secured his mother beneath worn leather straps that dangled from the underside of its aluminum frame. Outside, the flashing red ambulance lights illuminated the faces of shocked neighbors as they milled and murmured in the darkness. The boy jumped into the hospital ambulance and wove his fingers through his mother's while the Paramedics prepared an IV and radioed their dispatcher. Racing into the dark with sirens blaring, the reflective blur of street lamps and traffic lights passed like a mosaic across his face.

Now, two weeks had passed since that ride to the emergency ward; fourteen days filled with school, homework and endless self-imposed household chores, done by reflex, in a futile effort to keep his mind and heart detached. During a quiet dinner meal his stepfather cheerfully reported on his mother's improving condition. She had been moved to room 506, a semiprivate room with a view of majestic Central Park. She was "doing well." The boy asked to visit, but the stepfather urged patience. In fact, she might soon "return home." He punctuated his sentence with a smile.

Coming home? Really? The cheery statement seemed too positive, even rehearsed. Skeptical, the boy decided he would visit his mother alone.

The following morning, in an effort to appear older, he dressed up for school: dark suit, white shirt, tie and polished shoes. "Class picture," he explained to his curious stepfather. Remaining on the bus as it passed his school, he traveled to the end of the line and transferred to a subway destined for the city, practicing to himself the lie he'd have to tell his mother about not being in school. Maybe, some kind of teacher's conference day.

Waiting for the train on the outdoor platform seemed to take forever. A young man standing several feet away listened to a salsa tune from a hand-held radio. That was his mother's favorite music. The boy closed his eyes and traveled back to a time when he'd come home unexpected from school during a lunch break. She didn't hear him enter because the sounds of salsa had filled the house.

From the living room archway beside the door, he watched his mother dance around the room, moving with an uninhibited, natural rhythm of agility and style. Suddenly she turned and noticed him. Startled, she began to laugh like a mischievous child caught playfully jumping on a bed. "Come here," she said through a smile, "I'll teach you to salsa." And, for some timeless moments in the light of a sun-drenched room filled with the echoing sounds of Tito Puente, she patiently taught him to salsa, holding his hands, leading him, twirling him and giggling at his "two left feet" while applauding his diligence.

Discreetly entering the hospital, he slipped past the visitor check-in desk, taking the steps on the emergency stairway two at a time. Once on the fifth floor, he passed the nurses station and entered the room corridor. It reeked of an odor he would try forever to forget: a mixture of strong disinfectant and medicine that overwhelmed the sounds of coughs and moans and the steady electrical pulse of life-support machines.

Each room looked the same; broken bodies and anonymous faces, drip bottles and oxygen feeds from green tubing that kept death at bay, at least for the moment. His eyes searched every room, but still no sign of the face that for thirteen years had nurtured and loved him. She was supposed to be in 506. Could he have missed her?

He ran back to 506 and surveyed the room from the doorway. Dreary light filtered through half-closed venetian blinds casting its linear shadows across an empty bed. Stripped of sheets, the bare mattress loomed as a visual testimony to all that's mortal and temporary—here today, gone tomorrow. Frantic, his mind assaulted him with questions: Had she been in that bed? Did they move her? Was he too late? In mid-thought, his eyes darted across the room to an opposite corner bed where, beside a web of intravenous lines, monitors and pumps, a young woman lay propped against several pillows, lifeless eyes fixed on the ceiling.

It was his mother.

Her vivacity and shapely figure, now sacrificed to the ravages of sickness and chemical treatment had become lean and frail. She lay quietly still. The bright hazel eyes which once had gleamed were now darkened orbits of torment. The silence of her presence felt deafening.

Thirteen years of memories flooded his mind; she was a gifted dancer, painter and poet and had struggled through a devastating divorce with a graceful resiliency sustained by a faith as constant as the sunrise. And the smile—it was something she always wore—a smile of radiant warmth that was both disarming and inviting.

He knew that her illness was considered *terminal*—from the Latin, *terminus*; a word to mean "finishing point; of an end; resulting in death." But, the child in him refused to accept the crushing reality of a life without her; the one person always available to confide his deepest thoughts to, the solace for his fears and whom he depended on for unconditional loving. He stood frozen, numbed by naive hope that had melted into despair and guilt—he had not recognized his own mother.

Of all things changeable and unsettling, the one thing, now painfully clear and certain, was that nothing would ever be the same.

This is a true story. In fact, it is my story. My mother, still young and beautiful at thirty-five, died one week later. Over the next thirty-five years, I lost numerous other family members, including my natural father, to cancer and a variety of degenerative diseases. They all died painful, disabling and traumatic deaths. Helplessly, I watched their weight and appetite decrease as life gradually slipped away. Deep beneath the exterior pretense of a tough and hardened adult, I still carried my boyhood fear of the same fate. I reasoned that if most of my family became sick, surely my turn was inevitable.

Repeatedly, I asked myself the same questions: What factors caused them to become sick? What, if anything, could prevent me from becoming sick? Are we all just victims of some mysterious master plan, or do we really have some choice in creating healthy, vital lives for ourselves?

At that moment, I made myself a promise; a promise to find a natural way to be well, a promise to learn from the mistakes of my family members so their deaths would not seem in vain. I discovered a renewed strength in thinking of their short lives as a sacrificial lesson in *what not to do*, or *how not to live*. If I couldn't save my mother, I could certainly try to save myself, and as a tribute to her memory, give myself the permission to experience the life she could not.

At sixteen, I left home and began my odyssey in pursuit of a healthy life. Over the years, this became my quest; a formidable quest of learning through the trials of education, observation and experience.

And what did I learn?

I learned growing older does not have to mean unavoidable sickness, senility or incapacitation. I learned of profound alternate therapies that might have saved, or extended, my mother's life had this information been more widely known in 1965. And, I learned things that have undoubtedly saved mine since. For over 30 years, I've dedicated myself to sharing this information through counseling and lecturing.

Now, in writing this book, I share it with you.

INTRODUCTION

What Everyone Should
Know About Cancer

*"If we are to effectively prevent cancer, we will have
to change our diets and our smoking habits; we're also
going to have to clean up our environment, change industrial processes, and do any number of things that will be
difficult, expensive, time-consuming and intrusive."*

—John Bailar, III, M.D.,
Biostatistician and former editor of
The *Journal of the National Cancer Institute*

We all have relationships we value—whether with family,
friends or associates. And we devote an enormous amount of
time to cultivating and nurturing those relationships. In turn,
these are the people who support us and help us grow.

Of all the relationships we develop in this lifetime, the most
important and intimate is the one with our own body. It is the
home of our psyche and spirit. It is the physical residence in
which we live.

If you're at home in your own body, in control of its functions
and familiar with its rhythms, you cannot help feeling connected. But many of us avoid thinking about our body and the
power we have over it. Such a separation from your own power
fosters a distinctive sense of loneliness.

One of the reasons you might avoid thinking about your body is because it sometimes behaves in ways that seem mysterious. If you're fatigued, do you understand why? What if you can't fall asleep, or you have indigestion, or have trouble thinking clearly? In all likelihood, your body doesn't give you immediate clues about why those things are happening.

To unravel the mystery of the body is, first, to understand how it works and, second, to develop a sensitivity to what's going on physically. If you have that physical sensitivity, you can begin to experiment with the way you nourish that body—and through experimentation, begin to confirm your beliefs. You'll come to *know* what works for *your* body. You'll become more intimately familiar with its strengths and its limitations.

NATURE'S CANCER-FIGHTING FOODS

In this book I offer a simple and wholesome approach to transforming your health by using the power of ordinary, everyday food. My approach is based on the premise that certain foods—that just happen to be affordable and readily available—have powerful medicinal value. In the medical traditions of many cultures throughout the world, the notion that food determines health is widely accepted. During the last 25 years, medical research has certainly validated this idea.

Through healthy eating, bowel function can be kept regular. Certain foods and specific dietary habits increase the amount of beneficial intestinal flora—that is, the bacteria that help your body to synthesize nutrients. With appropriate dietary practices, blood sugar can be regulated. Certain foods can help you minimize, or control, tumor growth. Immune function can be maximized by eating foods that increase the activity of natural killer (NK) cells that "fight off" invasive microbes such as harmful viruses and bacteria. By careful selection of foods, you can significantly reduce inflammation and pain. And you can enrich your diet with certain nutrients that help reduce the cell-damaging actions of dangerous "free radicals"—the unstable molecules that are blamed for harm that can afflict even the core, genetic material of your body cells.

Nutrition can prevent, halt further progression of, and in some cases, reverse cancer. A statement of that kind might have been considered controversial a few years ago. Now, there's ample research that provides incontrovertible evidence that cancer and the environment—including, certainly, everything you eat and breathe—are intimately related. Large populations have been studied, and we know that certain kinds of cancer are far more prevalent among some people than others, largely due to their dietary habits. In lab experiments, researchers have observed tumors that are caused or that proliferate because of specific components in diets that are high in animal proteins. Even at the cellular level, scientists are seeing how certain food components have an immediate and direct impact on the way living cells remain healthy or, conversely, suffer irreversible damage.

Much of the information in this book is drawn from ongoing research in world-wide prestigious medical facilities. That research is pointing to some inescapable conclusions. Nutrition has preventive powers. It also, in some circumstances, has redemptive power—the ability to stall or reverse the damage that has been done.

When I work with clients one-on-one, I review their diets in great detail before providing extensive nutritional counseling. When they experience positive health transformations in a relatively short period of time, invariably they ask, "Why didn't my doctor tell me about this?"

No wonder they ask! The practical advice about eating habits—advice that clearly reduces the risk of disease and increases the chances of good health—does not come from any medical school. With few exceptions, these practical nutritional guidelines are not even *taught* in med school, except in the most cursory manner. While many medical schools are now beginning to wake up to the critical importance of nutrition and starting to expand their curricula, nutrition emphasis has been anemic; the average U.S. physician, in four years of medical school, typically gets only two hours of course work in nutrition. Only 25 percent of the accredited medical schools in the country have a single required course in nutrition.

Even if a medical doctor were to have thorough training in nutritional therapies, the schedule of the typical M.D. precludes in-depth work with individuals. Most doctors are, by necessity, afflicted with huge caseloads. They're overbooked. That not only leaves them less time for individual patients, it also means that keeping up with journal articles is a supreme challenge. Nutrition, among the lowest of priorities in medical school, remains the least-urgent topic for attention afterward. Sooner or later, some dietary knowledge does trickle down, but, often, doctors are only aware of the nutritional findings that are publicized in the popular press. So, the problem that began with medical-school education is often perpetuated during the years of practice.

But there's another, less subtle reason why nutrition news gets short shrift. Food, the great healer, found on the shelf of your local supermarket, farmer's market, or health food store, does not have the backing of multibillion dollar marketing campaigns.

Neal Barnard, M.D., President of the Physician's Committee for Responsible Medicine in Washington, D.C., and author of *Foods That Fight Pain*, notes what happens when each new drug is developed, patented, and promoted by the company that makes it:

> *"Then the drug company will hire a public relations firm, pay for massive mailings to physicians, and advertise in medical journals. The company will sponsor medical conferences that highlight the role of the drug and pay speakers to discuss it. Drug companies, motivated by potentially millions of dollars in profits, are skilled at getting a busy doctor's attention. But no industry makes money if you stop eating a food that causes your migraines. No surgical supply company makes a cent if you open your arteries naturally through diet and lifestyle. A pharmaceutical company's bottom line does not improve if you use natural anti-inflammatory foods instead of expensive drugs. And without the PR machinery paid for by industry, some of the most important findings never make their way onto a doctor's desk. Patients with arthritis, migraines, menstrual cramps, or even cancer who ask their doctors what they*

should be eating to regain their health get no answers, simply because no one has brought new information to the doctor's attention."

It is not surprising that modern medicine has put little emphasis on prevention. Disease prevention offers meager profit. It's certainly more profitable and expedient to authorize a sophisticated diagnostic test than it is to educate someone on a preventive diet and lifestyle. A fifteen-minute MRI scan can cost $800 to $2000. Fifteen minutes of nutrition education might lead to a more effective resolution of a health problem. But imagine what an insurer or a private patient would say if a physician charged this much for a ten- to fifteen-minute doctor-patient chat on illness prevention.

HABITS DIE HARD

Of course, *knowing* how to change your diet and *doing* it are two different things. There's no guarantee that you would suddenly stop eating "junk food"—as we almost gleefully call it—even if a doctor declared unequivocally that it would increase your risk of certain kinds of cancer by twenty or thirty or forty percent.

For the best example of failure to change habits, just see the research on smoking. Thousands of well-publicized studies showing the health risks of smoking, along with warnings on packages and mountains of publicity, and millions of people are still lighting up every day.

In a similar way, our addictions to "favorite goodies" can keep us hostages to the kinds of food we've always eaten, even when clear evidence and good research is directing us along a different path. Secretly afraid of change, of substances unfamiliar, or of deprival from our comfort "treats," we may see a simple change of diet as a threat to the very essence of a comfortable, convenient, and familiar lifestyle.

Thinking of dietary change as a "short-term experiment" often eases the fear that you might feel deprived if you don't get food that is familiar or ritually comforting. If you find that your craving disappears for foods that are not health-supportive and that you feel better without them, saying good-bye (or managing an occasional hello) to them is fairly effortless. So, think about the short-term, and when you're making a change, view it as an "experiment."

Fortunately, you can experience the results of good eating. Where education can motivate us, offer a clearer understanding of how the body works and what it requires nutritionally, the ultimate test is simply how we respond. Our own convictions are truly enforced not by theoretic argument, but by the experience of change.

FACTS OF THE MATTER

As I have revealed in the preface to this book, I have a very personal reason for pursuing a "war on cancer." I want to offer some clear, effective, cancer-preventive and cancer-fighting techniques to anyone who is looking for ways to help protect themselves. Obviously, I'm not alone in fighting this war. But unfortunately, all of us who are trying to find answers— whether in conventional medicine or in nutritional and holistic approaches—know that we're up against a powerful foe.

I could cite many statistics about the steadily growing risks of various kinds of cancer—and the costs in life and health. But, to me, the most telling statistic is the way the risks have increased for every one of us.

According to the US Bureau of the Census, in 1900, 47 people out of every 100,000 died of cancer, making it the sixth leading cause of death. Today, 173 people out of every 100,000 will die of cancer, ranking it the second leading cause of death, exceeded only by heart disease.

In 1992, a statement signed by 69 highly respected medical and scientific experts in the USA stated, "Over the last decade, some five million Americans died of cancer and there is growing evidence that a substantial proportion of these deaths was avoidable."

Our modern diet of refined foods laden with chemicals and deficient in many nutrients is *currently thought to be the great-*

est single contributor to cancer development. According to the World Cancer Research Fund, you can reduce your risk of cancer by up to 40 percent just by lowering fat and consuming a higher percentage of wholesome vegetable foods.

Current research suggests that 80–90 percent of all cancers occur as a result of poor nutrition, lifestyle (smoking, alcohol, etc.), chemical ingestion, and other environmental factors. This information has now been corroborated by other major agencies, such as: The National Academy of Sciences, The National Department of Health and Human Services, The Cancer Institute, and The American Cancer Society.

Researchers agree that most cancers have a ten- or twenty-year interval between their carcinogenic stimulus and the appearance of a developing tumor. So the food that you're eating today—in addition to other lifestyle habits—are likely to influence the state of your health a decade or two from now.

It is true that the incidence of some cancers is decreasing, but what is particularly concerning is the rise in hormone-related cancers. These are cancers of hormonally sensitive tissue. (In men, that means cancer of the prostate and testes; in women, cancer of the breast, womb, ovaries, and cervix.) Not only is the incidence of these cancers more frequent than a decade ago, statistics also show that these cancers are occurring earlier in people's lives. It is also known that dietary changes, along with exposure to environmental toxins, plays a significant role in development of these particular cancers.

Five of the most common cancers—lung, breast, stomach, colorectal, and prostate—were practically unheard of before the early 20th century. Population studies have revealed that the escalation of cancer parallels the industrialization and chemicalization of our world. The more developed a country, the higher its cancer ratio. As per capita income increases, so does the incidence of cancer.

Ironically, this is because most cancers are primarily the result of the changes we've made to our total chemical environment—what we eat, drink, and breathe. In the short space of only two generations, ten million new chemicals have been invented and randomly released into our environment. Many are known to be carcinogens—poisons that we inevitably end up ingesting through food, air, and water—but a good number of these are easily avoidable.

BAD INFLUENCES—AND GOOD AGENTS

Carcinogens are not new kids on the block. They exist in nature and even in common health-promoting foods, but they rarely present a problem because our bodies have unique mechanisms to help detoxify them. It's only when our body's defenses are vulnerable, when we're repeatedly exposed to many types of carcinogens, that our risks sharply increase. This is why it's essential to increase the health of your entire immune system and to make a habit of avoiding dietary and lifestyle factors that can weaken immunity.

It is also well known that certain intestinal bacteria can activate substances such as bile and ingested fats to mutate into cancer-producing carcinogens. Over time, these carcinogens initiate cell division and change the surface of the colon in a way that can eventually lead to cancer. The DNA of a normal cell appears to be permanently altered into a cancer cell anxious to divide.

In the last twenty years, a staggering amount of scientific information has clearly demonstrated that certain compounds in foods provide significant protection against cancer and can slow, interrupt, or even reverse its development. Many of these compounds have been shown to stop normal cells from becoming rebel cancer cells, and some can actually reverse cancer cells back into normal cells.

Specifically, the natural plant substances, known as *phytochemicals* or *phytonutrients* (*phyto* = plant), seem to have hidden potency that is being revealed by testing. Phytonutrients have been flawlessly crafted by Nature for millions of years in response to challenging stresses such as drought, temperature variation, plant-eating insects, and fierce sunlight. These phytonutrients are simply not present in processed foods. And you simply can't rely on getting necessary phytonutrients from the hoards of "anti-cancer" supplements currently on the market.

Whole grains, vegetables, beans, and fruits can provide a genuine feast of these cancer-fighting substances that number in the thousands.

A SELF-HEALING PRIMER

First and foremost, this is a book about the healing power of food. It is not within the scope of this book to exhaustively detail numerous alternative treatments, environmental concerns, stress management techniques, relationship conflict, or the role of faith in spiritual guidance, other than to mention that the healing puzzle consists of many pieces which fit together to comprise a whole picture.

Being able to prevent or at least lower your risk of cancer, the focus of this book, can reduce the fear and sense of helplessness that is inspired by this dreaded disease. The old adage that an ounce of prevention is worth a pound of cure accurately applies to cancer. The solution begins with nutritional education and progresses by learning to make healthier choices in the way we feed ourselves.

Interestingly, many of the measures that reduce cancer risk resemble the way many cultures lived and took nourishment in over 150 years ago; people were more physically active, had less exposure to toxins, and consumed fresher, better quality whole foods before the labor-saving technology and food-processing arrived to "save" us time as it warped our taste buds.

In attempting to stall, reverse, or prevent cancer, *Nature's Cancer-Fighting Foods* offers a practical formula for achieving four health strategies that serve as a foundation with which additional therapies (conventional or alternative) can be incorporated:

1. *Strengthen Blood Quality*—This is accomplished through the daily consumption of a wide variety of nutritious whole foods from plant sources. These foods include: whole grains, grain products, beans, vegetables, sea vegetables, fruits, vegetable quality oils, nuts, seeds, fruits, and small quantities of animal protein (optional).

Additionally, minimizing foods high in acid residue contributes to a more alkaline mineral status which also optimizes metabolic functioning.

2. *Strengthen Immunity*—In *Nature's Cancer-Fighting Foods*, you'll find practical strategies for reducing sugar, fat, and chemicals which have a tremendous impact on immune health. Learning to regulate activity and sleep are also crucial steps toward keeping immune health in maximized condition. Proven immune enhancing supplements and herbs are detailed for their valuable influence on immune health.

3. *Regulating Blood Sugar*—The Nature's Cancer-Fighting Food Plan helps evenly stabilize blood sugar while increasing one's sensitivity of what foods help or hinder this balancing act. Ultimately, this gives you more control over your physical and emotional health.

4. *Strengthening Your Detox Ability*—The balance in our carbohydrate, fat, and protein ratios, as well as food quality, dramatically influences our body's ability to detoxify. Nature's Cancer-Fighting Food Plan strengthens the organs of elimination (intestines, liver, kidneys, lymph, and skin) as it promotes better circulation to make the natural process of detoxification more efficient.

These four factors constitute the blueprint for strengthening health and cancer prevention. One mouthful at a time, the power of good food offers us an essential key for transforming our health and the health of generations to come.

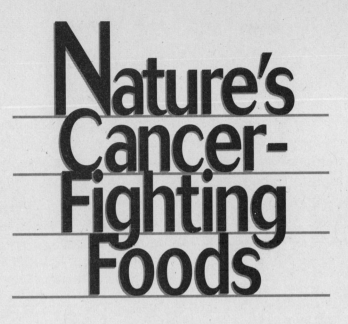

Nature's Cancer-Fighting Foods

EATING HABITS, FOOD QUALITY, AND CANCER PREVENTION

WHY "MMM, MMM, GOOD" IS NOT ENOUGH

Over the last 150 years our eating patterns, food quality, and nutrition ratios have dramatically shifted to a packaged, mass-produced, adulterated, and refined fare that has sacrificed wholesome nutrition for consumer convenience and corporate profit. You can almost hear the marketing logic being fed to a gullible public: "Hey, we're selling you refined food with high sugar content and lots of additives, but don't worry, we've forti-fied it so you'll get the nutrition you need. We care!"

Some of the changes marking our eating patterns and food quality seem like trading diamonds for pebbles. Here are seven key shifts that have occurred in the last 100 years:

1. *Refined Sugar Increase / Whole Grain Decrease*
   We've witnessed a dramatic increase of simple sugars from refined white sugar, syrups, fruits, fruit juices, milk, and artificial sugar sources. At the same time, there's been a decrease in eating complex carbohydrates from whole grain, grain product, and bean sources. Ironically, a deficiency of whole complex carbohydrates is one of the reasons for sugar cravings.

1

ROBBING THE NUTRIENTS

I once heard physician Joe D. Nicols, tell a humorous story illustrating the idiocy of enriching refined food. He gave the analogy of an armed mugger who emerges from the shadows of an alley on a cold, snowy night to accost a man who walks alone on a barren street. He robs the man's wallet and then, admiring the man's winter coat and suit, demands he remove everything he's wearing. Minutes later, with his clothes in a heap on the wintry sidewalk, the bare-naked man stands shivering. Suddenly, the mugger begins to feel some remorse and decides to show his generous side. He hands the man one of his socks (at this point, Dr. Nicols would call out: "That's vitamin A!"). Then, he gives him back his belt ("That's vitamin B!"). The man continues to shiver, so the kind mugger gives him back his tie ("That's vitamin C!"). After a moment of consideration, the mugger returns the man's hat ("That's vitamin D!"). Dr. Nicols concluded his story with a question: "Food suppliers strip out hundreds of valuable nutrients and micronutrients through food refinement and then after putting back in four boast about it! Let me ask you, do you think that man on the street has been enriched, or robbed?"

2. *Animal Source Protein Increase/Vegetable Protein Decrease*

   Intake of animal source proteins from beef, poultry, eggs, and dairy foods has risen, while consumption of vegetable proteins such as grains, beans, and bean products has decreased.

3. *Saturated Fat Increase/Unsaturated Fat Decrease*

   The intake of saturated fats from animal proteins has increased, while intake of unsaturated fats from vegetable oil sources has decreased.

4. *Increase of Fiber-Absent Foods/Decrease of Whole Fibrous Foods*

   A dramatic increase in the consumption of nonfibrous foods as in dairy products, fatty sauces, and most grain products (flour cereals, breads, pastas, crackers, etc.) is contrasted by a decrease in consumption of unbroken fiber chains (whole grains, vegetables, and fruits).

5. *Increase of Artificial Additives / Decrease of Foods Naturally Containing Them*

   We are becoming more reliant on vitamins, minerals, hormones, and other vitamin industry supplements, as we continue to consume deficient, chemicalized food from nutrient-depleted soils.

6. *Increase of Synthetic Chemicals / Decrease of Natural Quality*

   Synthetic chemicals in the form of fertilizers, insecticides, preservatives, emulsifiers, artificial dyes, and stabilizers have increased, while natural textures, colors, tastes, and odors have decreased.

7. *Increase of Fast-Paced Lifestyle / Decrease of Meal-Time Rituals*

   From regular home-cooked meals to store-bought, prepackaged meals, we eat faster and read or watch television while eating. We place priority on convenience instead of nutrition, and we frequently eat "on-the-go," making sensory satisfaction the primary goal.

Not All the Food News Is Bad

In response to this general decline in food quality, eating habits and nutrition, there is also a growing trend in the opposite direction. Over the last thirty years the alternative health movement has blossomed. The traditional large supermarket, home to retail sales of packaged, frozen and canned foods with only a single aisle dedicated to produce, has evolved to include expanded produce sections of nonorganic and organic varieties and bulk items such as whole grains and legumes. Low-fat meats and larger seafood sections reveal America's newfound zeal for reducing red meats and emphasizing poultry and fish. Whereas health-food specialty items were once relegated to import or dietetic sections, they now have their own aisles and provide increasing competition for more standard and familiar fare.

Nutritional supplements, once found on the shelves of pharmaceutical sections, now merit their own display sections in markets, convenience stores, and drugstores. Outdoor farmers' markets offering low-cost organic produce have sprung up in every large metropolitan city. With the national expansion of exclusive natural food markets, our changing tastes have become more than just a trend. As revenue streams for natural products increase, big business takes interest. Suddenly, we see promotions like "free packet of Saint John's wort with every stick of Grandpa's Natural Butter" and "free vitamin C packet with every beef jerky bar at participating stores."

In the face of conflicting claims and opposing viewpoints, your nutritional choices go beyond quality to the meaning of balance. Balance is not theoretical; it's practical. It's how you individualize your diet by understanding your needs, experimenting with different percentages of carbohydrates, fats, and proteins, and developing a sensitivity for what works and what doesn't.

STAPLE, SUPPORTIVE, AND PLEASURE FOODS

Staple Foods: Whole Grains, Beans, and Vegetables

The concept of a principal or staple food, to most Westerners, is a foreign one. A staple food is a food consistently eaten with every major meal, or at least once daily. This practice of eating staple foods is still followed throughout the world, although predominantly in Third World cultures. Eat a meal in the orient, India, Ethiopia, Mexico, or Tibet, and you can bet cereals, beans or bean products, and vegetable side dishes will be central to the meal. The word *meal,* in fact, means "cereal." Mealtime means time for grain.

Factors that make a food worthy of being considered a principal food are as follows:

- *Availability*—A food available locally.
- *Taste*—A food that is naturally sweet the more it is chewed.

- *Economics*—A food that is affordable. This is a sociological consideration.
- *Sustainable*—A food that one can live on for short periods of time, healthfully.
- *Versatile*—A food that can be prepared with great variety.
- *Nutritious*—A food with nourishing quality that helps to regulate blood sugar.
- *Storage*—A food that can be stored for long periods of time without spoilage.

Whole cereal grains, beans, and vegetables, all principal foods, contain abundant vitamins and micronutrients and good long-chain fiber quality, promote stable blood sugar, offer storage capacity (vegetables were typically dried for winter seasons), and naturally contain a sweet taste. These factors easily qualify whole grains, beans, and vegetables as ideal candidates for staple foods.

For the last 10,000 years whole cereal grains and vegetables have been the principal food of humans. Traditionally, these plants were revered as the sacred source of life. The Bible does not say "Give us this day our daily chocolate-chip cookies." The reference is to whole grain bread, the "staff of life."

Every culture that had a developed agriculture cultivated corn, rice, wheat, barley, millet, rye, buckwheat, and numerous other native grains as principal foods along with various types of beans and vegetables.

WASTED FOOD ENERGY

According to the U.S. Department of Agriculture, half of the present world's supply of food energy comes from cereal grains and more than 70 percent of croplands are devoted to their cultivation. Unfortunately, today much of this harvest is used to feed livestock. Considering that it takes nearly 8 pounds of grain to produce 1 pound of meat, our obsession with animal protein seems to be the definitive concept of waste. Ecologically, socially, and economically, this does not make good sense.

Vegetables can be classified in three categories: root vegetables (e.g., carrots, onions, radishes, parsnips, turnips), ground and round-shape vegetables (e.g., squash family, cauliflower, broccoli, pumpkins, mushrooms, cucumber), and green leafy vegetables (e.g., bok choy, kale, collards, mustard greens, endive, watercress). For many coastal cultures, vegetables from the ocean (also known as seaweeds), with important mineral, trace mineral nutrients, and anticancer qualities, were standard fare.

Supportive Foods: Animal Proteins and Fruits

This category is composed of secondary foods that support staple foods. Animal protein was used by most cultures as more of a condiment, consumed less frequently and in small volumes. In some cultures it was of minor importance due to economics or availability, while in others its lack of importance might have been due to ideology.

Meat is not a staple food. Our tooth structure was designed primarily for grinding, with twenty molars, eight cutting teeth, and only four canines for tearing. If we desired to eat meat, we were equipped to do so—but only a small percentage of our diet. For people living in temperate climates, meat was not to be consumed as a staple food, especially two or more times daily.

Fruit, too is a supportive food, not a staple. While fruit contains many vitamins and some fiber, it is still a simple sugar source and best taken in moderation, according to craving, for optimum health.

Pleasure Foods

The category of pleasure foods can be misleading. If we enjoy good health, we should feel free to eat whatever we want with a spirit of joy and in moderation, as on social occasions. There should be no guilt involved if we have a basically healthy lifestyle.

Recently, I was dining with a friend in an upscale, beachfront restaurant. The menu was full of interesting choices from a number of culinary styles. I noticed a colorful advertising tent on the table promoting the restaurant's featured dessert. The copy read, "Enjoy Our Guilty Pleasure: Chuck's Chocolate Decadence Cake—Make Your Day Deliciously Sinful!" An ad like this is trying to appeal to our inner rebel by telling us in advance that the dessert is sinful and decadent but will bring us pleasure. Of course, a little bite of this and that, here and there, won't make you spin your head 360 degrees and spew green bile. However, you need to keep a larger perspective on so-called pleasure foods. In this case, intuition might be your best guide.

CANCER: DETECTION VERSUS PREVENTION

The war on cancer in the United States has been mainly focused on detection. Detection has become our method of prevention. Medical organizations and the media routinely publicize the benefits of cancer detection by promoting breast, skin, and testicular self-examination as if they were methods of prevention, encouraging this deception.

The amazing variety of detection techniques, which are constantly being revised and developed, no doubt save lives, especially if a tumor can be removed before it spreads. Generally, this is accomplished through surgery, radiation, and/or chemotherapy. However, once a mass of tumor cells has been diagnosed, prevention is after the fact.

A cancer cell is an out-of-control invader setting its own course of gradual multiplication in any organ, gland, or body

---

STEALTH ATTACK

Nearly 75 percent of a cancer's growth occurs before it is medically detectable. This rate of growth is slow, but progressive, often taking up to twenty to thirty years to announce itself. Most detection instrumentation, as of this date, cannot identify a tumor until it reaches a weight of nearly 1-gram—roughly 1 billion cancer cells. Most imaging equipment can only detect a tumor of a size approximating 10 billion cells! A tumor of this density will weigh close to 10 grams.

system. It continues to divide until, as a mass, it breaks apart to invade other parts of the body. This process of spreading is called metastasis. Cancer devastates the most important part of the cell—the DNA, which controls the cell's functioning.

The only logical and immediate line of defense is to employ a self-healing lifestyle with a dietary focus targeted to reduce the possibility of developing or nurturing cancer cells. Prevention is still the only approach possible to "win the war on cancer." This does not mean that you have to deprive yourself of everything that you like or crave, but that you become more moderate in your indulgences, more educated in your choices, and more experienced with the positive benefits of a healthy way of eating.

CANCER AND DIET

Faulty diet encourages the growth of cancer cells. Lung, stomach, colon, uterus, ovary, prostate, and breast cancer fall into this category. It has also been documented that certain foods will increase the volume of hormones that elevate the risk of cancer. Cancers such as breast, uterus, ovary, and prostate are directly associated with an excess of sex hormones.

A number of foods also carry carcinogens that can stimulate the production of free radicals. A free radical is a reactive atom with unpaired electrons within the cell that damages cellular functioning.

The increase in cancer is lower in countries where more traditional diets of complex carbohydrates and minimum animal protein and fat are still being followed. In fact, The National Cancer Institute estimates 80 to 90 percent of cancers originate from environmental causes, which include diet and tobacco smoking.

Much of the research on diet and cancer can seem conflicting. However, the most reliable and promising research comes from population studies where dietary and lifestyle patterns broadly differ. The most common cancers linked to faulty diet are those that develop in organs governed by sex hormones, such as breast, prostate, ovary, and uterus, as well as cancers that involve the pancreas, liver, colon, esophagus, and stomach. On a broader scale, dietary factors also influence many other cancers.

THE CHINA PROJECT

One of the best summaries of population studies associating faulty diet with cancer is a major research project called The China Project (CP). It was developed by Professor T. Colin Campbell and Dr. Chen Junshi during 1983–1984 and again in 1989–1990. The CP study intensively surveyed 6500 individuals from 65 counties (100 from each county) for dietary disease patterns. The discoveries of the CP have vigorously challenged and altered existing conceptions about nutrition and health.

According to Professor Campbell:

The China Project offered a rare opportunity to study disease in a precise manner due to unique conditions that exist in rural China. Approximately 90% of the people in rural China live their entire lives in the vicinity of their birth. Because of deeply held local traditions and the absence of viable food distribution, people consume diets composed primarily of locally produced foods. In addition, there are dramatic differences in the prevalence of disease from region to region. Various cardio-vascular disease rates vary by a factor of about 2-fold from one place to another, while certain cancer rates may vary by several hundred-fold.

These factors make rural China a "living laboratory" for the study of the complex relationship between nutrition and other lifestyle factors and degenerative diseases. As a result, the China Project is the first major research study to examine diseases as they really are, multiple outcomes of many inter-related factors.

Chinese diets are much lower in total fat (generally, 6 to 24 percent of calories), much higher in dietary fiber (10 to 77 grams daily), and approximately 30 percent higher in total calorie intake while substantially lower in foods of animal origin.

Differing widely from American diets, the Chinese diets contain approximately 0 to 20 percent animal-based foods, while American diets typically comprise 60 to 80 percent animal-based foods.

The CP findings showed dramatic differences in cancers of the breast, ovary, uterus, and prostate. These cancers are significantly associated with dietary fat and higher levels of reproductive hormones, such as estrogen and testosterone, which typify the meat- and diary-rich diets found in Western countries. Estrogens are part of the family of chemical messengers called sex hormones.

In regard to dietary fiber, the average Chinese intake was three times the Western diet ratio. According to the study, "consistent reductions in cancers of the colon and rectum were found with higher intakes of these various fiber fractions." Large-bowel cancer has been associated with lower intakes of a wide variety of dietary fiber components in plant-based foods.

PROSTATE HEALTH

American statistics estimate that one out of every ten men will be diagnosed with prostate cancer. This figure does not apply to Chinese men, who have the lowest advanced prostate rates in the world—one in every 100,000. Although not conclusive, it is well known that testosterone can be a triggering factor in prostate cancer. Animal protein can stimulate testosterone production.

Numerous studies have shown that men consuming diets high in foods containing *phytoestrogens* have reduced chances of developing cancer. Isoflavonic phyto-estrogens ("plant estrogens") help to normalize the proportion of testosterone to estrogen in the body. Phytoestrogens are weak estrogens that displace normal estrogens from their receptor sites on breast cells, reducing estrogen's potentially harmful effects. Two additional studies, cited by Professor Campbell, show that men who ate the most fat (increasing testosterone levels) had 79 percent more advanced prostate cancer than the men who kept to low-fat diets. It was suggested that the worst offenders were red meats, mayonnaise, and butter.

OTHER FINDINGS THAT SHOULD CHANGE APPETITES

There have been several other studies that support the conclusions of the CP, with the bottom line being that diets high in fat, protein, and calories but low in fiber increase the risk of cancer. Here are some confirming studies:

- The vegetarian Seventh-Day Adventists have prostate cancer mortality rates about 30 percent less than those of the population in general in California.

- The incidence of prostate cancer has been related to the consumption of dairy products, eggs, and meats.

- In a case-controlled study at Roswell Park Memorial Institute, high milk consumption, a chief source of American dietary fat, was found to be associated with higher risk of breast, mouth, colon, stomach, rectum, lung, bladder, and cervical cancer, relative to consumption of no milk at all.

- Alcohol also plays a featured cancer-nurturing role: One drink per day can increase breast cancer risk by more than 50 percent, compared with nondrinkers.

- Animal fats seem to pose a greater threat than vegetable oils. Researchers at New York University compared the diets of 250 women with breast cancer to those of 499 women without cancer from the same province in northwestern Italy. Both groups consumed a good deal of olive oil and carbohydrates. The striking difference with the cancer patients was in the volume of animal products consumed. Those who ate the greater amount of meat, cheese, butter, and milk had about three times the cancer risk of other women.

- When animal proteins are heated, they produce cancer-causing chemicals called heterocyclic amines that are implicated in colon and breast cancer. Although this has been known to occur in beef, it was not until recently that a report by the National Cancer Institute revealed that the same phenomenon occurs in chicken. However, it appears in a greater degree in chicken than beef. A well-done hamburger contains 33 nanograms per gram of the carcinogen PhIP, the same as grilled steak. The picture grows dimmer with chicken: It contains 480 nanograms per gram, a total of fifteen times higher than for beef.

PROTECTING YOUR COLON

The influence of bile acids in the colon is another factor in cancer development. Bile acids, released by the gall bladder into the duodenum to emulsify fats, flow into the small and then the large intestine. Unfortunately, bacteria in the digestive tract change these bile acids into cancer-promoting chemicals called secondary bile acids. These secondary bile acids are formed from the growth of bacteria encouraged by a meat-based diet. Vegetarian-based diets form a harmless bacteria that does not pose the same risk. In societies with a high consumption of grains, vegetables, beans, and fruits, lower rates of colon cancer appear. Plant roughage, devoid of animal protein complexes, bonds to toxins while moving food through the intestine quickly. The fiber absorbs and dilutes bile acids, altering the quality of intestinal bacteria to a less harmful one.

In addition to preventing colon cancer, fiber can help the individual already diagnosed with colon polyps, intestinal growths that can become cancerous. Surgeon Jerome J. DeCosse, from Cornell Medical Center, experimented with dietary bran on patients with recurrent polyps. Within a period of six months, the polyps became smaller and fewer in number.

The benefits of a diet focused on whole grains, beans, vegetables, and fruits come from abundant long-chain fibers that absorb toxins and expand to keep the intestinal tract clean and free of harmful bacteria without the addition of animal fat and cholesterol, which stimulate colon cancer.

2 CARBOHYDRATES, FATS, AND PROTEINS: MYTHS, TRUTHS, AND HEALTHY ADVICE

CARBOHYDRATES: FUEL FOR YOUR BODY

Intricately manufactured by plants as a way of storing energy from the sun, carbohydrates provide us with most of the energy we require for everyday functioning. For some people, the word *carbohydrate* sounds like a nutritional swear word; it conjures images of impossible-to-remove fat and memorable images of favorite treats from times past. Suddenly, you feel guilty for even thinking about such foods.

The truth is simple, yet complex. Literally.

Your body requires a constant supply of carbohydrates for all of its metabolic activities. There are two basic types of carbohydrates, some with very simplified molecular structures (simple sugars) and others with more complex forms (complex sugars). Eventually, for the body to utilize carbohydrates (also generally known as "sugar"), they have to be broken down into their simplified form—glucose. Glucose is the only form of sugar that is transportable in the bloodstream. It is also the sole source of energy for the brain. Any lack of glucose, or of oxygen to burn the glucose, could result in permanent brain damage.

13

Digestion of simple sugar is analogous to tending a fire. You can use newspaper which has a quick-burning effect and has to be added constantly, or you can use wood, beginning with fine splintered shavings (kindling) until you have a steady flame that will then penetrate thicker branches and eventually logs of wood. Logs will burn for long periods, providing a consistent and enduring heat.

This is the story of carbohydrates; some burn quick, some burn slow. Quick-burning carbohydrates (simple sugars) are usually sweet to the taste, lose most of their taste when chewed, and flood the bloodstream with sugar, elevating hormonal levels, producing potentially harmful anaerobic bacteria, and producing strong acidity.

White and brown sugar, honey, maple syrup, molasses, fruit, rice syrup, barley malt, milk sugar, dextrose, high-fructose corn syrup, and maltose are all simple sugars. The blood can only maintain approximately 2 teaspoons of sugar at one time, and excess sugar is converted into a large branched molecule called glycogen and stored in liver cells. When the 60- to 80-gram capacity is reached in the liver, the sugar is converted into fat and stored in the body tissues—a fact that sweet lovers find endlessly annoying.

Complex sugars are found in whole grains, grain products, beans, and vegetables. They burn slowly and evenly, regulating blood sugar and promoting abundant energy. Nearly every culture that had a developed agriculture used whole grain as a dietary staple. The white rice you see in a Japanese restaurant was originally brown rice, with its seven layers of vitamins, minerals, and trace minerals intact before it was polished off in the name of uniformity, unquestioned tradition, and mechanical habit. Whole grains, with their covering intact, provide necessary fiber, which is known to lower the risk for cancer, heart disease, hypertension, diabetes, and numerous digestive problems. Initially, whole grains might taste somewhat bland; however, if thoroughly chewed, they'll begin to impart a subtle sweetness that is both satisfying and healthier for digestion.

"THE WHOLE GRAIN AND NOTHING BUT THE GRAIN ..."

To combat heart disease, diabetes, obesity, and cancer, the public has been repeatedly told to eat plenty of whole grains. Indeed, this is mentioned in countless books and magazines. But what does this mean? Bread? Pasta? Bagels? Flat bread? Popcorn? Cold breakfast cereal? Muffins? Cookies? What these products have in common is that they all were created from original whole grains. However, they are no longer considered whole grains. They are grain products, products made from whole grains. Bury a bagel and it will not sprout a bagel tree. This dramatic difference is sadly misunderstood.

Unsuspecting consumers buying a loaf of bread feel a false sense of security when seeing the bold print on the package that says, "Made with whole grain goodness!" Actually, this is a marketing strategy. Maximum protection comes from whole grains and not grain products. If we ground up whole wheat and from its flour make bread, we'll have unrefined whole grain bread. Refine that wheat flour by taking out the bran and you're left with refined flour—ordinary white bread.

Breaking the grain structure and making it into flour particles allows the grain much quicker access to the blood than the whole grain digestion normally would. In some sensitive individuals, refined flour enters the blood just as quickly as simple sugar. The glycemic index has documented this. The glycemic index is a rating system for foods that enter the blood quickly and raise sugar levels enough to create insulin excess.

Western culinary techniques tend to rely on refined or flaked grains for quicker cooking times. For example, the word oatmeal literally means "oats that have been cooked into a meal." You can cook the whole oat groats, which takes hours, or a steel cut version that is about one-fourth the size of the groats and cooks in thirty minutes. Still short on time? You can cook the rolled version of the groats, which, by the rolling process, resembles a flake. Rolled oats cook in fifteen minutes. Some manufacturers steam cook the rolled oats, dry them, and sell them as "instant oats." So, there are actually many versions of whole grains. However, as long as they are unrefined and the bulk of your grain eating is not floured, you can enjoy all the benefits of whole grain.

WHAT ARE WHOLE GRAINS?

Whole grains are cereal grains with their bran intact. They have seven layers of protective fiber with hundreds of nutrients and micronutrients locked in. Botanically, wild rice and buckwheat are classified as seeds; however, for the sake of simplicity and due to their fiber content, I've listed them as a whole grain. There are also many varieties of native corn, traditionally know throughout the world as maize. General knowledge of corn today is limited to grits and the hybrid variety that is actually considered a vegetable. Dried versions (grits and dried whole kernels) qualify more as a grain.

Examples of common whole grains are as follows:
- Brown rice
- Barley
- Millet
- Oats (rolled, steel cut, instant flaked)
- Buckwheat
- Rye
- Whole wheat/cracked wheat (a.k.a. bulghur)

Examples of Native American whole grains are as follows:
- Quinoa ("keen-wa")
- Corn grits
- Amaranth
- Wild rice

Five Reasons for Eating Whole Grain

Here are five benefits you derive by eating whole grains:

1. *Regularity*

   Eating whole grain means you'll be getting long-chain fibers, which take up water in the colon and expand to create bowel regularity. Often, when people first begin to eat whole grain and reduce foods and substances that stimulate bowel function (caffeine, sugar, tobacco, etc.), they complain that whole grain causes them to become constipated. Quite to the contrary! In the beginning, you may experience several days of your bowels acting sluggish as they become accustomed to purging themselves without the help from stimulants. Within days, you'll be amazed at your body's adjustment to whole grain and a new kind of regularity you've probably never experienced.

2. *Blood Sugar Stability*

   The complex sugar chains of whole grains' molecular structure slowly break apart and, as they enter the blood, gradually raise blood sugar in a way that is even and consistent, as opposed to the wild up-and-down swings of refined sugar. This creates more sustaining energy and mental calm. Wide swings in blood sugar create the release of stress hormones and can initiate the build-up of arterial plaques.

3. *Vitamin B and E Group*

   The bran covering of whole grains contains many B vitamins, such as niacin, vitamin B6, pantothenic acid, riboflavin, and thiamin, as well as Vitamin E. These water-soluble vitamins are essential for immune health, protection from diseases such as beriberi and pellagra, cardiac strength, DNA health, the building and maintenance of body tissues, skin and eye health, cholesterol reduction, appetite regulation, prevention of depression, certain hormone formation, red blood cell development, and gum health.

4. *Toxicity Discharge*

   Whole grain's bran covering bonds to different toxins and escorts them out of the body via the bowel. Because of the bran's tendency to absorb water, possible toxins within the bowel do not remain long enough to become absorbed into the blood.

5. *Decrease of Cravings for Sugar and Fat*

   For its nutritional value as well as its ability to stabilize blood sugar, whole grain consumption will automatically reduce your cravings for sweets and fatty foods. This makes your change of diet less of an effort and means that you need less willpower to avoid foods that are not health supportive.

"But Do They Go Well with Hot Dogs?"

A skeptical client once asked me, "If whole grains are so good for you, why isn't everybody eating them, and why aren't they on the menu of my favorite fast food restaurant?" From my experience, I'd suggest the following reasons for why whole grains are typically avoided:

1. *Lack of Education*

   The closest many of us ever got to brown rice was by eating white "minute rice." The closest most of us get to millet is by noticing it in birdseed formulas. We might have a mushroom-barley soup in a deli, have a tabouli salad (made with cut whole wheat particles called bulghur wheat), or have some buckwheat pancakes on a Sunday morning (loaded with artificial syrup), but that's about the limit of our whole grain exposure. Only in the last twenty years have nutrition experts discussed whole grains. Typically, they refer to grain products. The hard-core truth about our relationship with whole grains is that we don't know what they are, why we need them, where to get them, how to cook them, or how to eat them. We lack education.

2. *Availability*

   Until recently, you had to go to specialty health food stores to purchase whole grains. While natural food markets offer the widest choices and bulk rates, whole grains are now available in some super markets.

3. *Time Constraints*

   For our fast-paced lives, the idea of daily cooking, much less cooking something that takes from thirty minutes to an hour to cook, seems practically primitive in the face of microwaves and our instant-mania about food preparation. Of course, there is a wealth of food preparation shortcuts, but "throwing something together" out of cans, frozen packets, or instant mixes does not create true health. Creating healthy meals requires planning and effort.

4. *Taste*

   "It's bland—Yeech!" I once heard this from a client about her first whole grain meal. Apparently, she forgot she had teeth. Whole grain begins its digestion in the mouth, with the alkaline elements of saliva enzymes working to break complex starches into smaller particles. These smaller particles of complex carbohydrate gradually raise blood sugar to provide us with more enduring energy. At first, grains might seem bland. However, as they are chewed, their taste becomes naturally sweet and delicious.

5. *Unfamiliarity with the Benefits of Whole Grain*

   Let's presume you frequently suffer from constipation, find yourself fatigued, are not satisfied with your meals, and seem to be always craving something sweet. Then, you begin to eat whole grains on a daily basis and suddenly your bowels regulate with precision, your energy picks up, and you discover a renewed satisfaction with meals while your craving for sweets automatically lessens. This experience allows you to witness the power of simple food, the power of whole grains to change your health. This experience will motivate you to continue to eat and appreciate whole grain.

THE GRAIN PRODUCT LOWDOWN

Grain products, particularly breads, are the Western version of whole grains. In the Orient the most popular forms of grain products are noodles and dumplings, usually both included as soup ingredients.

In the West, we like our bread dry and usually toasted—we're a nation of carbon lovers. The dry texture of bread or crackers makes an ideal companion with sauces, soups, sandwiches, or spreads, as in jams, nut butters, and pates.

There is a downside to our toast fanaticism. Different mutagens are formed with prolonged toasting, or baking, of flour. A diet of toast, regardless of its beneficial whole grain quality, is not health supportive.

Grinding a whole grain (or bean) into a flour increases available calories and the tendency to store fat, since the fiber is removed during processing. Fiber contains virtually no calories, so its removal increases calorie concentration. With flour, specifically with refined flour, a greater rise in blood insulin levels occurs during digestion as compared with the blood sugar stabilizing effect of whole grains.

POPULAR GRAIN PRODUCTS

Aside from the obvious advantage of convenience, the most appealing factor about grain products is their texture. This adds a sense of variety to the daily diet.

Here are some common examples of grain products:

- Breads
- Pasta
- Bagels
- Muffins
- Rice cakes
- Crackers
- Flat breads
- Corn chips

Since individual tolerances often vary, no hard-and-fast rules apply. Some people are energized by flour, while others exhibit allergic symptoms. Unyeasted whole grain breads made without stabilizers, conditioners, chemical preservatives, sugar, molasses, honey, coloring, and so on, are the best choices when you desire bread. Real bread shouldn't taste like a sweet roll. For pastas you may want to try Japanese soba, artichoke, corn, brown rice, quinoa, or whole wheat pasta versions.

Just short of needing a support group for my own bread addiction ("I am here tonight because I am powerless over toast ..."), I happily discovered that when I began eating whole grain, my bread cravings were significantly reduced and meals suddenly became more satisfying. Previously, I always left the table feeling bread deficient. When I travel and am unable to eat grain because of availability, I make sure to at least have several slices of unleavened, unsweetened, whole grain bread for a fiber source. In a pinch, it'll do.

FIBER: FRIEND OR FOE?

Good news/bad news—it never seems to fail. A new study comes out triumphantly heralding the miraculous benefits of a particular product and is soon followed by news alerts that warn of its dangers. This was the case with fiber during the early 1970s.

When missionary surgeon, Dennis Burkitt, M.D., returned to England from working in Africa with native tribes, he brought dramatically impressive observational research about the length of time it took food to travel through the natives' digestive systems. This information rocked the nutritional world and popularized the word *fiber* for the world-wide lexicon. Dr. Burkitt concluded that constipation and intestinal cancers were rare in native societies due to the heavy fiber content of their natural diet. The Africans studied had active lifestyles and lived chiefly on whole grains, vegetable, bean, fruits and low-volume, low-fat animal proteins. Transit time, from mouth to bowel discharge, was approximately 17 hours, maximum. Immediately, "fiber" became the new buzzword in the national lexicon. It became a featured marketing slogan ("Now, with more fiber!"), featured supplement ("Get your fiber in convenient pill form daily!"), and the newly embraced cause of every ill imaginable ("Death begins in the colon!").

Then, the inevitable happened. Phytates were discovered and, almost overnight, fiber became the bogeyman of natural food diets. Suddenly, fiber was a no-no.

Phytates are the storage forms of phosphorous compounds found in the fiber of whole grains, legumes, nuts and seeds, and numerous other plant foods. Nutritional researchers warned the public to avoid phytates because of their ability to bind minerals and decrease the breakdown of proteins. This conclusion came from studies in which raw wheat bran (a concentrated source of phytates) or baked goods high in wheat bran were given as a primary source of dietary fiber. However, these conclusions have little relevance to vegetarians or whole grain eaters whose intake of dietary fiber comes from a variety of cooked, raw, and processed sources.

Phytates have recently been applauded because they bond to excessive iron elements and carry them out of the body, protecting susceptible individuals from iron overload. There is some research that links excessive stored iron to cancer development. So, suddenly phytates are our friends. Additional research suggests that phytates provide benefits by regulating the absorption of glucose from starch.

In a World Health Organization (WHO) report summarizing the effects of fiber and phytates on the availability of minerals from plant foods, phytate fears were explained:

> *Studies from the eastern Mediterranean region suggest that very high intakes of unleavened bread, where the cereal phytate has not been destroyed by the endogenous phytate in the grain, do lead to problems of mineral absorption. However, this seems to be a problem of food preparation rather than of the diet as such. In human physiological studies, exchanging full grain cereals for refined starches low in fiber does not lead to calcium zinc or iron malabsorption, because the whole grain provides an additional intake of the minerals that compensates for any reduced mineral availability. Oxalate-rich foods such as spinach do, however, limit mineral absorption.*

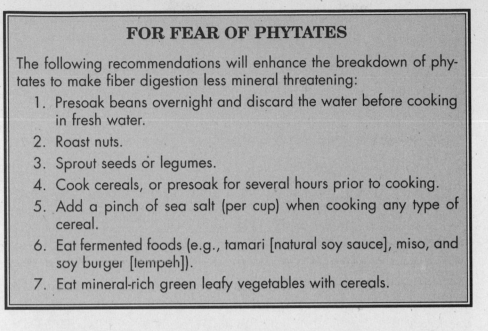

FOR FEAR OF PHYTATES

The following recommendations will enhance the breakdown of phytates to make fiber digestion less mineral threatening:

1. Presoak beans overnight and discard the water before cooking in fresh water.
2. Roast nuts.
3. Sprout seeds or legumes.
4. Cook cereals, or presoak for several hours prior to cooking.
5. Add a pinch of sea salt (per cup) when cooking any type of cereal.
6. Eat fermented foods (e.g., tamari [natural soy sauce], miso, and soy burger [tempeh]).
7. Eat mineral-rich green leafy vegetables with cereals.

The WHO study further states that there appears to be no advantage to intakes of dietary fiber in excess of 40 grams per day and even proposes 54 grams as a healthy limit.

Fiber is best consumed from whole foods (long-chain carbohydrates). A diet of whole grains, grain products, vegetables, beans, and other plant foods will supply abundant fiber that will not compromise your mineral status.

SWEET NEWS WITH A BITTER TASTE

In the early 1900s two-thirds of the carbohydrates in the U.S. diet came from complex sources such as whole grains, grain products, and vegetables. Today, half of all carbohydrates consumed come from refined and concentrated simple sugars. Since 1990, the average American consumed over 150 pounds of sweeteners per year. Add noncaloric sweeteners to that number and it leaps to 165 pounds. If you compare these numbers to the consumption of less than 10 pounds of sugar per person per year in the late 1700s, you'll find that sugar consumption has risen more than 1500 percent in the last two hundred years!

FIBER FIX-UPS

- A 1977 study that examined women eating a low-fat, high-complex-carbohydrate diet over a two-year period found that the women had changes in breast tissue composition that were linked to a reduced risk of developing breast cancer.

- The fiber that comes with whole grain, commonly referred to as roughage, is actually the indigestible part of the carbohydrate. The outer covering of the grain absorbs water in the digestive tract, making the stool bulkier as it sweeps along the intestinal walls to be discharged. A bulkier stool passes quickly through the digestive tract, allowing less exposure (and thereby absorption through the gut) to carcinogen-containing foods. The fiber bonds to these carcinogens, so they do not have time to ferment within the intestine.

- A study from Uruguay examined the diets of over 700 women and uncovered a strong link between dietary fiber intake and a reduced risk of breast cancer in both pre- and postmenopausal women.

- A study by the National Cancer Institute examined the different roles nutrients played in cancer prevention and tumor inhibition. The study looked at the different ways a variety of fibers attached to different colon carcinogens (such as 1,2-dimethylhydrazine, or DMH). Wheat and corn bran, alfalfa, citrus pulp, and citrus pectin were evaluated for their pH. The pH readings ranged from 1 (highest acidity) to 12 (highest alkalinity). Results showed that as the pH of each fiber tested increased in alkalinity, the percent bound to the carcinogen was increased. This study revealed how dietary fiber inhibits cancer by binding to chemical carcinogens and removing them from the colon. The pH factor, in this case, appeared to be an influential factor in the fiber attraction and binding to the carcinogens.

How concentrated are simple sugars?

The industrial process can take approximately 3 feet of sugar cane, wash, cut, crush, industrially evaporate it, and end up with 1 teaspoon of white sugar. The average piece of cherry pie, cut into eight pieces, contains nearly 10 teaspoons of sugar. Add one large scoop of ice cream (5 teaspoons of sugar) and you have a grand total of 15 teaspoons of sugar! So, through the efforts of modern technology we can, in the course of about six minutes, consume 45 feet of concentrated sugar cane and call it a "little snack."

Honey, regardless of its quality, is also a very concentrated food. One of my nutrition professors claimed that 1 teaspoon of honey was equivalent, in sugar concentration, to five or six medium-sized apples. To make 1 gallon of maple syrup you may have to boil approximately 35 to 40 gallons of tree sap. And if you've ever squeezed oranges to make juice, you already know it takes three to four oranges just to fill a small cup.

This does not mean that these substances are bad across the board; it just emphasizes their concentration. By the design of our intestinal tract, digestive secretions, and tooth structure, our bodies require complex-carbohydrate fuel on a daily basis. We might all have varying needs, but our physiology demands that this food group make up a central part of our daily eating. Lack of complex sugar in the daily diet is one of the most common reasons behind simple sugar cravings.

"As the Blood Sugar Rises ...": An Internal Drama

When we eat simple sugar, its simplified molecular structure allows it to become absorbed into the blood almost immediately as it leaves the mouth and enters the esophagus. This is why, in most cases, you feel like tap dancing immediately after eating sugar—it's already in your blood. When the blood sugar level increases abruptly, the pancreas shoots off insulin as a protection response. If the blood sugar is too high, you can end up in coma. Before a high-blood-sugar coma can occur, the pancreas saves the day by responding with swift and plentiful amounts of insulin. However, since most of the blood sugar is being shuttled into the liver, you soon end up with a low (hypoglycemia) blood sugar condition.

A low blood sugar condition can happen between 1½ and 2½ hours after eating something sweet. Two hours after your 8 A.M. breakfast, while at work, you have that 10 A.M. sweet break.

After your noon lunch (with dessert) you seek a sweet relief for that 2 P.M. break—perhaps a cola. Then, you leave work between 4 and 5 P.M. and suddenly find yourself in the company of a number of very happy people who, after consuming a liquid sugar together, poorly sing top forty songs. This is aptly called "Happy Hour." You go home, have dinner (with another dessert), and find yourself nibbling again two hours later. This is referred to as "prime-time snack." Finally, before you retire to bed, ritual practice takes you into the kitchen, where you stand in front of the freezer and take several tablespoons of ice cream before bed—or indulge in that childhood memory of milk and cookies.

If we were to diagram these blood sugar waves of high and low, it might look like the chart below.

What you've done is continually tease your blood sugar throughout the day—elevating it, making it drop, over and over until you finally fall into bed and call it a day. The well-known consequences of such blood sugar hopscotching are a lack of energy, mood swings, weight gain, tumor growth, immune weakness, mineral deficiency, lack of mental clarity, and, most notoriously, fatigue.

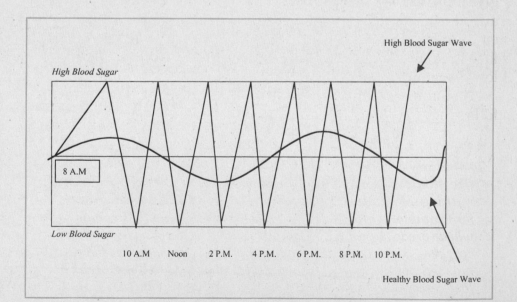

GLYCEMICALLY INCORRECT: THE POLITICS OF BLOOD SUGAR

"Pasta makes you fat." Eating carrots can be worse than eating refined sugar." "Eating 2 ounces of noodles has the same effect on blood sugar as a chocolate bar."

If you've ever heard these confusing claims and scratched your head in bewilderment while feeling overwhelmed with this "new science," you're not alone.

For the past sixteen years, The Glycemic Research Institute has been conducting research on what dietary factors trigger insulin changes in the body. Scientists believe that by determining how the body metabolizes foods, they can gain insight into the varying effects of different foods on an individual. Insulin elevated by a particular food is calculated by a clinical rating system called the glycemic index.

The glycemic index (GI) measures how much a person's blood sugar rises over a certain period of time (approximately two to four hours) after the ingestion of 100 calories of a food. The higher the glycemic index, the higher the blood sugar. Scientists conclude that the most important factor in predicting glycemic ranges is the surface area of the food. The more finely a food is ground, or the more highly refined a food is, the higher its high glycemic rating since grinding it increases its surface area. Foods that have a small surface area typically have a low glycemic index.

A summary study by Tomas M. S. Wolever, M.D., offered the following:

> The GI does not necessarily relate to food factors that are *popularly expected to make a difference, such as the dietary fiber content, the amount of sugar, or the degree of cooking or refining. Many diverse common foods have similar GI values; for example,* melba toast®, *bagels, white bread, 100% whole wheat bread, angel food cake,* graham crackers®, *whole wheat crackers, couscous, corn chips, oatmeal muffins, french fries, mashed potatoes, and canned green pea soup, and the break-fast cereals* Cream of Wheat®, Cheerios®, *and* Golden

Grahams®, *have almost identical GI values (range 94–106). On the other hand, the GI values of some foods can vary markedly, depending on variety, processing and preparation. This does not invalidate the GI concept, but may make it more difficult to apply in practice.*

Glycemic researchers found that every food tested produced a unique glycemic response. Their continued testing produced a few surprises:

- Lentils and beans yielded very low glycemic responses (confirming earlier studies on soluble fibers).
- Ice cream and yogurt also produced low responses (due to fat content).
- Bread and corn produced sharper responses than rice.
- Pasta produced much less of a glycemic reaction than breads; yet breads taken together with beans resulted in a lower reaction characteristic of beans (far lower than pasta) rather than the high response of bread alone.
- The texture of foods affected their glycemic rating—a wetter, creamier texture produced a faster rise in glucose (e.g., "rice slurry" and pureed apples both cause a more rapid response than rice grains and whole apple).

Based on this research, which can and has been easily misinterpreted, many diet book authors are recommending that "bad" carbohydrates (e.g., bananas, carrots, brown rice, millet, corn and sweet potatoes, rice cakes, parsnips, and apricots) should be avoided because of the speed with which they are converted into glucose when eaten and, therefore, elevate insulin levels.

Taken out of context, if this were true it would mean that ice cream and potato chips are as good as lentils and superior to brown rice and carrots. Many researchers were quick to point out that this indexing was a serious oversimplification.

Studies had already shown that although adding fat to carbohydrates (as many protein-oriented diet books recommend) produced a flatter glucose curve by slowing absorption, it had

THE VALUE OF THE GI

It is important to remember that the glycemic index is determined by taking concentrated foods in isolated trials and observing their effects on blood glucose and insulin. While this might be factual in isolated studies, we rarely eat large concentrations of one food in such a static manner. The important factors that easily influence the glycemic index are cooking, use of sodium, mixture with other foods, fat content, manner of eating, and individual biochemical conditions.

I think the glycemic index has been helpful for drawing attention to the fact that refined (and even some unrefined) flours can elevate blood sugar and frequently result in fatigue, sweet cravings, acidity, and so forth. The unfortunate ramification of this important discovery has been misunderstood and used to further assorted dietary agendas by labeling traditional foods, eaten by cultures for thousands of years, as "no longer good for you." If anything, the importance of depending on whole complex carbohydrates, such as brown rice, barley, millet, and oats, as opposed to grain products has been one of the most valuable findings of glycemic index research.

no such effect on the person's actual insulin response. Moreover, high-fat, low-glycemic index foods such as buttered potatoes, potato chips, or ice cream actually impaired glucose tolerance in the subsequent meal.

WHAT HAPPENS TO SUGAR IN THE BODY?

As anyone who has a passion for donuts will confirm, an excess of sugar easily turns to fat in the body. This is the ingredient insanity of many low-fat foods. They may contain a low percentage of fats, but the amount of sugar (added to make the food more palatable) ends up producing the very condition consumers are trying to avoid in the first place—weight gain.

Excess sugar eventually affects every organ in the body. The excess is stored in the liver as a form of glucose called glycogen. If the liver storage capacity (limited to 60 to 90 grams) is exceeded, the liver can swell. This can happen simply by eating too much fruit. Some evidence for this exists in medical literature, which has shown that fruit sugar actually causes liver cells, as well as the endoplasmic reticulum (a series of membranes within the cell that carries proteins to different parts of the cell), to take up water and swell. This disturbs, and ends up compromising, the cell's natural detox functions.

With the liver at maximum sugar storage capacity, excess glycogen is returned to the blood in the form of fatty acids. These acids are taken to various parts of the body and stored, first in the most inactive areas such as the belly, buttocks, thighs, and breasts. Once filled, excess fatty acids are distributed among the active organs, such as the heart and kidneys, in the long term hindering their function. Eventually, their tissues turn to fat.

We have to be careful when pointing an accusing finger at fat as other hidden fingers collectively point to sugar. However, sugar's agenda is just a bit more sly. It's a fine food in any form to enjoy occasionally, when healthy, as a treat or during social functions. But, for healing purposes, sugar should remain as a rare indulgence. When you do indulge, eating it in small volumes is the safest bet.

The Wrath of Sugar

There are many debilitating conditions that excessive sugar can create, or at least aggravate. It seems ridiculous to hear so-called nutritional experts screaming about the dangers of fat when, in many cases, the problem is an excess of sugar that turns to fat, fostering acidity and triggering immune breakdown.

Some French statistics seem to illustrate this point. Despite the fact that the French diet is higher in fat than the American diet, the French have lower levels of obesity and heart disease than American counterparts. In addition to having a more active lifestyle, this could chiefly be due to their sugar consumption; the French per capita sugar consumption is five and a half times less than that in America.

We do not require sugar as a dietary nutrient, which it is not, anyway. There is no recommended daily allowance (RDA) for sugar. If there were, you'd hear this: "Hey, Marie, it says right here on the wrapper: 'One chocolate bar provides all the essential non-nutrition sweet lovers need for the next 24 hours!' Cool!"

The list of degenerative conditions excessive sugar produces is exhausting. Most notable are mineral deficiency, excess of anaerobic intestinal bacteria, inflammation, tooth decay, obesity, candida, heart disease, diabetes, irritable bowel syndrome, gall stones, and tumor growth.

The solution to sugar cravings is first to understand what our basic nutritional needs are and how to adapt them into our lifestyle so we can enjoy natural sweet treats without developing the addictive feeling that requires a sweet after every meal.

THE CARBOHYDRATE–CANCER CONNECTION

Cancer cells feed directly on blood glucose, similar to a fermenting yeast organism. Swings in blood sugar, where the blood becomes flooded with glucose after sugar consumption, are like tossing gasoline on a smoldering fire. Here are some of the studies that support cautious use of sugar for a precancerous or cancerous condition:

- There is a well-accepted association between elevated insulin levels and cancer potential.

- Cancer cells show a three- to five-fold increase in glucose uptake compared to healthy cells. Modest ingestion of glucose (75 grams) caused a measurable decline in cell-mediated immunity in seven healthy human volunteers.

- Healthy human volunteers ingested 100-gram portions of simple sugars from sucrose, fructose, white sugar, honey, and orange juice. The simple sugars significantly impaired the ability of the white blood cells to engulf bacteria for up to six hours. Complex-sugar ingestion did not have this reaction.

- An epidemiological (population) study of twenty-one countries indicates that a high sugar intake is a major risk factor for breast cancer.

- In a study where animals were fed isocaloric diets of carbohydrates, the group consuming more sugar developed significantly more mammary tumors than the starch-fed group.

- Women who drank two to five servings of alcohol per day had a 40 percent higher risk of breast cancer than nondrinkers did.

- According to a profile of Medical Director, Darryl See, M.D., of The Immune Institute in Hungington Beach, CA, the institute's low sugar diet for Cancer protocols ". . . doesn't just include avoiding refined and natural sweeteners, but also high sugar-content fruits, alcohol and refined carbohydrates such as white flour. Normal cells utilize fats and proteins as fuel in addition to utilizing glucose (blood sugar). Adhering to a low-sugar diet not only robs cancer cells of the nutrition they need, but also prevents sugar's deleterious effects on the body that encourage cancer growth. These effects include suppressing the immune system, creating an acidic environment and stimulating prostaglandin E2 production that promotes tumor growth."

FAT: THE DIETARY "F" WORD

Our love affair with dietary fat has complex social, lifestyle, nutritional, and psychological grounds. Fat holds in the taste of food; it has a chameleon quality that absorbs flavors without imparting its own taste. Fat is a common fast food, from french fries (80 times the amount of fat contained in a baked potato) to chicken fried steak, fish (as in fish 'n chips), salad dressings, hash browns, fried eggs, ice cream (with nuts), and so forth.

Fat does not really become digested until it leaves the stomach after three hours. Once fats enter the first section of the small intestine, the duodenum, bile salts from the liver are poured from the gall bladder to emulsify them before they travel the intestines for absorption. Therefore, fat provides a sense of fullness, of solidity, of a "stick to your ribs" kind of feeling. Fat has a stabilizing effect on blood sugar, which makes it a common food to eat in place of sugar since it can sometimes delay cravings. Fat's texture and lack of fiber make it similar to a baby food; no doubt there is some association with fat (particularly dairy food) as a "comfort food."

Zoned Out

If the 1980s and 1990s were low fat, the millennium has birthed a renewed interest in fat. Not just any old fat, but animal fat. Suddenly, best-selling diet books, putting their own spin on science, are recommending animal protein as it they've discovered youth's elixir, justified by the dichotomy of "good fats and bad fats."

Nothing could be farther from the truth. Population studies, years of established medical research, and the experience of thousands of individuals have borne this out. We went from 40 to 50 percent total fat diets in the 1960s and 1970s to the recommendations of nutrition and heart specialists, who suggested 10 percent fat diets. When this did not prove satisfying, along came recommendations for "the right kind of fats," and suddenly we're eating (and celebrating) high fat (30 to 40 percent ratios) again.

Moderation has always been the hallmark of good health. The real work is to find the balance and reduce the foods that trigger cravings for fats or that make a body experience continual blood sugar drops. From most research, the probable dietary culprits for these problems and those that can influence the growth of cancers are refined foods, sugar, excessive fat, and excessive protein—everything we claim to love.

During the 1950s, when Japan's cancer rates were very low, fat intake represented about 7 percent of the calories in the Japanese diet. In rural China, the average fat intake is now approximately 19 percent of daily calories. The China Project examined provinces with fat intakes ranging from 6 to 24 percent of calories and found that breast cancer was more common in those provinces at the higher part of the range. This would make the current American Cancer Society recommendations of a 30 percent fat intake too high to be of maximized protective benefit.

Fatty Acids

All fats have different amounts of saturated, monounsaturated, and polyunsaturated fatty acids. Fatty acids are the building blocks of fats. Although I discuss briefly these individual categories, no naturally occurring fat has just one or two of these types of fatty acids, but combinations of each.

Rich monounsaturated or polyunsaturated fatty acids are liquid at room temperature, while saturated fatty acids remain solid. The standard American diet contains combinations of these types, although for many years there has been an emphasis on saturated types. Saturated fatty acids are usually found in animal products, such as whole milk, cheese, butter, egg yolks, beef, lamb, and pork. Some of these might contain small amounts of monounsaturated and polyunsaturated fatty acids as well.

On the other hand, vegetable oils, such as corn, sesame, safflower, sunflower, soybean, and cottonseed, are fairly high in polyunsaturated acids. Monounsaturated fats can be found in olive, canola, peanut, and avocado oils as well as in nuts and seeds.

An exception to the rule is coconut and palm oil. These oils are highly saturated and, strangely enough, a common ingredient in many processed foods. Saturated fats will raise blood cholesterol levels. Currently, there is no positive data on the benefits of saturated fats but reams of research on its negative effects.

Regardless of the type of fatty acid you consume, it's worth remembering that all fats can be potentially harmful if eaten excessively. Diets high in any kind of fat (with the exception of fish oils) have been associated with cancer.

WHAT ABOUT FISH OILS?

Research with native Greenland Inuit populations has shown that the oils in cold-water fish can lower serum triglycerides (blood fats) and prevent blood clotting. This has spawned an entire industry of fish oil supplements, which are hawked to consumers for cardiovascular health and blood clot prevention. However, fish oils do not effectively lower the low-density lipoproteins (LDLs), the so-called "bad" cholesterol. Some studies reveal that fish-oil supplements can increase LDL cholesterol.

If desired, a small amount of seafood with omega-3 fatty acids, in place of red meat and poultry, can be eaten several times weekly in 4-ounce portions.

Monounsaturated fats (fats that contain a higher percentage of monounsaturated fatty acids) have a neutral lowering effect on cholesterol and can be eaten in moderate amounts of 2 to 4 teaspoons daily.

OXYGEN BANDITS

The sole purpose of the approximately 11 to 14 breaths we take every minute, over 17,250 daily breaths and well beyond 6,000,000 per year, is this: to obtain oxygen. Our lungs will process this oxygen and send it via the circulation to all body cells, whose function is dependent on this fuel. Oxygen cut off from the brain for four minutes can produce irreversible brain damage.

As you inhale, millions of oxygen molecules attach themselves to red blood cells and travel to cell structures by way of progressively narrowing vessels called arteries, arterioles, and finally, capillaries. The red blood cells have a slight electromagnetic charge that repels them from each other, keeping them separate so they can flow smoothly through the capillary.

In the narrow diameter of the capillary, the oxygen molecules disengage from the red blood cell and pass through the capillary wall to enter cells. In exchange, cellular waste (carbon dioxide) enters the capillary, attaches itself to the red blood cell, and hitchhikes to the lungs, where it is discharged through exhalation.

The best way to upset this flow of red cells is by consuming a fatty meal. Fat, by various mechanisms, makes the blood sticky. In digestion, fats are broken down and emulsified into small droplets called chylomicrons. Different from other nutrients, such as glucose and amino acids, which are carried directly to the liver by the bloodstream, fats are absorbed into the lymphatic system, a slow-moving auxiliary circulation to the blood system. The lymphatic system bypasses the liver and empties the fat into the blood at the heart level. Now, the heart pumps the fat throughout the body. The bottom line: Consuming an excessive amount of fat means a bloodstream full of fat.

Fat coats the cells and makes them bond together. The cell sticking, or clumping, traps them. This picture of red blood cells clumping together and slowing the general circulation is called rouleaux formation, or red blood cell aggregation. Most frequently it's described as "sticky blood cell syndrome." This gumming of red blood cells prevents oxygen molecules from entering the cells. The result is a deprival of oxygen. Estimates of such oxygen loss have been calculated at 30 percent.

Dr. Timothy Regan, at the cardiovascular research laboratory of Wayne State University College of Medicine, studied the way one high-fat meal prohibited oxygen supplies to the heart tissue. Healthy volunteers without a history of heart trouble consumed a high-fat meal. At peak levels of fat in the blood, the oxygen uptake by the heart was reduced by 20 percent.

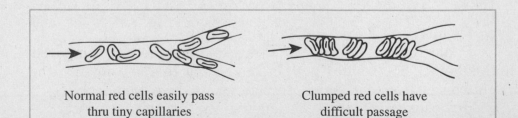

Normal red cells easily pass   Clumped red cells have
thru tiny capillaries   difficult passage

Cancer cells will thrive in a deoxygenated environment. Any substance that diminishes cellular oxygen can foster the growth of cancer cells.

CANCER RISKS WITH A HIGH-FAT DIET

China, Japan, and Singapore, where the majority of the population consumes a low-fat diet, have the lowest incidence of breast cancer. Countries that have a higher percentage of fats, such as England, Scotland, Wales, and Finland, have a greater incidence of breast cancer. Finnish women on higher-fat diets showed greater estradiol levels than Asian women—and a higher degree of breast cancer. Estradiol, one of the most powerful natural forms of estrogen is increased in the body by 30 percent when a high-fat diet is followed. Many breast tumors are fueled by estrogen.

While estrogens are normal and essential hormones for both men and woman, the higher the production of estrogen, the higher the chance of stimulating certain kinds of breast cancer. On high-fat diets, estrogen levels increase; on low-fat diets, they decrease. This pattern is also found in prostate cancer. Men who consume diets that emphasize animal proteins tend to have more testosterone and higher levels of estrogen when compared with men who have lower levels of animal protein and fat. This could also be due to the way fiber will bond to sex hormones and help discharge them from the body before they can become reabsorbed within the intestine.

In dozens of animal studies, a high-fat diet has been shown to stimulate the growth of cancers. Another study from the *British Journal of Cancer* showed that a 15 percent low-fat diet, strictly followed for two years, lowered estradiol levels by 20 percent. Animal fats seem to be a bigger problem than vegetable oils.

Paulo Toniolo, of the New York University center, compared the diets of 250 women with breast cancer to 499 women without cancer from the same province in northwestern Italy. Both groups consumed identical amounts of olive oil and carbohydrates. The distinguishing factor among the cancer patients was that this group had eaten more meat, cheese, butter, and milk. Among the women who consumed more animal products there was a three times higher cancer risk compared with the other women in this study.

The power of a vegetarian diet can be undermined by the inclusion of milk, cheese, and other dairy products. Some studies of lacto-ovo-vegetarians (vegetarians who eat milk and egg products) have found that their cancer risk is comparable to meat eaters. While these vegetarians were avoiding meat, they were eating considerable amounts of diary products, which, like meats, contain animal fat and are devoid of fiber.

However, vegetable oil is not exempt. Vegetable oils have been shown to affect estrogen levels while increasing cancer-causing free radicals. More than substituting deep-fried onion rings for fried chicken, the wisest preventive, as well as healing choice, would be to eliminate, or dramatically reduce, animal protein and consume a minimum amount of vegetable oils.

PROTEIN PROPAGANDA

The word protein usually conjures instant associations with meats, dairy food, and, most recently, protein powders. There was as time when people believed they could never get enough protein. Americans in the early 1900s were advised to eat over 100 grams of protein daily. When I was in high school during the 1960s there wasn't a coach worth his salt that didn't advise varsity athletes to boost their protein. "Get that steak in before the big game!"

Weight trainers went a long way to perpetrate this exclusive meat–protein association. When I was in my twenties, I went to a famous West Coast bodybuilders' gym for an evaluation. The owner, a well-known 1950s muscle man who graced many a cover of the muscle mags, looked at my thin body and said, "If you want muscle, ya' gonna haf' to eat a lotta meat!" He also wanted me to drink a protein liquid blend he'd "created" that had four to six eggs mixed in. This was a part of his training protocol. I asked, in my youthful naivetè, whether it was really necessary to eat that much animal protein. His face scrunched up. I watched the words, "Don't be stupid!" fly from his lips as he leaned close to me with his bicep an inch from my nose. "See this?" he said, pointing to his bulging bicep. "Meat! Workin' out, rest, and clean living! That's the formula. You wanna healthy body? You gotta work for it." Words of irony from a man with perfect-appearing proportions who later succumbed to colon cancer.

While there are many myths surrounding protein, the idea that protein is vitally important is not a myth. Protein is a crucial component of every cell and most of the chemicals necessary for life. We build the proteins of our bodies from amino acids, which are provided from the protein in our diets. Protein is essential for blood vessels, skin, bones, muscles, cartilage, lymph, hair, digestion, enzymes, antibodies, and some hormones. Hundreds of other body functions depend on protein. However, this does not mean we must have a high degree of protein to sustain these functions.

The current recommended allowance for protein is 0.8 grams per kilogram (2.2 pounds) of body weight for adults, or 44 grams for the average woman and 56 grams for the average man. Routinely, many Americans eat over 100 grams daily.

I have often seen clients who later told me that when they increased their protein percentage, they felt "better." While the protein I predominently suggest is vegetable quality such as beans and bean products, for certain clients I will recommend fish, and sometimes poultry, but still in percentages of 10 to 15% of the total diet. Invariably, after further questioning or review sessions, I realized that as clients reduced their fat or increased their dietary sweets, they would crave more fat or seek fat via a protein source (nuts, meats, etc.).

For some clients who were previously on high-fat diets, I found that gradual transitions, in the long run, were more consistently effective. Sometimes, just adding 1 to 2 teaspoons of flax or olive oil per main meal or a sprinkle of nuts on grains did the trick.

With clients who had advanced cancers and were on conventional therapies, a greater amount of protein was necessary. I have observed that cancer clients on very strict macrobiotic diets with a maximum of 20 to 30 grams of daily protein are rarely satisfied with their diets. They constantly crave a variety of other foods, frequently overeat, lose muscle mass, and inevitably become depressed by their diminishing body image, equating it with cancer progression. This doesn't negate the effectiveness of a macrobiotic approach; however, it does address the need to individualize a dietary program and maintain some flexibility.

The bottom line is that there are always dietary variables, which can only be dependent on individual physiology, previous diet, daily energy demands, and individual disposition.

PRACTICAL PROTEIN POISONING

Excess protein has been linked with osteoporosis, kidney disease, urinary tract calcium stones, and some cancer development.

After almost a century of nutrition, the best advice is to eat a well-balanced diet, not a high-protein diet. Research from Willard J. Visek Professor Emeritus (retired), University of Illinois at Urbana-Champaign suggests that an excess of ammonia is the result of a high-protein diet. Cell culture experiments revealed that ammonia slows the growth of normal cells more than that of cancer cells. Ammonia can alter the character of RNA, the cell's regulator of protein production. It also changes the rate at which thymidine is used for DNA, the cell's genetic material. These qualities of protein metabolism make cells less able to protect themselves from infection and from malignant transformation.

Visek believes that cells inside the human body act the same way as they do in laboratory tissue cultures. Cells in the body are exposed to ammonia whenever protein is broken down. The higher the protein volume, the greater the possibility of producing damaging quantities of ammonia.

The kidneys take the worst beating from having to eliminate the breakdown products of urea, uric acid, and sulfur. Excess protein creates an acidic condition of the blood, requiring the body to mobilize minerals such as bone calcium to neutralize increasing acidity. When the kidneys eliminate these breakdown products, the mobilized calcium goes with it.

Although fat is portrayed as the underlying cause of male cancers, protein has a definite role. Populations that eat meat on a regular basis seem to be at an increased risk for colon cancer. Researchers believe that fat, protein, natural carcinogens, and the absence of fiber in meat all play significant roles. In 1982, the National Research Council noted a link between cancer and protein.

Beans have been noted to lower bile acid production by 30 percent in men with a tendency toward eleveated bile acid. Bile acids are necessary for proper fat digestion but in excess have been associated with causing cancer, especially in the large intestine. Case-control studies showed that pinto and navy beans were effective in lowering bile acid production in men at high risk for this condition.

It has also been observed that a high protein meal results in a greater increase of prolactin levels than an isocaloric high fat meal. The research indicated that the high protein diet typically consumed by the average American can contribute to an ele-

---

A HEALTHY PERSPECTIVE ON PROTEIN

- Your protein needs can be met by eating a wider variety of plant foods without the dependency of animal protein. The healthiest, cancer-preventing sources of protein are beans, bean products (Tempeh soy bean burgers, tofu, natural soy sauce, miso soup bouillon paste), whole grains, and vegetables.

- Only 12 to 15 percent of your daily calories should originate from protein. Excess protein turns to body fat.

- Many types of animal protein contain high percentages of fat, which can be responsible for numerous disease conditions related to a high fat intake.

- For athletic performance, complex carbohydrates are the most effective and clean-burning fuel. Most frequently, athletic needs are based on greater volumes of foods.

- For extremely active individuals or those on conventional cancer therapy (chemotherapy, radiation, etc.), more protein might be required.

vation of prolactin levels. It has been established that high prolactin levels accelerate the growth of human breast cancer
under experimental conditions.

The Nature's Cancer—Fighting Food Program (see Chapter
10) includes a varied diet of whole grains, beans, and vegetables
that contain all the essential amino acids. Years ago, many
health books advised eating certain bean and grain combinations to create more "complete proteins." Nutrition experts
eventually concluded that this type of combining is unnecessary with each meal since a varied diet of grains, beans, and
vegetables can meet all protein needs within the course of a
day. Occasional animal protein, during a dietary transition or
when weak, might be recommended; however, this must be
based on individual considerations, not a blanket rule.

3
PHYTOCHEMICAL SUPER HEROES AND AMAZING ANTIOXIDANTS

SHOWDOWN ON THE CELLULAR FRONTIER: ANTIOXIDANTS VERSUS FREE RADICALS

Oxygen is considered vital to life, but scientists are also finding that this essential element could contribute to aging and illness. When oxygen is metabolized, or burned by the body, the cells form byproducts called free radicals.

Free radicals are not political upstarts, but an atom, or groups of atoms, with at least one unpaired electron. This makes them highly reactive. On a positive note, free radicals promote beneficial oxidation that produces energy and kills bacterial invaders. Sometimes the body's immune system purposely creates them to neutralize viruses and bacteria. However, environmental factors such as pollution, radiation, tobacco smoke, and herbicides can also spawn free radicals. Normally the body can handle these reactive atoms, but if antioxidants are unavailable, or if free radicals suddenly multiply, the cell's functioning becomes disrupted and cell components become damaged. Such damage is believed to contribute to the aging process and assorted health problems. It has been shown that free-radical damage normally accumulates with age.

Antioxidants to the Rescue!

Antioxidants can protect cellular components from damage by neutralizing the free radicals. People who consume adequate amounts of foods high in antioxidants (vegetables, fruits, etc.) have a lower incidence of certain cancers, heart disease and cataracts. The most popular phytochemicals (plant chemicals) with antioxidant properties are vitamin C, vitamin E, and beta-carotene (converted by the body into vitamin A).

ANTIOXIDANT-RICH FOODS

Vegetables	Vitamins:	A	C	E
Carrots		* * *	* * *	
Cauliflower			*	* * *
Cabbage		* * *		
Squash			* * *	
Broccoli		* *	* * *	
Pumpkin		* *		* *
Watercress		* * *		* * *
Peppers		*	* * *	* * *
Sweet Potatoes		* * *	*	* * *
Peas		*	* *	* *
Tomatoes		* *	* *	
Beans	**Vitamins:**	**A**	**C**	**E**
Beans				* *
Seeds/Nuts	**Vitamins:**	**A**	**C**	**E**
Seeds/Nuts				* * *
Fruits	**Vitamins:**	**A**	**C**	**E**
Lemons		*	* * *	
Melons			* *	* *
Grapefruits		*	* *	
Oranges		*	* *	
Apricots		* *		
Strawberries		*	* * *	
Kiwis		*	* *	
Mangoes		* *	* *	

Carrots, broccoli, sweet potatoes, cantaloupe melons, and apricots are particularly high in beta-carotene. Eating these foods appears to prevent DNA damage (halting the initiation of cancer) and to stop cancer from developing.

Vitamins—The Antioxidant Solution?

The best sources of antioxidants are fruits and vegetables. In 1999, scientists from John Hopkins University in Baltimore compared various diets in 123 people during an 11-week study. During the first three weeks of the study, participants ate diets with varying amounts of fruits, vegetables and dairy products. Some groups consumed a maximum of four servings of vegetables and fruits daily.

Scientists measured the breath ethane levels of the participants. This measurement indicates how well the body neutralizes harmful free radicals (the lower the breath ethane level, the better). The study's conclusions revealed that the participants consuming the most fruits and vegetables had the lowest breath ethane levels. Lead study author Dr. Edgar R. Miller claims that a natural antioxidant-rich diet provides the body with naturally occurring antioxidants, which protects the body against cancer and heart disease.

THE PHYTOCHEMICAL SUPER HEROES

Phytochemicals (*phyto* = Greek for *plant*) are plant chemicals from whole grain, bean, vegetable, fruit, and nut/seed sources. These chemicals protect the plants from disease. Produced by the hand of Nature, these biologically active compounds have also proved to augment the body's defense against disease and aging. Some phytochemicals have shown promise in inhibiting tumor growth while others can stop the chain of events in the body that leads to cancer, heart disease, diabetes, and hypertension. Some phytochemicals have antioxidant properties (protecting against harmful cell damage), anticancer properties (preventing the initiation and promotion of cancer), and anti-estrogen properties.

Although the way in which plant compounds specifically help combat disease is still being researched, the mechanisms are as complex as the molecular structures themselves. Some may work as antioxidants, others as enzyme inhibitors. Each chemical class could contain components that number in the hundreds, making individual classification complicated, if not painfully boring. The most popular class of phytochemicals researched to date is the phenolic group. This includes monophenols, polyphenols, and flavonoids, which are found in most cereals, vegetables, and fruits.

VEGETABLE SOURCES

The following table breaks down the vegetable sources of key phytochemicals and nutrients.

Plant Family	Types	Prime Nutrients
• Whole grains	Brown rice, oats, barley, millet, buckwheat, wheat (also bulgur), rye, quinoa, etc.	Soluble and insoluble fiber, B vitamins
• Legumes	Lentils, black beans, chick peas, aduki, pinto soybeans, peas, etc.	Protein, B vitamins, fiber
• Allium	Onions, scallions, leeks, shallots, chives, garlic	Anticancer elements, heart-disease fighter
• Leafy green	Kale, collard, endive, swiss chard, root vegetable tops (turnip, beet), lettuce, bok choy, etc.	Vitamins A, B, and E, iron, calcium, magnesium
• Cruciferous	Broccoli, cabbage, turnips, Brussel sprouts, cauliflower, bok choy, watercress, rutabaga, sprouts	Vitamins A, C, calcium, iron, magnesium
• Umbelliferous	Carrots, parsnips, parsley, celery, fennel, cilantro	Beta-carotene, vitamins A and C
• Cucurbitaceous (gourd family)	Squash, pumpkins, watermelons, muskmelons, cucumbers	Vitamins A and C, iron, fiber, phosphorus, beta-carotene
• Convolvulacoeus	Sweet potato	Vitamins A and C, potassium
• Solanaceous (nightshade family)	Tomatoes, eggplant, potatoes, peppers, capsicum	Vitamins A and C, potassium
• Fruit	Apples, pears, peaches, apricots, bananas, oranges, etc.	Vitamins A and C, fiber, potassium

Consuming a whole foods diet (whole grains, vegetables, beans, fruits, nuts, and seeds of numerous plant foods will provide a wide mix of phytochemicals (phenolic compounds, terpenoids, pigments, and other natural antioxidants such as vitamins A, C, and E), as well as some nonnutritive substances that have been associated with protection and/or treatment of chronic diseases such as heart disease, diabetes, hypertension, cancer, and other medical conditions.

There are hundreds of phytochemicals, only a smattering of which has been studied to date. Current scientific research has identified approximately fourteen different classes of phytochemical compounds. With names like *isoflavones* (found in soy and other beans), *sulphoraphane, lycopene, lutein, xanthene, anthrocyanin, isothiocyanates, allium, glutathione, beta-carotene, quercetin, carotenoids,* and *glucosinolates,* they sound more like *Star Trek* terminology than substances that are fast

PHYTOCHEMICAL SOURCES

Phytochemicals	Food Sources
• Flavonoids	Cruciferous, umbelliferous, solanaceous, and cucurbitaceous plants, most vegetables, garlic, green tea, soybeans, cereal grains, licorice root, wine, most fruits (especially citrus), onions, kale, flax seeds
• Carotenoids	Dark yellow, orange, and green vegetables and fruits
• Isoflavones	Soybeans, legume family
• Phenolic compounds	Cruciferous, umbelliferous, solanaceous, and cucurbitaceous plants, green tea, garlic, soybeans, flax seeds, cereal grains, licorice root
• Monoterpines	Unbelliferous, solanaceous, and cucurbitaceous plants, citrus fruits, garlic, sage, camphor, dill, basil, mint
• Organosulfides	Onions, leeks, scallions, shallots, cruciferous plants, garlic
• Indoles	Cruciferous plants
• Isothiovyanates	Cruciferous vegetables, mustard, horseradish

becoming the new research frontier in the battle against America's deadliest diseases. Finally, the wisdom of "eat your vegetables" is being documented.

The most popular class of phytochemicals that has nutritional research is focusing on is the phenolic group. This group includes monophenols, polyphenols, and flavonoids, which are found in most whole grain cereals, vegetables, and fruits.

"Waitin' 'til all the lights turn green ..."

Numerous studies support a diet centered on whole grains, vegetables, beans, fruits, herbs, nuts, seeds, and small quantities of animal protein, if desired. When I first began lecturing in the early 1970s, much of this information was not available. In addressing academic groups as a speaker, I could hint, or offer theoretical science; however, there was still little scientific "proof."

I was limited to scant references of population studies or pseudoscience of early-twentieth-century theorists, who did not have the vast scientific resources available now. Cultural folk medicines offered interesting reasoning for disease conditions based on energetics, but this would not satisfy an academic audience. Such audiences want tangible facts—"proven" information.

When such research and reference was not available to me in my early speaking career, I had to rely on a different tact. I stressed economics ("Reduce your food bill by one-third!"), spoke about how to make natural food actually taste good, and hammered the point that one could feel better in a short time without negative side effects. I'd urge participants to let this "harmless experiment" be an adventure for discovering the power of food.

Many of the people who I counseled, either privately or in groups, would call back later, elated that their long-standing constipation was no longer a problem, that their lower back pain disappeared, or that their tumor had become noticeably smaller when scanned three to four months later. If their commitment level was high, their efforts usually proved quite positive. They learned, and confirmed, from their own experience.

The academic approach would be to offer verifiable research. However, beneath the need for "scientific proof," most people, academic or otherwise, usually want the same thing: to feel better, look better, live longer, and enjoy life without enduring pain or feeling deprived.

Remember that science is still in its infancy. We are somewhat stuck in reductionism theory, isolating parts and assuming that the independent activity of a part does not influence a whole. Unfortunately, it's not as simple as this.

Example: We isolate phytochemical catechins from green tea and discover that they have promise as an anticancer substance. So we recommend green tea—across the board. Glance in any nutrition cancer book and you'll see green tea recommendations. True, catechins may have anticancer properties; however, what about the caffeine content? Some research has shown high caffeine intake to weaken immunity, and other studies show that it inhibits the liver's detox mechanisms, producing structural changes in animal DNA. Yet, some research shows black tea extract to inhibit tumor growth. So where do we stand? What do we do in the face in contrary research? Who do we listen to?

Our viable options are either to continue doing what we've been doing all along, at the possible risk of further harm, until the final research comes in, or to make some adventurous lifestyle and dietary changes that may result in an increased sensitivity. With the second option, we know by our own experience that our path is, at least, in the right direction.

I once had a friend from the South who was a crack salesman full of Southern charm, descriptive metaphors, and country proverbs that he'd rattle off with a liquid tongue and an easy smile. His closing comment to anyone waiting for more research was in the form of a homespun traffic analogy: "If you keep waitin' 'til all the lights are on green, you'll never get out the door."

PHYTOCHEMICAL CANCER PREVENTION RESEARCH

For the more academically inclined, the following data, based on a variety of research studies, supports my overall theme from the scientific side of the field:

- While fruits and vegetables are often mentioned in the same breath as the cancer-prevention twins, scientists at the Fred Hutchinson Cancer Research Center in Seattle think this is only half right—the vegetable half.

  In a study on prostate cancer, Fred Hutchinson scientists reported in the January, 2000 issue of the Journal of the National Cancer Institute that a diet rich in vegetables—particularly cruciferous varieties (so named because their flowers have four petals suggestive of a cross). Examples of cruciferous vegetables are: broccoli, cabbage and brussel sprouts and they are thought to reduce the risk of prostate cancer by nearly 50 percent. The popular notion of tomatoes are as especially protective against cancer wasn't borne out by the study. Fruits did not offer any preventive advantage.

  "We found no protective effect at all from fruits," said Dr. Alan Kristal, an investigator with the center's cancer prevention research program. While their study only looked at prostate cancer risk in 1,230 middle-aged men, Kristal said a growing body of evidence from other studies of diet and cancer indicates this may also hold true for other cancers as well.

  "We think it's all in the vegetables," he said. "Go ahead and eat fruit as well," Kristal remarked, "but do it because it tastes good."

- The results of an early 1990s twenty-million-dollar study that spanned five years, researching the anticancer potential of plant foods, showed that the foods and herbs with the highest anticancer activity include garlic, soybeans, cabbage, ginger, licorice, and the umbelliferous vegetables (such as carrots, celery, cilantro, parsley, and parsnips). Foods with a modest level of cancer-protective activity include onions, flax, citrus, tumeric, cruciferous vegetables (broccoli, brussel sprouts, cabbage, and cauliflower), solanaceous vegetables, (tomatoes and peppers), brown rice, and whole wheat. Other foods that were found to contain a measure of anticancer activity include oats, barley, mint, rosemary, thyme, oregano, sage, basil, cucumber, cantaloupe, and berries.

- New phytochemical research has identified a host of active substances in specific foods that provide protection from cancer. These substances include ally sulfides in onions and garlic; phytates in grains and legumes; glucarates in citrus, grains, and solanaceous vegetables; lignans in flax and soybeans; saponins in legumes; indoles, isothiocyanates, and dithiolthione in cruciferous vegetables; ellagic acid in grapes, strawberries, raspberries, and nuts; phthalides and polyacetylenes in the umbelliferous vegetables; and a complete range of flavonoids, carotenoids, and terpenoids in numerous plant foods. These powerful phytochemicals have been shown to block the many hormone actions and metabolic pathways associated with cancer development.

- Some have claimed that phytochemicals may be diminished in the process of cooking. However, research has shown that most of the compounds are heat stable and are not significantly lost in the cooking water. Although vitamin C might be reduced through cooking, carotenoids and indoles (broccoli source) may actually be increased during the cooking.

- A complete variety of phenolic compounds, which include flavonoids, are contained in whole grains, vegetables, herbs, and fruits, so that you already may be ingesting as much as one gram of phenolic compounds per day. These phenolics can influence the quality, digestibility, and stability of foods by acting as flavorings, colorants, and antioxidants.

- Glutathione *S*-transferase (GST), a cancer inhibitor, is stimulated by the phthalides in celery seed, the sulfides in garlic and onions, the dithiolthiones and isothiocyanates in broccoli and other cruciferous vegetables, the bitter liminoids in citrus, and the curcumins in ginger and tumeric.

- Flax has also been proven to be an extremely rich source of lignans, which have been shown to be anticarcinogenic. The lignan metabolites bear a structural similarity to estrogens and can bind to estrogen receptors to inhibit the growth of estrogen-stimulated breast cancer.

- Soybeans have very high levels of numerous compounds with established anti-cancer activity. Those compounds include, phytates, protease inhibitors, phytosterols, saponins, and isoflavonoids. Soybeans are thought to be a contributing factor in the low incidence of breast and prostate cancer in Japan. Chinese who regularly consume soybeans and/or tofu have only one-half as much cancer of the stomach, colon, rectum, breast, and lung compared with those Chinese who rarely consume soy or soy products. Decreased prostate cancer has also been observed in Hawaiian men of Japanese descent who regularly consume grain (rice) and bean products (tofu, tempeh, etc.).

- Whole grain is not without its powerful phytochemical members, containing ample amounts of plant sterols, phytases, phytoestrogens, rocotrienols, lignans, ellagic acid, and saponins. These powerful substances reduce the risk of cardiovascular disease and cancer. Of particular importance is that the active phytochemicals are concentrated in the bran and the germ, confirming that the health benefits of grains truly come from eating grains in their whole form. The refinement of whole wheat illustrates this point clearly: Refinement causes a 200 to 300-fold loss in its phytochemical make-up.

BURDOCK: THE GARDEN PEST YOU'LL LEARN TO LOVE

Native to Europe and Asia, burdock now grows wild throughout the United States, thriving in backyards, overgrown fields, and parks. Its leaves, which grow up to two feet, are large and heart shaped. Its carrot-like root is dark brown.

Burdock stimulates the flow of bile by improving liver function. Anything done to aid liver function will improve blood quality and general health. Another detoxing bonus is burdock's diuretic properties. It contains a compound called inulin, which is believed to enhance immunity by encouraging white blood cell activity. A 1984 study in *Mutation Research* showed that burdock protected cells exposed to carcinogenic chemicals from mutations, which can lead to cancer. Another 1996 study published in Pharmacology Letters found that burdock extract has antiviral—in particular, anti-HIV—properties.

Recommended by herbalists and used in numerous cultural folk Medicines, burdock is generally considered to be a blood cleanser and is an essential ingredient in many herbal cancer formulas. It was a staple in Japanese monasteries, where monks were given side dishes to increase stamina.

With a mild, earthy flavor, burdock can be added to soups and stews and combines well with sweet vegetables such as carrot or onion. It can be purchased in many natural food stores, as well as in Asian markets. The Japanese call it, "Gobo."

THE FIVE-STEP RX FOR "VEGGIE-PHOBIA"

When former President George Bush made national front-page news with his "I do not like broccoli" statement, he opened up a controversial public dialogue on the American love–hate relationship with this frequently maligned vegetable. News media debated the topic for days, nutritionists rallied with defensive assertions on broccoli's abundant value, and broccoli growers sought to capitalize on this negative publicity with a positive spin and all-out campaign.

THE VEGETABLE RAINBOW

I once read a Japanese culinary book that explained the value of "psychological appetite." This term implies visual arrangements of foods and color to inspire the appetite in your mind. Considering the variety of plants available to us, different pigments in our food not only lend unique health benefits, but also enhance our enjoyment of the eating experience.

Estimates have calculated there are approximately 200 known plant pigments in our food. Contained within this amount are over 800 flavonoids, 450 carotenoids, and 150 anthocyanins. Fortunately, it's not necessary to memorize every single one of these chemicals before your next meal, but the importance lies in understanding that these pigments do more than just provide pleasant sensory appeal. They protect us from disease by combating free radicals to offer protective oxidative damage and stimulate immune function.

Overnight, Bush became the poster boy for vegetable haters throughout the United States. I recall seeing a news cartoon that showed an adult pushing away a restaurant broccoli plate with the caption "If the president won't eat it, I won't either." However, Bush's remark is the tip of the veggie-phobia iceberg: The average American eats only about one and a half servings of vegetables per day and less than one serving of fruit per day.

A recent survey of American eating habits showed that less than 10 percent of the population met the guidelines for eating at least three servings of vegetables and at least two servings of fruit daily. This survey also revealed that one in every nine Americans ate no fruit and no vegetable on the day of the survey, and 45 percent reported eating no fruit that day.

I think that vegetables have played such a small role in most of our diets chiefly due to a lack of education. The importance of vegetables in the daily diet has never been really explored other than with general lip service, and we lack the skills for selection, preparation, and cooking vegetables. Here are five simple ways to create greater appeal and enjoyment from vegetables:

1. *Reduce consumption of refined and simple carbohydrates.* The frequent eating of concentrated sugar lessens the desire for and taste appeal of vegetables. A child who loves soda pop won't get excited about eating squash, just as an adult who consumes a bowl of ice cream has little inclination to eat oatmeal afterward. The solution? Eat less sweets, and stick to small amounts of fruit, fruit-juice-sweetened treats, or natural syrups and malts such as barley malt, rice, or maple syrup.

2. *Eat more vegetables.* Consume a wide variety of colorful vegetables on a daily basis. Make vegetables more familiar to your tastes. Different cooking styles create a greater sense of texture for meals. Try steaming, water-sautèing, baking, and making soups to avert boredom. Many vegetables are delicious eaten raw.

3. *Avoid eating between meals.* While it might be a good general suggestion to eat more frequently throughout the day, allow approximately 3 to 4 hours between meals. Constant snacking can reduce the desire for vegetables.

4. *Chew your food.* This might sound insulting, but, few of us really chew our food. We gulp, bolt, and wash food down. Watch people eat for five minutes in a restaurant and you'll see diners virtually inhaling their food. Are you any different? Being carbohydrates, vegetables begin their digestion in the mouth. Chewed thoroughly, they will impart a natural sweetness you'll never forget.

5. *Learn to cook.* Believe it or not, this can be invaluable. I'll never forget my first garden and the joy at being able to go into the back yard, pick some carrots and greens, and then go prepare them. At times when I did not have a garden, I'd find out where the farmer's markets were in my city and visit them, talk with the growers, and buy fresh, quality vegetables whenever possible. It became my Saturday morning ritual. After taking a short cooking class and learning the basics, I'd invite friends over as a weekly ritual and cook a meal. Learning simple food preparation can take the fear out of cooking, make your

RAW VS. COOKED?

Research has shown that the vitamins and minerals in raw vegetables may be much less available to the body than those present in cooked vegetables. Cooking carrots can enhance carotenoid absorption by as much as 500 percent. This holds true for other vegetables rich in phytochemical carotenoids.

A study released in the June 1999 issue of *Scientist* reported that cooking and mashing the vegetables increases carotenoid absorption from 4 percent to 20 percent. By softening the plant's cells, cooking allows for better intestinal assimilation of the carotenoids. Carotenoids, such as the beta-carotene in carrots, the lutein in yellow peppers, and the lycopene in tomatoes are all known to offer cancer protection. This doesn't mean to avoid raw carrots, but to make sure of getting a mixture of cooked vegetables into the daily diet.

Some roots, seeds, stems and leaves contain natural toxins that can be eliminated through cooking. According to Andrew Weil, M.D., "most raw beans are in this category, along with sprouts. Alfalfa sprouts, the omnipresent health sandwich ingredient, are actually high in the natural toxin, *canavanine,* which can damage the immune system. Ordinary button mushrooms may contain *agaritine,* which is a natural carcinogen. Even celery has its dark side: it tends to produce *psoralens,* compounds that sensitize the skin to the harmful effects of ultraviolet radiation in sunlight.

While our body's immune system can often bear these toxins out, a system that is overly taxed might respond reactively. Moderation, the hallmark of health, also applies to our cooking styles.

food more enjoyable, reduce the compulsion to eat out all the time, benefit your budget, and increase your sense of self-worth, simply by the action of a healthy self-care effort.

WHAT ABOUT SUPPLEMENTS?

Some marketers would like potential consumers to believe that phytochemical and antioxidant protection can be delivered via supplements. The benefits of long-term phytochemical supplementation are still premature and require verification from large-scale intervention trials. We do know that regular consumption of these phytochemical super heroes (whole grains, vegetables, legumes, fruits, etc.) produce substantial health benefits, and while some of these foods have high levels of

---

VEGETABLE RECOMMENDATIONS

The following recommendations are generalized but worthy of making a daily goal. (Additional detail and vegetable lists are featured in Chapter 5.)

- Eat enough to maintain a healthy and consistent weight.

- Eat a variety of vegetables from leafy green groups, root vegetable groups, and ground/round vegetable groups. Make sure your vegetable selection is colorful and cooked in a variety of styles, including raw. For those prone to any kind of stomach acidity, anemia, irritable bowel syndrome, or ulcers, raw can be quick boiled or lightly steamed, softening for better digestion but still crisp and vitamin rich.

- I have found recommending cups easier for clients than traditional "servings." I recommend a minimum of 3 cups of vegetables daily.

- A frozen garden mix is always a great quick addition to add color and sweetness to any grain dish.

- Have precut vegetable and fruit slices on a tray in the fridge or an easy-to-reach-place for quick snacks.

- Fibrous seasonal fruits are usually lower in sugar content and can be enjoyed once to three times daily. For individuals prone to fatigue, acidity, gas, or mineral deficiency, fruit recommendations are encouraged to be minimized to your sugar cravings. Juice, a concentration of sugar minus the fiber, is recommended infrequently. Better to enjoy the whole fruit. In cases of digestive weakness, fruit can be slightly cooked into compotes or baked (as in baked apple) for reduced acidity.

- Have a soup-making night once or twice weekly. This can last several days and will satisfy the most finicky of palates. (See the recipe section for soups such as Barley Vegetable, Sweet Vegetable Miso, Lentil-Leek, and Native Corn Chowder.)

antioxidants, many of them are thought to act synergistically. Therefore, a pill or potion may exert a different physiological effect in the body compared with the effect of naturally occurring phytochemicals available from whole grains, legumes, vegetables, and fruits.

A compelling argument for cancer prevention based on diet, as opposed to supplements, can be found in the natural, yet still unidentified compounds contained in food. It is thought that these compounds magnify the effects of identified phytochemicals. Foods generally contain many phytochemicals and compounds whose effects are not entirely understood. However, newly emerging research from laboratory and human studies suggests that phytochemicals do their most powerful work in combination with each other and a mixture of assorted plant nutrients could help the efficacy of certain cancer drugs.

The advantage of whole foods over supplements is not only in unidentified compounds but in their valuable fiber, fat, protein and carbohydrate content.

At this point, the best, safest, and most economical advice would be to eat real foods in their whole forms.

4 THE HEALING POWER OF ACID AND ALKALINE

ACID/ALKALINE BALANCE

The acid/alkaline balance of our body's fluid and blood levels is highly relevant to controlling health. Typical American diets are highly acid producing. Acids are also a waste product of the metabolic process, and unless properly eliminated, they accumulate in the connective tissue and in organs, where they can lead to premature aging and disease conditions.

Much of the acid/alkaline theory, first popularized by a number of the vogue diets of the 1930s, has insufficient medical research to support its basis. However, it is well known that any sudden acid or alkaline extreme can immediately impair health, particularly digestive, kidney, and immunity function. The increased acid load of refined simple sugars has also been demonstrated to diminish cellular immunity. In contrast, complex sugars do not have this effect.

This chapter clarifies the concept of acid/alkaline as it relates to diet while explaining how the acid/alkaline quality of foods can be measured and balanced. Research indicates that cancer cells feed directly on blood glucose, like a fermenting yeast organism. Elevating blood glucose in a cancer patient, thus causing a rise in acidity, has been equated to throwing gasoline on a smoldering fire.

The acid/alkaline concept may be fairly new to the general public, but it's old news to alternative health writers and holistic physicians. Mainstream nutrition researchers now seem to be finally catching up with the ideas behind acid/alkaline theory.

Acid/alkaline balance is critical to cancer prevention. But it has many other benefits to general health as well. I'm going to elaborate them in this chapter, too, because the better your all-around health, the stronger your ability to fight cancer.

With all of this in mind, let's cover some of the evolving acid/alkaline dietary theory.

THE ACID TRUTH ABOUT OUR ALKALINE HERITAGE

I once audited an advanced biology class in which the professor began his lecture standing completely still behind the podium and staring at the class. He didn't move a muscle. After a minute that felt like three days, he said something in a monotone voice that broke the class into a spasm of laughter:

"To you, it may look like I'm doing nothing, but on a cellular level, I'm actually very, very busy."

His statement was true.

As you read this paragraph, your body is involved in the complicated process of homeostasis. Homeostasis is defined as the process of maintaining constant physical and chemical conditions within the body despite external change. Our blood sugar levels, blood oxygen, carbon dioxide, and blood acid/alkaline levels are in constant fluctuation. These fluctuating levels are based on our stress exposure, daily diet, physical activity, and environmental influence. At this very moment you are secreting and eliminating acid waste products from your breath, nose, bowel, urinary tract, body cell metabolism, and skin pores. Imagine that.

However, while the acid waste produced by our cells is constant, it's fairly weak compared with the potentially toxic acid generated by refined, processed foods we choose in the name of nourishment.

The human body contains fluids inside and outside the cells of all muscles, bone, brain, bloodstream, urine, saliva, digestive fluids, and the spine. On the average, we carry nearly 10 gallons of fluid in our bodies. All of these fluids have different levels of acid and alkaline percentages, with their values expressed in terms of pH, representing the *p*otential of *H*ydrogen. The pH scale indicates the relative acidity, or alkalinity, of a solution.

Acids have a tremendously wide range of potency. You can eat a citrus fruit, containing citric acid, with no ill result, but the hydrochloric acid from a chemistry lab class could burn a hole right through your stomach if permitted direct contact with your tissue.

An acid/alkaline imbalance can instigate many disease conditions. Excessive acidity can breed yeast growth, nurture viruses, stimulate tumor growth, feed parasites, throw off mineral ratios, reduce helpful intestinal bacteria, and cause general fatigue. Many of these conditions are prevalent today because the standard American diet is dangerously high in acid-forming foods. These foods leave an acid residue after digestion, which influences blood balance.

Chemically speaking, an excess of hydrogen ions indicates a more acid pH condition, while less hydrogen ions indicate an alkaline condition. Acids are missing hydrogen atoms, and to compensate for this they rob electrons from wherever possible. This thieving nature makes them corrosive.

THE pH SCALE

...........*Healing Zone Area*............													
ALKALINE													ACID
High Alkaline			Low Alkaline			**Neutral**		Low Acid				High Acid	
Total	*Very*	*Moderate*	*Slight*			*Slight*		*Moderate*		*Very*		*Total*	
14	13	12	11	**10**	9	8	7	6	5	4	3	2	1

Commom Food/ Substance pH Values:

						Coffee	Orange Juice
						4.9	.4-3.8

Lye	Baking Soda		Pancreatic	Human	Cow's Milk	Beef/Pork	Vinegar	Soda	Stomach
13.5	12.0		Juice	Blood	6.6	5.0	3.5	2.8	Acid
			8.8	7.35-7.45					1.0-3.5

Soap	Sea Water	Water		Cottage Cheese	Beer/WIne
9.1	8.1	7.0		4.6	4.4

62

TIPPING THE SCALE

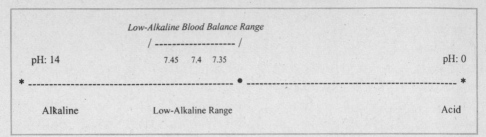

The pH of a substance is measured on a scale from 0.00 to 14.00, with neutral being 7.00—neither acid nor alkaline. The lower the pH number, the more acidic the solution; the higher the pH number, the more alkaline the solution.

In biochemistry, it is taught that the blood pH must be slightly alkaline to maintain normal metabolic functions. This slightly alkaline margin, on a scale from 0 to 14, could range anywhere from 7.35 to 7.45. A deviation in either direction beyond these narrow margins could prove fatal.

An acid pH of 6.95 can result in a diabetic coma and death, while an excess alkaline pH of 7.7 may cause tetanic convulsion, with eventual death. A more acid blood pH can slow your heartbeat, whereas more alkaline plasma will speed it up, thereby irritating your nervous system.

In the body's attempt to maintain acid/alkaline balance, there are some industrious mechanisms that are at constant work to decrease or increase either end of this spectrum. Here are four ways the body controls acid/alkaline levels:

1. *Physical Movement*

   As muscle fibers move, lactic acid from stored carbohydrate (glycogen) is created. This elevates the body's acid levels. This also explains why excess movement of muscles that have not been previously active results in soreness the following day—remember how you felt the morning after you helped a friend move and carried a zillion boxes up and down stairs all day? That soreness is from a build-up of lactic acid.

2. *Exhalation*

   Cell metabolism produces a waste product called carbonic acid, which is expelled though our lungs exhaled as carbon dioxide. This process helps to keep acid levels at a tolerable minimum. While stress can increase acid levels, deep breathing helps alkalize the blood by eliminating acid waste. This accounts for the "centered" feeling that breathing exercises accomplish.

3. *Kidney Function*

   One vital function the kidneys perform is the excretion of excess acid, or alkaline elements, into the urine for balancing purposes. When urine reeks of ammonia, this could be an indication of an overly acid metabolism with insufficient buffering elements (sodium, calcium, magnesium, etc.). These alkaline-buffering elements rely on the strong alkalizing back-up system of ammonia to help reduce excessive acidity.

4. *Daily Nourishment*

   Once the food we eat is broken down and metabolized, acid or alkaline elements will predominate. Foods high in carbonic and sulfuric acids, iodine and chlorine are considered acid forming, while foods that leave the buffering minerals of calcium, iron, potassium, sodium, and magnesium are alkaline forming.

THE EXTRACELLULAR CESSPOOL

Electrolytes carry essential oxygen to the cell for its survival. In a healthy digestive system, nutrients provide much-needed electrolytes to the fluid surrounding tissue cells. This fluid is called extracellular fluid and accounts for approximately 15 percent of our body weight—5 percent being blood and 10 percent extracellular fluid.

The extracellular fluid absorbs acids and other waste products from all cells. If acidity levels of this fluid increase, electrolyte imbalances (the primary nutrients of sodium, potassium, magnesium, and calcium ions) are sure to follow. When this electrolyte imbalance occurs, the extracellular fluid becomes toxic and waste product removal from the extracellular fluid becomes burdened. With poorly balanced amounts of minerals and nutrients, oxygen transport to the cells is compromised. When cells cannot receive the oxygen they require, they begin a slow death. It has been suggested that cancer can be accelerated by an acid condition of body fluids. Cancer cells are acidic, while healthy cells are alkaline. It is well known that cancer cells survive longer than normal cells in the acid and low-level oxygen environment of extracellular fluid.

For good nutrient health, the chemistry of extracellular fluid must remain fairly stable. Our organs of elimination— large intestine, kidneys, liver, lungs and skin—support this extracellular fluid. The health and discharge ability of these organs are dependent on being able to eliminate poisonous wastes from our body.

THE POTENCY OF ACID AND ALKALINE

All foods can be classified as having an acid or alkaline nature. The acid or alkaline pH of food is determined primarily by its mineral content.

WIDE RANGE OF PH LEVELS

In the following chart, notice the variety of pH levels within the body:

Digestive System		Elimination System	
Saliva	6.50–7.50	Urine	4.80–8.40
Stomach fluid	1.00–3.50	Feces	4.60–8.40
Duodenum fluid	4.20–8.20		
Pancreatic fluid	8.00–8.30	**Miscellaneous**	
Liver bile	7.10–8.50	Blood	7.35–7.45
Gall bladder bile	5.50–7.70	Spinal fluid	7.30–7.50
Small intestine fluid	6.50–7.50		

ALKALINE-FORMING MINERALS
Calcium, potassium, sodium
Magnesium and iron

ACID-FORMING MINERALS
Sulfur, phosphorous,
Chlorine and iodine

If your daily food leans more toward the acidic end, alkaline quality minerals will be required to neutralize acidity. These minerals, originating from bone and digestive secretions have neutralizing power. Think of this "buffering" procedure as a form of biochemical autoprotection. The typical American diet pushes the boundary of acidity. Our modern diet is a one-way ticket to Acid Land, chock full of strong acid elements (caffeine, sugar, alcohol, spices, excessive protein and fat, vinegar, and refined grain products) and seriously deficient in alkaline factors (such as vegetables and salt). This may be one of the reasons people become so hooked on salting (alkaline-forming source) everything that touches their lips. It may also be another reason why many people find vegetarianism difficult to maintain—meat cravings, due to salt contained in animal tissues become overwhelming. This is just not due to habit, as many claim, but could be from meats being a potent source of sodium, which occurs naturally within the meat tissue.

However, animal meats are a poor sodium source. Through daily urination and perspiration, salts within the meat soon leave our body and we are left with high residues of sulfuric, phosphoric, and uric acid—byproducts of meat breakdown. We compound this acid overload by indulging in large amounts of refined sugar (high acid), living fairly stressful lives (acid producing), overeating (acid indigestion), and consuming lots of acid-forming flour products and high-fat foods. On top of all this, we add insult to injury by gorging ourselves on highly concentrated artificial and other acid-based foods such as tomato juice, peppers, and spices. The rationale for eating these foods is nutritional. However, the larger view sees that the end result, despite nutritional gains, could be an excess of acidity, beneficial to some and weakening to others. The benefits are always relative to an individual's present condition.

DEMYSTIFYING ACID AND ALKALINE

The concept of acid/alkaline remains one of the most misunderstood concepts in nutrition. It is commonly referred to as *terrain medicine*, a reference to treating the whole individual. It has been established that pH in the blood, saliva, urine, and other areas is a critical factor for building health.

How does one determine an acid or alkaline condition? Through blood work? Saliva tests? Hair analysis? Muscle resistance? Urine? These are some of the tests being recommended by current nutrition authors. Most of these tests can show relative amounts of acid or alkaline, which is always interesting to compare. But there are so many varieties of acid and alkaline appearing in the system that to get any conclusive results about your acid/alkaline status it might be best to read the intracellular fluid—a test rarely performed. Most current diagnostic tests show the acid wastes present in the body fluids of blood, lymph, urine, mucus, or saliva. The problem with such tests is that they don't read how much acid waste is within the cellular fluids since these fluids are running through tissues and removing acid wastes. While it might be possible to measure the relative acid or alkalinity of body fluids, it is rare and more complicated to evaluate the acid or alkaline quality of body tissues such as skin, organs, glands, muscles, ligaments, arteries, and vessels. The majority of standard tests focus mainly on saliva, urine, or blood.

The tissue quality of skin, organs, glands, muscles, ligaments, arteries, and vessels is the real determining factor of our health. When acid wastes are not eliminated, they become reabsorbed through the colon, get filtered through the liver, and end up being re-released into the general circulation. In this case, you're recirculating waste, as opposed to cleansing and rejuvenating.

Even measuring a person's blood for acid/alkaline variations can be a difficult task. When acid is introduced into the blood, alkaline minerals from other parts of the body (digestive fluids, bones, etc.) are immediately mobilized to maintain a crucial pH balance of 7.35 to 7.45. The blood cannot tolerate elevated acidity. It must alkalize. To do this, it goes on an alkaline borrowing

FINDING THE BALANCE POINT

Moderation, the middle road, the balance point, has always been considered the hallmark of health. In support of this, how can you maintain a healthy balance of acid and alkaline in your daily meals?

Modern science tells us that our blood must be slightly alkaline. For balancing purposes, it would make sense to have the bulk of our food as centralized as possible in the following scale. To do this, you need an eating plan that's predominantly composed of low alkaline and low acid foods, with a slight emphasis on the alkaline side. You can achieve this by relying on the healing zone area diagramed in the following chart and permitting small quantities of strong alkaline foods. This mimics many cultural eating plans of the last 10,000 years.

Small Amounts .... Healing Zone .... Special Occasion

ALKALINE   **ACID**

High Alkaline   _Low Alkaline_   _Low Acid_   _High Acid_

Salt   Miso/Soy Sauce   Seaweed Land Vegetables   Grains Breads Beans Fish Fruit Sugar Vinegar Alcohol

.... MAIN FOODS ....

Along with vegetables, fruits are actually considered to be alkaline forming. However, I have taken the liberty of listing this category in the acid end of the scale due to the acidifying nature of sugar. While there may be minerals to classify fruit as an alkaline substance in lab diagnosis, what is almost always overlooked in acid and alkaline writings is sugar's resulting acidity in the digestive process. Simple sugars promote the growth of yeasts and leach the body's mineral sources, compounding an already acid environment with additional acidity. For some individuals, the acid effect of fruit might to help balance an overly alkaline condition. This gives the impression that fruit creates a low-end alkalinity. Again, in some individuals this may be so, but for cancer cells, candida growth, and compromised conditions of reduced intestinal flora (usually due to antibiotics, excessive animal protein, and sugar excess), minimum fruit, as a medicinal suggestion, is recommended.

spree, indiscriminately and immediately, with no intention of paying back the bone, tissue, and digestive juice mineral donors. This means that to do a blood test for an accurate acid/alkaline reading, testing would require your doctor to take blood samples at numerous intervals throughout the day and only after eating one particular food to obtain a true reading.

This could be very exhausting, costly, and still not reliable.

A number of nutrition writers suggest testing acid/alkaline levels with litmus paper (saliva) or urinalysis sticks (urine). Thinking you can determine acid/alkaline pH through such testing is assumptive, simplistic, and misleading. Saliva or urine is not reflective of your overall acidity. Such arbitrary and unpredictable testing does not read the cellular fluid or tissue quality of skin, organs, glands, muscles, ligaments, arteries, and vessels. It can only yield a partial evaluation.

The best barometer for evaluating your general acid/alkaline levels is your overall well-being.

CARBOHYDRATE DIGESTION—THE TORTOISE AND THE HARE

Recently, a biochemistry student attending one of my public talks complained that "whole grains eventually turn to glucose, just like white sugar, so they really have the same effect."

He was partially correct.

In the long run, both simple and complex carbohydrates turn to the simple sugar glucose. Both share a common acidity, but in different degrees; sugar is a high-acid food and grains/grain products are low-acid foods. However, I explained that the real difference has to do with the rate of absorption. It's like claiming that newspaper and wood logs burn identically in your fireplace. Of course, they don't. One burns quickly and the other has a more enduring and consistent flame. The tortoise and the hare both reach the end of the race, but at different speeds.

Recent studies have shown that refined grain products, *despite* being classified as complex carbohydrates, in many cases digest almost as quickly as simple sugars. Whole grains, such as brown rice, barley, and oats, digest more evenly and at a slower speed. Complex-sugar digestion does not cause high and low swings in blood sugar levels. It's stabilizing.

Making "healing zone" choices will encourage good, sustaining health. This doesn't mean you should never eat food from the strong acid category; it means you should respect the power of strong acid and freely indulge as your health and sensitivity permits. Otherwise you run the risk of becoming fatigued, less emotionally stable and with diminished immunity. This can set you up for sickness.

I've met and counseled many vegetarians who live on daily diets of high acid-forming foods (honey, fruits, sugar, etc.) and lack in whole grain, sea salt, or some of the blood-strengthening fermented foods (naturally brewed soy sauce, tamari, or miso). For vegetarians, whole grains and fermented soy products, such as tamari and miso, although seemingly exotic, offer essential value and taste appeal, which quickly results in more energy and better digestion. The typical high acid-forming vegetarian diet can cause muscle weakness, fatigue, poor memory, inability to gain weight, decreased sexual desire, and diminished immune function.

For years, in private counseling practice, I've successfully advised vegetarian clients to reduce strong acid foods while adding small amounts of high-alkaline foods. Within a week, positive differences become positively noticeable.

ACID/ALKALINE CONFUSION

An acid- or alkaline-forming food refers to the condition food causes in the body after being digested—and herein, lies the problem: Most charts, books, and explanations on acid and alkaline categorize food by ash content.

This perspective creates a broad misunderstanding since scientists are estimating a food's acid- or alkaline-forming capacity through a controlled laboratory procedure called *titration*. As a first step, this titration process burns the food (attempting to duplicate digestion). Next, about a liter of pure water is added to

100 grams of the resulting ash, producing a solution that is then tested to estimate the degree of relative acidity or alkalinity.

What occurs in vitro during lab experiments cannot substitute for what occurs in human digestion. Burning a lemon to ash leaves alkaline elements and no trace of its natural acidity, which is why lemons are usually classified as an alkaline-forming food. The same applies for honey, maple syrup, malts, and most fruits. The natural acidity and simple sugar content actually make lemon an acid fruit. Even if you're left with mineral ash, after digesting the fruit, the residual acidity of sugar's metabolism has a sustaining influence in your sugar and insulin levels and cortical hormone output.

Frequently, you'll hear nutritional experts recommend that we "eat lots of fresh fruits and vegetables." They're always lumping fruits and vegetables together. Why? There is a vast difference between these food groups. In most individuals, fruits have an acid effect, whereas most vegetables will tend to alkalize, since their sugar structures are complex and not simple. In our great reverence for science, we've overlooked the fact that trying to replicate human digestion under artificial lab conditions, performed outside the body, cannot possibly yield the same result that occurs with natural digestion. In many acid and alkaline writings, authors wax eloquent about the "alkalizing effect of fruits" to support their recommendations. Again, if someone is registering a high alkalinity, a little fruit can be highly beneficial and reduce the high alkalinity to a more mild status. Confusing as it may be, this is relative to an individual's condition.

How Sugar Produces Acidity

Simple carbohydrates are small numbers of sugar units that get absorbed into the blood immediately on contact with the mouth. Before you can say "fruitcake!" they've entered your blood and with lightning speed are distributed to body cells. This is where the problem begins: Simple sugars flood body cells with glucose so quickly that the oxygen necessary for effectively burning and metabolizing the sugar is not available.

The end result of this incomplete burning generates acidity. This is why so-called alkaline fruits actually acidify the blood.

Refined sugar, the "empty nutrient" food, has been stripped of virtually all minerals and vitamins. The minerals that have been processed out are essential for the building of tissues and bones, nervous system functioning, and blood filtering. Without a constant renewal of iron and sodium elements from this powerfully concentrated nonfood, the blood cannot take up sufficient oxygen. Metabolic waste products then fail to be neutralized and eliminated. The result is a bloodstream burdened with various acids (lactic acid, butyric acid, pyroracemic acid, acetic acid, carbonic acid, etc.). As acid levels in the blood elevate, a general drowsiness and sluggishness occurs—typical symptoms of sugar's carbonic acid toxicity. Therefore, the end result of sugar metabolism in the human body is acid forming.

Sometimes you'll hear the argument that unrefined simple carbohydrates (honey, maple syrup, rice syrup, barley malt, raw brown sugar, evaporated organic cane sugar, molasses, etc.), unlike refined white sugar, "contain some minerals" that "help balance sugar's acidity."

Don't bet on it.

While honey might contain some alkalizing minerals to classify it "alkaline forming," chemically, its overwhelming sugar content (approximately 86 percent) keeps it acidic in the human body. The same applies for maple syrup, barley malt, corn syrup, and other sweet concentrates. Natural quality sweet syrups with some mineral content, such as barley malt, rice syrup, maple syrup, and molasses, are healthier choices when you desire a sweetener, however, they can still be highly acid forming. Moderation, again, is the key.

MINERAL THEFT

You're being swindled. Yes, it's a harsh truth to face, but on a daily basis, from right under your own nose, grand larceny occurs with almost every meal you consume and it's happening in your very own body—your mineral bank is being blatantly robbed!

CHAPTER 4

ACID INDIGESTION? REACH
FOR . . . AN UMEBOSHI PLUM?

What do holiday meals, late night eating, party snacks, food-tasting expos, and the World Champion Contest for Highest Number of Hot Dogs eaten, have in common?

If you guessed indigestion, you probably have some past experience with indigestion you'd rather forget. We're told, in endless commercial advertisements that the solution lies in a simple over-the-counter antacid.

However, it's not so simple.

Antacids, while popular, can do more harm than good. First of all, they are a symptomatic remedy and merely bandage the real cause of the problem: excessive consumption—which creates acidity—excessive food acidity and often, stressful or rushed meals that are not conducive to digestion.

The second point is that antacids are ineffective for bloating or gas and contain a number of dyes, preservatives and often, sugar. Aluminum, commonly used in these products, can cause constipation and even lead to intestinal problems. Combinations of calcium carbonate and sodium bicarbonate cause the milk-alkali syndrome: electrolyte imbalance, irritability, headache, nausea, weakness, kidney, and possible immune damage.

While hydrochloric acid is normally produced in the stomach to aid digestion, it's destroyed by the regular use of antacids. The stomach responds by making more acid. This causes a rebound effect, which may cause you to take more antacids, causing further suppression of the acid your stomach requires for digestion. Studies have shown continued use impairs the stomach's ability to digest protein and can cause erosion of the esophagus.

While prevention is the most sensible approach, the odd time digestive upset may present itself and would better warrant a small piece of the Japanese Umeboshi plum, a slightly-sour tasting, salted apricot-like fruit that has been dried. It's available at most natural food markets and works well with gas, indigestion, grain digestion, and for enhancing immunity.

I never travel without them.

And all you can say is "What's for dessert?"

Here's the frightening internal drama that might be occurring every time you eat food that tips the acid balance: If we cannot maintain an alkaline condition of body fluids, it becomes difficult to maintain healthy cells. When cells are not healthy, organs become sick, and body fluids become more acidic and toxic as weakened cells turn into sick cells. Eventually, this can develop into numerous degenerative conditions. The normal pH for all tissues and fluids in the body, except the stomach, centers on neutral or slightly alkaline.

It may seem insignificant that the blood borrows minerals from the bones; however, if continued, it could eventually lead to osteoporosis—porous bones from loss of minerals. Since there are over 206 bones in the human body, the bones represent the largest storage of usable minerals, making them a reliable source for "borrowing." It's actually more like remorseless theft because the blood ends up defaulting on the loan—those minerals are never replaced. *Borrowing* is just a cosmetic term.

Mineral loss will also affect the ability of your immune system to function at an optimal range. In using diet to support the healing process, minerals are vital elements for a strong, resilient immune system.

THE DIRTY TRUTH

The soils used for growing our crops have become highly deficient for a variety of reasons:

- The widespread use of N-P-K (nitrogen-phosphorous-potassium) fertilizer in modern agribusiness farming methods
- The common practice of overfarming, which diminishes protective ground cover and trees
- A general lack of humus
- The natural erosion factors of drought, wind, and floodings

The unfortunate result is plentiful crops with reduced nutrient content. We are sacrificing quality for quantity.

N-P-K fertilizer is highly acidic, and in the same way that acid rain affects soil quality, this acidic fertilizer disrupts the acid/alkaline pH balance of the soil. Such acid conditions destroy valuable soil microorganisms. The primary job of these microorganisms is to transmute soil minerals into a usable form for plants. However, in the absence of these microbes, the minerals become neutralized and unavailable to the plant.

While the fertilizer will stimulate plant growth, the plants will grow deficient in vital trace minerals. In the absence of these trace minerals, the plants compensate by absorbing heavy metals (aluminum, mercury, and lead) that exist within the soil. These toxic metals are then passed on to us through the food chain and assimilated into the body deficient in protective nutrient minerals.

Alkaline trace minerals, rapidly disappearing from our soils, play a vital role in electrolyte formation in the body. Electrolytes are mineral salts that conduct electricity when dissolved in solution. Normally, the bloodstream provides the fluid medium for electrolyte formation. Electrolyte deficiency can result in energy loss and fatigue, disrupting the body's natural homeostasis and invariably leading to disease.

Most important, the real solution for soil demineralization does not lie in adding trace mineral supplements to the diet, but in remineralizing the soil, which begins with our farming practices, and insisting on foods that are not chemicalized or otherwise treated.

Foods that are certified "organically grown" offer greater nutritional value and extra flavor. Chemically grown foods burden our filtering organs (liver and kidneys). Toxins will tend to concentrate in fatty acids. Therefore, avoid commercial-quality, nonorganic meats, dairy, oils, nuts, seeds, and grains whenever possible.

CAFFEINE: THE DAILY ACID FIX

The social ritual of drinking caffeinated beverages is an accepted global addiction, exceeding an estimated 4 billion cups sipped daily. Americans alone consume over 100 billion cups yearly

THE CAFFEINE KICK

Barely ten minutes after caffeine is consumed on an empty stomach, it reaches most body tissues. Even after a full meal, blood levels peak in about a half-hour. When that "lift" kicks in, your heart, breathing rate, blood pressure, stomach and kidney secretions, and central nervous system orchestrate their own little Indy 500 bio-race.

The Food and Drug Administration (FDA) estimates that a 5-ounce cup of coffee can contain anywhere from 75 to 155 milligrams of caffeine. Percolated coffee represents the low range and drip coffee the upper range. Black tea contains approximately 50 to 60 and oriental green tea from 30 to 40 milligrams. Some sodas, particularly orange and yellow varieties, may contain around 55 milligrams per 12-ounce bottle. I once had a client who consumed 20 colas a day. He never sat in my office chair—he'd pace. That was easy to understand.

Although caffeine itself is considered an alkaloid, there are numerous other chemical properties within coffee or tea that contribute to its high acid content. There are more than 208 acids in coffee that contribute to indigestion and a variety of health problems caused by overacidity. These acids eventually drain the body's alkaline balance.

In order to neutralize these acids, our bodies must use calcium, among other minerals, as a buffering agent. Coffee depletes available calcium by excreting it through the kidneys. This reduces calcium reserves while adding to bone porosity. One medical researcher I spoke with suggested that one cup of coffee required over 25 milligrams of calcium in order to be neutralized. So, in an accumulative sense, caffeine can be a major mineral leach. Caffeine also stimulates secretion of nearly twice the amount stomach acid. In sensitive individuals, irritation of the gastric lining could lead to ulceration and decreased protein digestion.

Decaffeinated coffee consumption paints a nastier picture; the chemical solvents used in extracting caffeine from the beans end up remaining as a residue in your cup. Even the Swiss-water process, which exposes the beans to a hot-water bath, leaves behind oils and acids. A 12-ounce cup of decaf typically contains at least 10 milligrams of caffeine, and possibly more, depending on brewing methods. Acidity levels in decaf tend to be higher because Robusta beans, which have a higher caffeine and acidity content than Arabica beans, are frequently used to produce decaf coffee.

Despite whatever "favorable elements" or advantages there might be in coffee, it's good sense to consider its overall effect on your metabolism. A 1975 British Lancet study found that one cup of coffee increased cholesterol up to 10 percent and three cups up to 14 to 15 percent. Often, this cholesterol can move undetected into the arterial lining and not show up as an elevated ratio in blood chemistry panels.

Green tea, promoted for its valuable catechin compounds usually destroyed in the fermentative conversion to black tea, is credited with anticancer and antibacterial effects and with lowering cholesterol and improving lipid metabolism. However, the most important issue here, beyond the wonder nutrients science finds by microexamination, is how your body reacts to caffeine and your total acid profile. The benefit of an ingredient within a food might be overshadowed by the total effect of that food. For some people, green tea might not be a good idea because of caffeine's demineralizing effects and possible tumor-enhancing trait.

Without a doubt, the daily caffeine habit is a practice that produces unnecessary acidity as it potentially compromises immunity—something anyone on a healing path, or just concerned about health, should limit.

without an understanding of caffeine's debilitating effects. The addiction to caffeine is best realized when one attempts to "kick" the habit. A wide range of painful and fatiguing withdrawal symptoms make it a very difficult habit to change.

Caffeine belongs to a group of alkaline chemical compounds known as methylxanthines (mteh-el-ZAN-theenz). Their close chemical cousins include theophylline, a prescription drug used to treat asthma, and theobromine, found in cocoa and chocolate products. Caffeine is also present in smaller amounts in black and green tea, kola nuts, guarana, and numerous soft drinks. Methylxanthines stimulate the heart and central nervous system, act as a mild diuretic, and, when combined with other drugs, can relieve pain. They are also found in surprisingly high amounts, in Excedrine®, Anacin®, Midol®, Vanquish®, Cope®, NoDoz®, Awuaban®, Vivarin®, Dexatrim®, and Codexin® tablets.

TRADITIONAL WISDOM DISGUISED AS WEIRD CULTURAL HABITS

My father, Cuban by birth, had an amusing way of eating an apple. He would sprinkle a couple of salt grains on each bite. Ironically, my maternal grandfather, who was born in Russia and raised in Turkey, had the same habit.

A similar act of balance is displayed in the Mexican tradition where the strong acidity of Tequila is taken with (alkalizing) salt prior to downing a shot. They lick the web of their thumb and forefinger, pour some salt on that area (saliva allows the salt to stick), down the shot, and immediately bite into a wedge of lemon to cut the sharp taste of salt and tequila.

Understanding acid/alkaline balance makes traditional customs more credible than assigning them as "pointless rituals." Traditional rural Japanese people cooked whole grain (weak acid) with various strong alkaline substances, such as a pinch of salt or a small piece of seaweed, or sometimes the grain was prepared with a small mineral stone (obsidian, also known as quartz trachycte) that was not eaten but simply cooked with the grain. A distant continent away, American Indian tribes would cook their staple food of corn (mild acid) with wood ash (carbon = strong alkaline) added to the water. In Mexico, a touch of the mineral limestone (strong alkaline) was added when preparing tortilla (grain product being mild acid).

These customs somehow recognized the need for maintaining a more alkaline blood status by adding minuscule amounts of strong alkaline substances to mild or strong acid foods.

In the early 1920s and 1930s, the problem of intestinal gas (acidity) was commonly remedied (neutralized) with charcoal (alkaline) in the form of charcoal pills. The Japanese use Umeboshi salted plum (alkalizing), to deal with digestive upset. Today, an antacid might be suggested, such as baking soda or Alka-seltzer® (alka = alkaline). As always, the goal is to neutralize acid and create a more balanced pH that leans toward mild alkaline.

Among caffeine's various acids, tannic acid interferes with mineral absorption and aggravates iron-deficiency anemia. This also holds true for black tea. Although few of these findings are conclusive, medical research has linked high caffeine consumption to fatigue, mood swings, premenstrual syndrome (PMS), hypertension, fertility problems, birth defects, irregularities in heart rhythm, anxiety, panic attacks, irritable bowel syndrome, migraine, tremors, restlessness, tension headaches, joint pain, lower back pain, fibrocystic breast disease, insomnia and other sleep disorders.

THE STRESS DEVIL NEVER SLEEPS

Acidity can also be induced psychologically. Emotional upsets produce subtle and immediate acidic changes. Anger, frustration, fear, resentment, feelings of victimization or other negative attitudes that keep us on edge, preoccupied, and absent from the present act as an unyielding form of internal stress.

Even that gentle and seemingly peaceful oblivion we call sleep fails to protect us from the acid-forming effects of stress. It has been observed from pH readings during sleep, when our body is influenced by subconscious thoughts, that acids generated by mental stress cause the body to work overtime. Therefore, it's a deception to think that sleep offers a peaceful stress refuge. Despite passive journeys in the dream world, you still cannot relax.

Of all body tissues, the brain is the most demanding blood consumer, occupying nearly 30 percent of our blood volume. This means that a brain nourished by good-quality blood is clear in thought and sharp in reflex. If our blood is even slightly acid (difficult to measure through ordinary blood panels), the lingering effects of excessive sugar and other stimulants can make us more susceptible to psychological stresses.

Since mental stress is acid inducing, deep breathing, which facilitates the discharge of acid-carbon wastes, can help alkalize the blood immediately. This is why yoga deep breathing exercises, singing, or chanting create such calming peace. Stress management, breathing exercises, prayer, psychotherapy, and exercise, which can be highly effective, are partial solutions for handling stress. A holistic approach must include an understanding of how our blood chemistry is influenced by daily food choices. Otherwise, we run the risk of going three steps forward with powerful therapies and five steps backward with poor nutrition.

TAMING ACIDITY WITH ALKALINE WATER

It may not be the fountain of youth but a unique water filtration process, backed by forty years of Japanese medical research and used in many Japanese hospitals is electrifying the medical community.

The process of "ionizing" water is the new antioxidant kid on the block. It helps to saturate body cells with more oxygen, fight disease, neutralize toxins, boost energy and improve wound healing.

The Hunza's are one of the longest-lived races of people in the world. Located in northern Pakistan, Hunza is situated in several high-altitude mountain valleys. While some claim to be 150 years old, many are documented centenarians (over 100), and amazingly still active in society but without the common infirmities we attribute to old age. According to scientists, one key to the Hunza longevity mystery is derived by the water they drink. The mountain water that flows into the Hunza villages comes from surrounding glaciers. Structured hexagonally, this water is filled with mineral solutes and tests as highly alkaline.

In the body, only perspiration, skin and stomach juices are acidic. Virtually all other organ systems and secretions are varying degrees of alkaline. The determinant is extra oxygen.

As is commonly known, water is H_2O, a binding union of hydrogen atoms and one oxygen atom. The water molecule is split into two ionized parts—an H+ ion and an OH- ion. The hydrogen-heavy H+ ion is acidic. The hydroxide OH- ion is alkaline, which means pH values beyond 7 mean more OH- ions (and greater alkalinity), while pH values lower than 7 contain more H+ ions and are considered acidic.

The addition of oxygen serves two important purposes: It makes alkaline water an excellent anti-oxidant that helps to neutralize free-radical cellular annihilater's and it also enables alkaline to dilute acidic body fluids and re-establish their natural balance.

The Western diet and lifestyle (sugar chemicals, alcohol, excessive protein, stress, etc.) instigates a high level of acidity. Acidity can rob your blood and tissue of oxygen, putting a burden on the heart and lungs as it drains your stamina. However, the real problem is that acidity prevents your body from neutralizing and disposing of harmful, poisonous toxins. *This can leave your more susceptible to the cell-damaging free-radical oxidation that leads to cancer.* In a newsletter mention regarding alkaline water, Robert Atkins, M.D. explains that, "...in an oxygen-rich environment, tumor cells can't survive."

When acid wastes enter the bloodstream, the blood, in order to maintain a necessary narrow pH range, has to store these wastes. If there are too many wastes to handle, they can be deposited in various organ systems or along arterial walls. The break-down of this waste disposal process is how the aging and disease process is defined.

Alkaline water, having a pH between 9 and 11, can neutralize these stored acidic wastes and help remove them from the body via the eliminative organs. Since the water is ionized, it will not leech out valuable alkaline minerals, such as calcium, magnesium, potassium, or sodium.

Japanese medical researchers believe that acidic wastes burden and compromise immunity. The process of using electrolysis to electrically split filtered tap water into alkaline and acid water was first developed in Japan during the 1950's, and approved for use as a medical device by The Health and Rehabilitation Ministry in 1966.

Combined with a moderate alkaline diet, alkalized water can be a great tool for an individual's healing arsenal of therapies.

WHAT HAPPENS WHEN YOU'RE TOO ACID

Current nutritional research links high acidity to numerous mental problems, arthritis, high blood pressure, diabetes, kidney disease, asthma, morning sickness, osteoporosis, indigestion, allergies, as well as the following conditions that are related to cancer:

NUTRITIONAL CONDITIONS

- An acidic condition hinders antioxidant activity. Free radical oxidation is encouraged in an acid medium.
- A lowered muscle pH leads to a decrease in muscle permeability, causing nutrients to become blocked from entering cells. Nutritional absorption, from food or supplement sources, becomes compromised.
- Cellular APT production decreases. This results in mood, stamina, and energy changes. Fatigue is a common sign of excess acidity.

IMMUNITY BREAKDOWN

- Excess acid hinders the breakdown of food within the small intestine. This occurs particularly in the area known as Peyer's patches, which are linked with longevity and produce lymphocytes to assist the lymph system in maintaining immunity. Excess acid weakens the production of these lymphocytes and negatively affects absorption.
- The immune system is impaired. An acidic condition decreases the beneficial bacteria within the intestine. Nutritional absorption of the B vitamin group is diminished.
- Fatigue, from failure to remove acid waste within and around the cell, is one of the most common problems from excess acidity.

ORGAN DAMAGE

- The heartbeat can be altered by acidic wastes when these wastes diminish tissue oxygenation. A moderate alkaline system creates ideal regularity.

- Excessive acidic wastes create added labor for the lungs, whose main job is to help rid the system of carbon dioxide.

- All nourishment assimilated by the intestines enters the blood via the liver. The burden on the liver is greater when acid blood wastes are excessive.

- In addition to regulating blood sugar, the pancreas produces alkaline enzymes and sodium bicarbonate. The physiological functions of the pancreas are designed to reduce excess acidity. To create optimal blood sugar balance, the pancreas requires an alkaline diet.

- Of all organs, the kidneys probably take the brunt of damage from acid wastes. In the last minute, over 1 liter of blood was filtered through your kidneys. The kidneys work ceaselessly to maintain blood alkalinity. Research has shown that kidney stones are composed of waste acid cells and mineral salts that have become adhesively bonded in an albuminous (waste acid) substance. Reducing acid-forming products from entering the body increases the likelihood of avoiding this painful condition.

- Toxins cannot be thoroughly removed via the kidneys, liver, and intestines. This creates greater susceptibility to infections and headaches.

SLEEP

The quality of your sleep becomes affected. You find yourself needing more sleep to compensate for poor-quality sleep. Difficulty in awakening is usually a sign of excess acidity.

LYMPH SYSTEM

Our bodies have about an equal number of lymph vessels as blood vessels, including over 600 lymph glands. The amount of lymph fluid we have is three times as much as blood, and this fluid has the dual function of transporting nutrition to the cell and removing acid waste products. Lymph flows best in an alkaline medium. However, if the lymph fluid is acidic, its movement is slowed, creating dryness and microscopic adhesions throughout the tissues. Acid wastes reach the tissues through lymph and blood toxicity. The scope of this problem can be responsible for numerous conditions, from inflamed nodes to lowered immunity and bowel irregularity.

CANCER AND THE GROWTH OF CANCER CELLS

German biochemist Dr. Otto Warburg had his own theories back in 1923 as to the cause of cancer. In 1931 he was awarded the Nobel Prize for his work. In his book *The Metabolism of Tumors,* Dr. Warburg explains that the primary cause of cancer is the replacement of oxygen in the respiratory chemistry of normal cell by the fermentation of sugar. After taking healthy cells and withdrawing oxygen, Dr. Warburg found that they would consistently turn cancerous. Without oxygen the glucose will ferment. Cancer cells live on the fermentation of glucose due to lack of oxygen.

A normal cell is surrounded by a membrane, which selectively allows materials such as oxygen and nutrients, including glucose, to flow in and cellular chemistry waste products to flow out. The cells are protected by the immune system, which in a well-functioning system, normally provides adequate defense against the formation of cancer cells. However, environmental toxins can overwhelm the system and weaken immunity. The process of cell breakdown strikes the membrane first; it loses its ability to exchange oxygen (a.k.a. respiration). Then the cell reverts to a primitive survival mechanism—fermentation. The newly formed cancer cell, which is anaerobic (without oxygen), cannot be repaired since fermentation is not reversible. The cell is now out of control and if not destroyed will continue to mutate and divide. In 1966, Warburg found that a 35 percent decrease in oxygen caused embryonic cells to change into cells with malignant characteristics.

In the 1950s, the National Cancer Institute verified Dr. Warburg's work. Unfortunately, little mainstream research has been done to determine the causes of a lack of oxygen in the human body. Most researchers have been attempting to halt the fermentation process through drugs, radiation, and surgery. Sometimes these therapies are temporarily successful. However, the goal is not only to find ways to bring oxygen to the system, but to understand what we are doing on a daily basis that robs valuable oxygen. Current research confirms that an abundance of acidity, whether it originates from excessive fat, free radical formation, or excessive dietary sugar, impedes cellular oxygen levels.

FINAL WORD ON ACID/ALKALINE

The "proof" of your body's acid and alkaline condition can best be determined by your own experience, not by peer-reviewed studies, medical establishment support, or static dietary guidelines. Without getting obsessively technical, the most practical advice would be to experiment for several weeks with a food plan that stays close to the middle of the acid and alkaline scale. You'll notice dramatic positive changes that can be attributed to your experiment. This will be your best teacher.

The negative symptoms associated with excess acidity are probably infinite. It's not the symptoms that need to be addressed (unless you're in severe pain); it's the root cause, the way we eat, our exposure to stress and its effect on blood chemistry, immunity, and daily vitality. I believe, in the near future, that acid and alkaline nutritional research will become an increasingly valid foundation for determining dietary safety and healing protocols.

5
THE MEAT AND DAIRY ISSUE

FOR THE LOVE OF MEAT

Americans love their meat. A leading hamburger chain adver-
tises "billions and billions" sold. Many American males take an
unquestioned pride in identifying themselves as "meat and
potatoes" men—associating themselves with staple food character qualities that are basic, simple, and solid. However,
despite American's love affair with meat and the meat industry's intensive marketing efforts, the necessity of meat in the
daily diet is being given serious reconsideration by leading scientific evidence.

There is no question that modern society's dietary habits
are excessive when it comes animal proteins. The average
American eats daily approximately 70 grams of animal protein
from a total protein intake of 107 grams or more. Compare this
with the daily Asian protein intake of 56 grams of protein,
where merely 8 might be from animal sources. While beef consumption has dropped more than 10 percent over the last 20
years, Americans are still eating nearly 65 pounds of red meat
per person annually. More alarming is the fact that a typical
American adult will eat the meat of seven 1100-pound steers in
his or her lifetime. This figure is based on 65 pounds of meat a
year and 659 pounds of dressed meat per 1105-pound steer.

EATING THE FARM

Each year the average American family eats half a steer, a whole pig, 100 chickens, 556 eggs, and 280 gallons of milk products. Using this figure, over an entire lifetime the average American would eat the flesh of 15 cows, 211 hogs, 900 chickens, 12 sheep, thousands of eggs, hundreds of gallons of milk and ice cream, and hundreds of pounds of cheese and saturated fats in the form of butter, margarine, and lard.

Due to their high fat content, meat and diary products provide the most significant source of dietary fat in the American diet. Because of this, their impact on dietary-related cancers cannot be ignored. Combine this with the common use of added fats and oils and you now have a potent recipe for cancer development, most notably of the breast, ovaries, prostate, and colon.

A 1992 Hawaiian study found that animal fat and protein, especially from sausage, processed cold cuts, beef, lamb and whole-milk diary products was associated with the highest rates of breast cancer.

Meat excess is also cited as a factor in escalating glandular cancers because its lack of fiber content contributes to increased hormone levels by reducing the fecal excretion of estrogen. Higher childhood animal protein levels have been cited as a primary reason for early menarche (first menstruation), increased body weight and height, and breast cancer.

Comparing chicken to beef yields some surprising nutrient percentages: 3.5 ounces of broiled lean flank steak is 56% fat, 42 percent protein, and contains approximately 70 milligrams of cholesterol. Light and dark chicken with the skin is 51 percent fat, 46 percent protein, and has 88 milligrams of cholesterol. They are nearly identical. Referring to *Bowes and Church's Food Values of Portions Commonly Used*, chicken breast without the skin is about 20 percent fat (total percentage of calories) while the highest-fat chicken (chicken franks) is fully 68 percent fat. Most commercial preparations run between 30 and 60 percent fat.

A HISTORICAL PERSPECTIVE

One of the early authors who related cancer to diet was an Englishman, William Lambe. In an 1809 book laboriously titled: *Report on the Effects of a Peculiar Regimen on Scirrhous Tumors and Cancerous Ulcers,* Lambe makes a then novel association between increased meat consumption and cancer development. Eighty-three years later, a January 1892 *Scientific American* article made the bold assertion that cancer was "most frequent among those branches of the human race where carnivorous habits prevail."

In 1907, the *New York Times* reported on an interesting study that contrasted the eating habits of numerous ethnic groups in the Chicago area. The Irish, Scandinavians and Germans were described as heavy meat eaters with high cancer death rates. By contrast, the Italians and Chinese, who were reliant on grains (rice, polenta, etc.) and grain products (pasta, noodles, etc.), had low meat consumption and reported lower cancer rates. This study included 4600 cases over a seven-year period that began in 1900.

Writing in his 1916 book *Notes on the Causation of Cancer,* Rolo Russell stated that cancer death rates were highest "in countries that eat more flesh."

During World War I, cancer rates fell by hefty percentages. Interestingly, during those times of economic belt tightening and diminished food production, meats and fats were significantly reduced due to unavailability. In Denmark, for example, the death rate from non-war-related disease was reduced by 34%.

In World War II, similar statistics were noticed, but by then documenting such information had become more sophisticated and conclusions were more widely accepted. The millions of European women who circumstantially were forced to reduce meats and fats had in the process greatly reduced both cancer and heart attacks. This lasted until a full seven years beyond the end of the war.

QUESTIONING MEAT QUALITY

Putting aside evolutionary, nutritional, philosophical, moral, sociological, agricultural, and economical reasons for drastic reduction in and/or elimination of meat consumption, there is the issue of quality—quality in the way meat affects the human organism, as well as its effect on the quality of our environment.

Pesticides and bacterial and viral contamination are too frequently present in the meat Americans consume. With increasing industrialization and changing farming practices, meat, poultry, fish, and dairy products now account for between 60 to 80 percent of the pesticide and organocholorine chemical residues in the American diet. This warrants serious consideration.

Organocholorine chemicals are a family of industrial chemicals heavily used in modern farming. Within the umbrella of this chemical compound group, PCBs and dioxins are known as potent immune-system poisons. Fortunately, only 10 percent of pesticide residues comes from grains, vegetables, beans, and fruits. Just changing your diet to a higher percentage of whole natural foods will help minimize your exposure to these powerful carcinogens.

Bacterial contamination of the national meat supply is a growing concern. Since 1906, when Upton Sinclair penned his book *The Jungle,* shocking Americans with detailed descriptions of the filthy conditions in slaughterhouses, unsanitary conditions have not been eliminated. When the media reports of people getting sick from contaminated meats, the U.S. Department of Agriculture (USDA) points its finger at the victims, the food preparers, or attributes blame to details about refrigeration or cooking.

The evidence of bovine leukemia present in American cattle herds is another concern. Viruses have been discovered in the milk and meat of affected cattle. Supposedly, these viruses are killed through cooking. However, while no proof exists for humans contracting cancer from meat viruses, it is more probable that a gradual reduction of resistance to lymphomas (a type of lymphatic cancer) would be of greater concern when meat and milk products are consistently ingested for many years.

Bovine growth hormone (BGH) is a genetically engineered hormone that, when injected into dairy cows, increases milk production by as much as 25 percent. However, it has a tendency to cause infections that demand antibiotic treatment. The residues from these antibiotics then show up in milk products and are absorbed into our bodies by ingestion.

This issue of meat quality only compounds the argument for the immediate reduction, or elimination, of animal products from the daily diet. Trying a three-month dietary experiment with reduced animal protein can show very positive and noticeable benefits. More than any research, this kind of personal test can provide the most enduring motivator for a permanent change of habit.

MEAT EATING AND CANCER RESEARCH

Available current nutritional research has consistently concluded that plant-based diets provide cancer protection whereas animal-based diets have the potential to stimulate and nurture certain cancers.

We have learned, repeatedly, that it is not necessary to depend on animal sources for our protein needs. Plant sources (grain, bean, bean product, miso, etc.) are equivalent in quality to animal sources minus the contaminated elements of saturated fat, hormones, excess cholesterol, bacteria, viruses, pesticides, and numerous other harmful substances previously mentioned in this chapter. The following is a portion of that research:

- In a large study on the meat–cancer connection, Dr. Takeshi Hirayama of Japan followed a group of 122,000 people for a number of years. Women from this group who consumed meat seven or more times each week had a nearly four times greater chance of developing breast cancer compared with women consuming meat a maximum of one time per week. It was established that those with an intermediate usage (2 to 4 times per week) were 2.55 times more likely to develop breast cancer than the low-usage group. The same exact trends were revealed for egg, butter, and cheese consumption.

- The digestion of meat produces strong carcinogenic substances, particularly deoxycholic acid, in the colon. Powerful carcinogens are created when deoxycholic acid is converted into clostridia bacteria in our intestines. It has been established that meat eaters generally have greater amounts of deoxycholic acid than vegetarians, which accounts for the higher rates of colon cancer present in meat eaters.

- There is some evidence regarding carcinogen production in cooked meat products. Charred meats, in particular, carry polynuclear aromatic compounds such as benzopyrene, which is a known carcinogen. There is also evidence that many meats carry viruses that might be a cause for the development of certain cancers, and that incompletely cooked meats could thus be sources of virally induced diseases; this line of thought, however, still warrants additional research.

- A diet high in animal fats will increase the concentration of saturated fat and arachidonic acid more than in individuals on a vegetarian diet. This would alter types of fatty acids available to tumor cells in a direction that increases their growth rate. Some evidence to support this is found in studies that show vegetarian diets associated with decreased tumor growth and longer tumor induction.

- Hawaiian researchers published a case control, multi-ethnic population study that examined the role of dietary soy, fiber, and related foods and nutrients on the risk of endometrial cancer. (The endometrius is the mucous membrane lining the uterus.) The researchers found a positive association between a higher level of fat intake and endometrial cancer as well as a higher level of fiber intake and a reduction in risk for endometrial cancer. They also found that a high consumption of soy products and other legumes was associated with a decreased risk of endometrial cancer.

THE POLYP PREVENTION TRIAL

A study in the April 20, 2000 issue of *The New England Journal of Medicine* reported that "the Polyp Prevention Trial provided no evidence that adopting a low-fat, high-fiber-fruit-and-vegetable-enriched diet reduces the risk of colorectal cancer. In an additional report on another trial in the same journal, the conclusion was similar: "A dietary supplement of wheat-bran fiber does not protect against recurrent colorectal adenomas." However, Dr. M. Robert Cooper, professor of internal medicine at Wake Forest University Baptist Medical Center, who was the principal investigator of the Polyp Prevention Trial, commented, "People should continue to eat a healthy diet, high in fiber and low in fat. It is good for diabetes, heart disease and obesity—it is good for everything."

Seconding this, Dr. Michael Thun, vice president for epidemiology of the American Cancer Society, said, "For the time being, our dietary guidelines won't change... A diet high in vegetables, fiber and fruit is still thought to be protective against a variety of smoking-related cancers and stomach cancer and also offers broader health benefits."

The American Institute Research offered the following in a bulletin in commenting on the Polyp Prevention Trial study:

> *Scientific evidence builds slowly, and each new published study must be viewed in relation to all previous findings. To date, well over 4,500 studies on the link between diet and cancer have been completed. These investigations were carried out across the globe by thousands of researchers using very different methods and measurements. Their results consistently point to the health-promoting, cancer-fighting benefits of diets high in whole grains, vegetables, beans and fruits. ... [these studies] cannot and do not close the discussion. If anything, they underscore the real need for further research and analysis. Both studies, for example, involved only short-term (four year) adjustments to the diet. We know that colon cancer is a disease that can take decades to develop. Convincing epidemiological evidence suggests that a healthy diet has its greatest preventive effect as a lifelong commitment, not a stopgap measure. ... Whether or not four years of whole grains, beans, vegetables and fruits protect against cancer, there is ample and growing evidence that a lifetime of these foods will do so.*

The bottom line for all these studies seems to be that you should reduce, if not eliminate, your consumption of animal-based proteins for cancer prevention and maximized health.

If you wish to keep animal protein in your diet, safer choices would be deep-water, low-fat fish, or occasional small amounts of non–hormonally fed, free-range lean fowl. Ideally, this would be eaten in small quantities, less frequently with a non-oil food preparation (steam, bake, or poach) along with an abundant amount of a variety of colorful vegetables.

UDDER NONSENSE?—QUESTIONING DAIRY FOOD

Dairy marketing has gone from Elsie the friendly cow to celebrities wearing milk moustaches and justifying dairy consumption because of calcium content. The dairy industry's attempt to recapture primary food status is rapidly becoming pointless as the scientific case against milk and other dairy products grows stronger. If anything, we should be reducing, or eliminating, our consumption of milk and dairy once we reach adulthood, not increasing it.

Terry Shintani, M.D., author of *Hawaii Diet,* writes:

Why is dairy recommended by many experts as a daily requirement in this country? Scientific studies are showing that dairy isn't the wonder food it was once touted to be. But there is so much money to be made that even the federal government, under the influence of commercial interests, promotes dairy. This is done despite scientific information that dairy fat promotes heart disease, that dairy protein is the leading cause of allergies in this country, and that dairy sugar cannot be digested properly by seventy percent of the adults in the world.

The basic dairy product, whole cow's milk containing a high percentage of fat, cholesterol, and protein, is low in carbohydrate and has no fiber. Popular products made from whole milk include cheese, cottage cheese, yogurt, butter, buttermilk, skim milk, kefir, ice cream, whey, cow-milk based baby formulas and "imitation milk."

> ## SOMETHING TO THINK ABOUT
>
> Milk is a food that is ideally designed for the growing nutritional needs of calves. Modern humans now have a unique distinction of being the only species that drinks milk after they are fully teethed—and from another species! We don't simply drink it for occasional refreshment; we've made it into a national principal beverage. Why pick the cow? Why not dog milk?

Comparing the fiber, cholesterol, and macronutrient (protein, carbohydrate, and fat) content of milk to meat reveals similar percentages of each, qualifying milk to be redefined as "liquid meat." Dairy products, like meats, are rich foods. Therefore, an excess of these foods can produce similar diseases found in affluent societies. While our focus is on cancer prevention, additional conditions that excessive diary consumption has been associated with, are the following: osteoporosis, diabetes, pesticide residue, antibiotics resistant bacteria, leukemia virus, vitamin D toxicity, iron deficiency, infant colic, constipation, childhood ear infections, cardio-vascular disease, lactose intolerance, cataracts, arthritis, colitis, enlarged tonsils, obesity, MS and food allergies.

The following research is part of the growing evidence that links excessive consumption of dairy products to numerous cancers, tumor growth, and immune dysfunction.

- *Ovarian Cancer*—Ovarian cancer rates parallel dairy-eating patterns throughout the world. The milk sugar lactose is broken down in the body into another type of sugar called galactose. Enzymes then take their turn and further break down galactose. In a Harvard study conducted by Boston gynecologist Daniel Cramer and colleagues, it was observed that when dairy-product consumption exceeded the enzymes' capacity to break down galactose, a build-up of galactose in the blood occurs, which is thought to affect a woman's ovaries. Many women have particularly low levels of these enzymes. When these women consume dairy products on a regular basis, their risk of ovarian cancer can be triple that of other women.

Yogurt and cottage cheese seem to be of the most concern because the bacteria used in the manufacture of these products increases the production of galactose from lactose.

In a July 19, 1985 issue of the *Journal of the American Medical Association,* Dr. John Snowden, epidemiologist at the University of Minnesota's School of Public Health, summarized a twenty-year study of diet and ovarian cancer: "Women who ate eggs … three or more days each week had a three times greater risk of fatal ovarian cancer than did women who ate eggs less than one day per week." Similar to other female cancers, ovarian cancer incidence rises not only with egg consumption, but also with the consumption of any form of animal fat.

- *Prostate Cancer*—Prostate cancer has also been linked to dairy consumption. This is thought to be related to an increase in a compound called insulin-like growth factor (IGF). Although a certain amount of IGF-I in the blood is normal, high levels have been linked to increased cancer risk. IGF-I is also found in cow's milk and has been shown to occur in increased levels in the blood by individuals consuming dairy products on a regular basis. Other nutrients that increase IGF-I are also found in cow's milk. Another study showed that men who had the highest levels of IGF-I had more than four times the risk of prostate cancer compared with those who had the lowest levels. According to a review published by the World Cancer Research Fund and the American Institute for Cancer Research, at least 11 human population studies have linked dairy product consumption and prostate cancer. In the United States as a whole, the incidence of prostate cancer is reportedly related to consumption of dairy products, eggs, and meat.

A 13-year look at 20,855 male doctors who took part in the *Physicians' Health Study* shows that men who enjoy lots of milk, cheese, and ice cream are 30 percent more likely to get prostrate cancer. The study is a long-term look at U.S. doctors who were aged 40 to 82 when the study began in 1982.

- *Breast Cancer*—Breast cancer is commonly called a hormonally driven tumor. The body's hormones stimulate the growth and development of a breast tumor. In breast cancer, the hormone estrogen chiefly drives a tumor's development and growth. Fat content in foods can encourage the growth of a certain species of bacteria that can split the complex molecule formed by estrogen. As a result, excreted estrogens are freed and readily absorbed back into the body. Inevitably, higher levels of these powerful hormones are found in women who eat foods rich in fats, which comes from the affluent Western diet of meats, dairy, and oil excess. High milk consumption was found in a case-control study at Roswell Park Memorial Institute to be associated with higher risk of breast cancer, as well as cancer of the mouth, stomach, colon, rectum, lung, bladder, and cervix, relative to consumption of no milk at all.

  Concluding a report in *Cancer Research,* Dr. Ronald Phillips indicated that the evidence is now overwhelming: Vegetarian diets strongly reduce the incidence of breast, uterine, ovarian, colon, and many other cancers.

- *Non-Hodgkin's Lymphoma and Lung Cancer*—A *Nutrition and Cancer* study in 1989 linked the risk of non-Hodgkin's lymphoma with excessive consumption of butter and cow's milk. Some medical research suggests that animal proteins, specifically dairy proteins, play a featured role in the development of this cancer of the immune system. Continuous overstimulation of the immune system by dairy proteins may eventually lead to weakening of immune function. Excessive levels of a milk protein called beta-lactoglobulin were discovered in the blood of lung cancer patients.

HUMAN BODY DESIGN AND FUNCTION

Our physiological design offers several indicators for what should constitute our basic diet. Our evolutionary history reveals that humans developed predominantly as herbivores (plant consumers) and not as carnivores (meat consumers).

Human salivary glands secrete carbohydrate-digesting enzymes into the mouth, where carbohydrates begin their initial breakdown. Our tooth structure is largely for grinding, as opposed to the sharp canines most animals predominantly have for tearing meats into smaller pieces. While we are equipped to eat meats (having four canines in the normal mouth, but still not resembling the canine teeth of true carnivores), our design indicates that animal protein should be a minor supplement, if included at all. This is one of the reasons thorough chewing is always emphasized for people who eat whole grains. Additionally, carbohydrates begin their digestion in the mouth, whereas protein digestion is initiated in the stomach.

Anatomically, the human is vastly different from natural carnivores such as cats and dogs, whose shortened intestinal length guarantees quicker bowel transit times. The contrasts are not only structural but functional as well; our bowel walls are deeply puckered and pouched, whereas theirs have smoother surfaces and are free of these pouches, similar to a stovepipe shape. Human intestinal lengths vary from 27 to 29 feet and resemble a winding mountain road full of angular turns, whereas carnivore intestines are from 7 to 9 feet long, without angular turns and structured like a chute. In the moist and warm environment of the human intestine, the putrefaction tendency is greater if meats are present at a higher percentage. Carnivore intestines have a great capacity to discharge the large amounts of cholesterol that their diet contains, whereas human livers can only process and excrete a limited amount of dietary cholesterol, leaving our tissues to deal with remaining amounts.

Human saliva has carbohydrate-digesting alkaline enzymes, which are absent from carnivores. Additionally, carnivores' stomach acids (for concentrated protein breakdown) are more powerful than human digestive secretions.

It is clear that the human physiological design is not suitable for large volumes of animal protein, despite nutritional recommendations from in-vogue diet books, enzyme theories, mega-conglomerate food recommendations, or Paleolithic references. We have become too dependent on animal protein as a staple food. Historically, aside from Arctic Inuit populations and some African and Middle-East Nomadic tribes, meat has never been a staple food.

The Vegetarian Option

The word *vegetarian* has an interesting origin. First coined in 1842 from the Latin *vegetus,* it means "one who is sound, whole, fresh and lively." If you are choosing to become a vegetarian, or plan to at least experiment with a plant-based diet, the following eight suggestions might make this choice easier and help produce better results. (They will also apply to individuals who have reduced animal protein in their diets.)

1. *The need for dietary sodium is crucial.* Sodium and potassium have a complementary relationship in the blood. As you increase the amount of vegetables, you need to have a source of good-quality trace mineral containing sea/salt, or salt contained within fermented products such as natural soy sauce (tamari) and soybean paste (miso). Among macrobiotic vegetarians, there has been a tendency to oversalt. Symptoms of oversalting are thirst, tendency to overeat, sweet cravings, irritability, and, in more exaggerated cases, elevated blood pressure. Whether an individual can benefit on a salt-free vegetarian diet is largely dependent on his or her previous diet. Someone with a dietary past heavy in meats, salt, and cooked foods initially does well on a more raw food and a low- or no-salt diet. However, this is for the short term. Over a long period of time, a no-salt diet might result in fatigue and meat or sugar (stimulant) cravings.

2. *Reduce simple sugars.* Vegetarians tend to use too many simple-carbohydrate products such as fruit juice, honey, maple syrup, barley malt, rice syrup, and molasses. These products, in excess, have been shown to cause blood sugar instability, fatigue, mood swings, suppressed immunity, compromised mineral values for blood buffering, and increased cravings for salt or meats. This can easily graduate into an addictive cycle: You're fatigued,

you crave something sweet as a stimulant, you eat the sweet, cause a blood sugar swing, and then find yourself fatigued again. For numerous reasons, vegetarians are more sensitive to the negative effects of acid-producing sugar.

3. *Fight meat cravings with moderate use of oil.* Transition to a low-fat and low-sugar diet often results in what is perceived as meat cravings. Increasing vegetable proteins (beans or bean products) and adding one to two teaspoons of daily oil from olive, sesame, or flax sources, either in cooking (except for flax) or in dressings, can make the difference between a satisfying meal or one that leaves you with mysterious cravings. Most often, vegetarians in this position will overeat to compensate for the lack of fat and reduction of protein.

4. *Be aware of possible deficiencies.* The most common deficiency vegetarians are warned about is for vitamin B_{12} and for the need to build healthy intestinal bacteria. The value of B_{12} supplements is questionable. Some sources claim that B_{12} pills contain breakdown sources of B_{12} and can even have an anti-B_{12} effect. Some fermented foods (miso, tempeh, and tamari) contain trace amounts of B_{12}; however, the degree of their bioavailability has also been questioned. Since actual deficiencies such as this are rare, it might be a good idea to have blood work done to determine a deficiency status before attempting to treat symptoms. While there are trace amounts of B_{12} in miso, tempeh, and sea vegetables, the question of bioavailability still remains individualized. Probiotic supplements for constant renewal of healthy intestinal bacteria would be recommended for those with recent medication and antibiotic history.

5. *Try for nutritional variety.* Consuming a wider variety of whole grains, bean and bean products, sea vegetables (for mineral insurance), vegetables (including daily portions of leafy greens), and fruits, plus small amounts of vegetable-based fermented products, will offer greater nutritional variety and healing power.

6. *Chew thoroughly*. Grain digestion begins in the mouth, temporarily stops in the stomach, and resumes again in the next digestive stage of the duodenum before being assimilated into the blood via the small intestine. Often, we'll change the quality of our food but hold on to old habits of rushing through meals as if the food were being inhaled. Thorough chewing ensures better assimilation of nutrients, less resulting acidity, and regulated bowel function.

7. *Avoid simple-sugar and complex-sugar combinations*. I've heard this repeatedly from clients over the years who might dine in a natural foods restaurant: "The meal was great, but I had gas for the next 12 hours—frankly, it's not worth it." There's a very simple reason for this: Simple sugars digest quickly, whereas complex sugars are broken apart more gradually. Clients will order a healthy grain-vegetable-bean meal and then enjoy a dessert immediately afterward. Within ten minutes there's a fireworks demonstration in their intestines. Generally, this gas attack could have several causes:

- Overeating

- Eating a dessert too soon after a complex sugar meal

- Eating unsalted beans or an excessive amount of beans

In this case, it would be advisable (unless you want to clear the room) to save dessert for a later time. A small amount of hot caffeine-free tea after a meal can often soothe dessert cravings and make for a satisfying meal closure.

8. *Eat whole grain daily*. The need for whole grain is important. I've met many vegetarians who don't know the difference between whole grains and grain products. An excess of grain products can result in fatigue and sugar cravings and sometimes produce allergic reactions, presumably due to the mixing of yeast, sugar, and refined flour.

These eight factors have proved very helpful to people trying to maintain a vegetarian program. They will also apply to individuals who have reduced animal protein.

THREE VEGETARIAN PITFALLS

Choosing to eat a predominant amount of plant foods is *not* simply a matter of steering clear of foods that are animal in origin. In addition to selecting good-quality food, we need to be mindful of the balance factors: a food's relative acid/alkaline ratio, the food's wholeness, and its fat and sugar content.

These are three pitfalls common to relying on vegetable quality foods:

1. *Concentrated sugar:* Check for ingredients such as white, brown, or any of the numerous sugar/molasses combinations of refined sugars. Additional concentrated sugars are honey, corn syrup, and fructose. When choosing a sweetener, it is best to do so infrequently and use small amounts of less refined sugars such as barley malt, rice syrup, fruit juice, and maple syrup.

2. *Refined flours and grains:* Limit your consumption of these categories. Sometimes you can mix a portion of these in with whole grains. I recommended this for several Hawaiian Japanese clients who were longing for their familiar white rice. I recommended 70 percent brown rice with 30 percent white rice, and this allowed them to obtain benefit while enjoying something that was familiar. Refined grains are white rice, white flour, couscous, flour (grain product) breakfast cereals, and wheat germ.

3. *Plant foods high in fat:* This category includes coconuts, avocados, olives, nuts, seeds, soybeans, tofu, vegetable oils. Many of these products can be included in the diet, but in limited amounts as you observe overall fat percentages of below 20 percent total calories from fat.

"SO, WHAT'S LEFT?"

A client once commented, "Everything I like and have been eating all my life is suddenly bad for me, so what's left?" This is an understandable sentiment. However, from the current evidence, it seems for the long term that neither meat nor dairy products are health supportive when consumed as principal foods.

For those desiring optimum health and noticeable benefit, it would be prudent to limit these foods severely, or eliminate them altogether, in the interest of "experimenting" in order to determine positive benefits. Sometimes just eating a little bit or "reducing" can foster cravings for more, escalating your daily eating into a battle of willpower to avoid the very foods you're trying to avoid. This can be enormously stressful. At best, an 85 to 90 percent reduction in these foods will still produce noticeable positive results, so if complete elimination proves too difficult, the alternate choice would be to eat less of these foods in volume and eat them less frequently.

6

NO-GUILT CRAVING STRATEGIES FOR ELIMINATING SUGAR, FAT, AND OVEREATING

WILL POWER AND HIS BAND OF EXCUSES

"Everybody's smart, only on different subjects," Will Rogers was fond of saying. Many people, despite having all kinds of healthy information in their heads, cannot stick to a healthy diet. Why is this?

From my observation, the key to eating consistently healthy is *not* about having more nutritional information. Dietary awareness in this country is definitely increasing—most people know, through the media, government reports, and medical studies, that whole grains, vegetables, beans and fruits are good for you and that we rely too heavily on animal proteins, dairy foods, and sugar. The most common excuses people offer for their dietary transgressions are the following:

"I have weak will power."

"It's not that bad for you."

"I just wanted it."

"Hey, you gotta live a little."

I have no problem with "living a little," just wanting something, or enjoying whatever, without fear that it's going to

103

strike you dead in your café chair. However, I do have a problem with thinking that it's "weak will power." In fact, breaking your diet rarely has to do with will. My contention is that it has to more to do with other factors that you unconsciously set up to engineer the craving than just mortal discipline.

The key is learning about balance; not just about low-acid and low-alkaline foods or nutritional elements, but the physiological and psychological reasons that make us crave strange foods or foods that cannot support long-term health. Otherwise, we feel out of control and find ourselves trying to justify the hypocrisy of our choices—and we know we're lying to ourselves.

The varied elements of the food scale are stronger than your will power. Eat excessively from one extreme and you will inevitably swing to the other extreme. Therefore, learning some fundamental information about cravings, and the substitutions we can make in an effort to achieve balance, is essential.

Internal Memo from the Body Department

Aside from sentimental associations ("Dad, remember how we used to have milk shakes every Sunday? Let's go get some ..."), most cravings indicate that your body is signaling a need to establish some kind of balance. It could be due to a number of physical or emotional reasons. Becoming more aware of these factors, the possible mechanisms behind your cravings, is the first step toward finding your own balance and creating good health without having to feel deprived or without creating a lot of mis-spent energy.

Actually, this is an issue beyond weak character or poor will power. The truth is, your cravings reveal valuable information about your health and its direction.

The process of homeostasis is how the body maintains its most desirable equilibrium. Your body has a number of automatic devices for regulating the fine balance of blood pressure, internal temperature, blood pH (acid/alkaline balance) blood sugar, and other hormonal secretions.

A number of our popular consuming passions wreak havoc with homeostasis: Alcohol, sugary foods, tobacco, caffeine, and various drugs all lead to gross imbalances that we attempt to counterbalance in more extreme ways. For example, excessive alcohol and refined sugar intake, due to their well-known mineral theft capability, often result in strong cravings for meats and salted foods; long periods of fasting (meal skipping) frequently give way to overeating; fatty food excess (which can produce fatigue as cells clump and bind oxygen) inspire cravings for foods that stimulate, such as spices, sugar, or caffeine.

While extremes can add an amusing bit of physiological and psychological drama to our lives, the negative long-term effects, both mentally and physically, pose inevitable consequences. By developing your awareness of the factors that create cravings, you can feel more in control of your body while acquiring an attuned sensitivity to your needs and body signals.

CRAVING WHAT THE BODY NEEDS

As is well known to farmers and ranchers, as well as to veterinarians, salt cravings are not uncommon among domesticated animals. Animals have been known to roam for miles in search of salt licks. As reported from various parts of the world for the past two centuries, some animals develop a distinct craving for bones. Presumably, these animals lack phosphorus, and bone consumption is an attempt to rectify this deficiency. Experiments with cattle who were phosphorus deficient revealed specific appetite preferences for ground bone or bird feces. These appetites disappeared when they were injected with phosphate, indicating a physiological basis for the craving.

Blood levels of calcium and phosphate have a definite influence on feed behavior. One study showed that calcium-deficient rats had a preference for high-calcium diets. However, on removal of their parathyroid gland, calcium intake increased to as much as 13 times the normal levels but returned to normal with treatment. In another report, calcium-deficient chickens ate eggshells whenever available. Not to be outdone, calcium-deficient pigs have been observed licking mineral-rich lime from the walls of their cages. These bizarre behaviors are simply an indiscriminate and driven impulse to overcome nutrient imbalance.

"MAKE MINE A DIRT SANDWICH WITH A SIDE OF PAINT CHIPS ..."

Another strange variety of animal and human craving is called pica. Described as an "appetite perversion," pica cravings are essentially the ingestion of strange, distasteful, or repulsive substances. *Pica* is a Greek word for magpie—a bird known for eating unusual objects. The physical rational for pica cravings is an underlying need for trace minerals or inorganic minerals absent from the current diet.

In animals, pica cravings run the gamut; cows have been known to eat nails, wire, and rusted objects; cats have been observed eating charcoal and ashes. Some other nonfood substances consumed by animals and humans are ice chips, dirt, laundry soap, chalk, starch, hair matches, antacids, paint chips, wood, plaster, pebbles, and wax. Striking all races and socioeconomic groups, pica cravings frequently indicate an anemic condition.

Another type of pica craving is called geophagia—the consumption of earth and clay. While geophagia is a cultural practice (typically using kaolin or white clay), its inherent toxicity has frequently resulted in death. Geophagia is most common during early stages of pregnancy. The clay is routinely consumed by pregnant women for symptoms of morning sickness, in Central Africa and the southern United States. Such cravings, according to one researcher, "fill a physiological need for missing nutrients." In Africa, the clay can be purchased at local markets in a variety of sizes with different content of minerals. After purchase, the clays are stored in a beltlike cloth around the waist of the mother-to-be and eaten as desired, most frequently without water. Geophagia's Western equivalent might be the pickle and ice-cream cravings attributed to hormonal fluctuation, which sharpens the senses and fosters nausea in early-stage pregnancies.

From an acid/alkaline perspective, strong cravings for certain forms of acidity during pregnancy (tomatoes, lemons, spices, peppers) draw minerals into the blood for neutralizing. While this acidity might adversely affect the mother, the developing fetus seems to be the probable benefactor. In a related example, Japanese physicians have suggested that alkaline water is another way to buffer the acidity of that dreaded early-pregnancy morning sickness.

The indigenous Pomo tribe of Northern California used dirt in their diet, mixing it with ground corn. Whether this could have been for reasons of tradition, superstition, wisdom, or intuition was not known, but this practice neutralized the corn's natural acid, making it easier to digest. A similar practice by some Southwest native tribes used wood ash in corn cooking water, presumably for the same reasons.

Finally, a brief on strange cravings would not be complete without mention of that most fascinating and feared pastime: cannibalism. Some scientists believe that cannibalism is motivated by circumstances of severe deprivation of minerals obtained from bone and blood sources. Other reasons for this practice might include territorial trespass, religious ritual, and general superstition.

Interestingly, native inhabitants of the Amazon Basin, noted for its plentiful rainfall, have a very low salt intake. Additionally, ground analysis of the area reveals very low levels of calcium and phosphorus. Endocannibalism (the eating of relatives or tribal members) was practiced there, particularly—according to physician and author, Douglas Hunt—the consumption of ground-up bones of relatives. The bone powder was added to *caxire,* an alcoholic beverage, to make the powder more palatable, or at least to help you forget what you were drinking.

THE EIGHT CATEGORIES OF CRAVINGS

Your desire for a particular food can be attributed to any one of these categories:

- Nutritional
- Acid/alkaline balance
- Blood sugar
- Emotional
- Genetics
- Allergy response
- Elimination/detoxification
- Expansion/contraction

These are all internal broadcasts the body uses to signal its different needs. It's important to give an ear to these signals, but equally important to recognize that there is a fine line between fueling dietary addictions and just following dietary intuition. Understanding the meaning behind different cravings can liberate you from feeling guilty or out of control with your eating. Self-mastery begins with awareness.

WHAT DRIVES OUR FOOD CRAVINGS?

There is very little conclusive scientific research on specific reasons for human food cravings; why you'd sell your first-born for exotic chocolate or drive 60 miles for a particular kind of cheesecake. Sometimes will is no match for reason.

The following information is not based on any established scientific documentation as a whole, but rather is based on my experience with 25 years of nutritional counseling, personal experimentation, and continued study. It is presented here for you to determine how it may relate to you and to support consistently good eating habits while reducing the common stress of needed dietary change. That stress can be physical, relating to nutritional needs, or psychological, relating to feelings of deprivation.

Let's look at some of the general categories of cravings. They will be referred to later on in outlining the specific strategies which will aid eliminating sugar, fat, and overeating with a minimum of effort.

1. Nutritional

Nutritional cravings can fall into two subcategories:

  a. Food group imbalance
  b. Specific nutrient excess/deficiency

A. Food Group Imbalance—The chief food groups are carbohydrates, fats, and proteins. Western nutrition, both clinical and naturopathic versions, seems to have a preoccupation with stressing the quantity of nutrients or watchdogging calories. The concern is usually about fear of deficiency. Do you have enough protein? Are you getting proper amounts of vitamins and minerals? Are you drinking enough water? These are all valid questions; yet it seems that most of our problems are due to excess and rarely deficiency.

A nutritional model proposed by some cultural folk medicines relates certain cravings to more proportional nutrient balancing. Using mother's milk as a human prototype for nutritional needs, the *ratios* of certain nutrients sequentially increase beginning with minerals. A developing infant receives the following:

100 grams	Minerals/Vitamins 120 mg.	Proteins 1,100 mg	Fats 4,000 mg.	Carbohydrates 9,5000 mg.	Water % 87.5	Oxygen (Cannot Quantify)
Mother's Milk	•	●	●	⬤	⬤	

The ratio of minerals to protein to fat to carbohydrate to water and oxygen ends up naturally progressing to increasing amounts.

Now, compare the difference with the two most popular categories of food in the western world: meat and sugar:

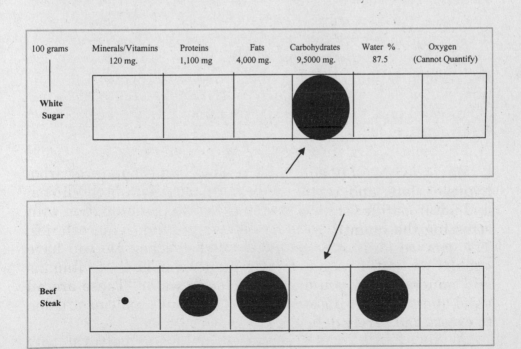

100 grams	Minerals/Vitamins 120 mg.	Proteins 1,100 mg	Fats 4,000 mg.	Carbohydrates 9,5000 mg.	Water % 87.5	Oxygen (Cannot Quantify)
White Sugar				⬤		

Beef Steak	•	●	⬤		⬤	

Note Imbalance: Sugar is virtually all carbohydrate, yet carbohydrate is absent from Beef protein.

What does this mean? If the bulk of our daily diet is made from food proportions that are not closely based on the mother's milk prototype, you might experience strong cravings for a variety of other foods. This is how we compensate for imbalance. For example, according to this model, if we have a large steak, this high amount of protein can stimulate cravings for minerals, which we take from a number of sources, but typically in a most concentrated source from ordinary salt. This is one of the reasons we reach for salt when we eat eggs, or meats or beans and bean products. The lack of carbohydrate in the beefsteak illustration also stimulates strong cravings for carbohydrates, such as potatoes and dessert, even though your dessert may contain water, it is still not enough. Sugar pulls water from tissues. Ever notice there's always a water fountain in an ice cream shop? Or that after a glass of "thirst-quenching" juice, you're still thirsty? This paradigm might offer a balanced understanding for such cravings. If we take a very concentrated amount of carbohydrate or water, our need for oxygen becomes greater. That's where that after dinner walk comes in—moving the circulation and oxygen to all cells. What can be observed by this model is the possibility that unbalanced dietary proportions can affect every subsequent nutritional factor in the order of its sequence, from minerals, proteins, fats, carbohydrates, water and oxygen.

This model, first proposed by author and educator Michio Kushi, in his numerous books on Asian medicine, might offer some explanation for meat- and sugar-based dietary patterns.

B. Specific Nutrient Excess/Deficiency—Another factor in the nutritional category of cravings might have to do with specific nutrient cravings based on vitamin, trace mineral, or mineral deficiency.

Pagophagia, the eating of ice, is often related to folic acid or iron deficiency and is popular among pregnant natives in Third World countries. When I've counseled clients who complain about having milk cravings, a recommendation for more mineral-rich foods or a mineral supplement will often eliminate these cravings. Smokers tend to crave foods with vitamin C (typically orange juice) since their vitamin C levels tend to fall below normal levels. Excess sugar or alcohol (both highly acidic) tend to eat up minerals, so it's not unlikely that both can cause cravings for more salt, pickles, meats (stored salt within animal muscle tissue), or other alkaline and mineralized foods.

Many woman experience strong cravings for sugar just prior to menstruation, presumably due to low progesterone levels. Hormones can be powerful initiators of numerous cravings; any diabetic who is insulin-dependent must have access to refined sugar in the event of the common occurrence of insulin excess. Tension, physical or emotional, can also create an imbalance in body chemistry that stimulates different cravings for foods, which provide comfort, either in the way they may relax you physically or psychologically by memory association.

Some chocolate cravings have been linked to magnesium deficiency, a mineral found in small quantities in chocolate. Magnesium is needed to make serotonin, a compound that is concerned with the process of sleep. In this regard, chocolate may be a means of acquiring much needed magnesium and elevating mood levels. However, with chocolate you have fat and sugar to contend with, which have their own problems. An alternate choice: dark leafy green vegetables, such as broccoli, kale, or spinach. These are excellent sources of magnesium and folic acid.

Some foods can work like a drug to suppress or stimulate cravings or appetite. Certain types of fat, called prostaglandins, help the body produce chemicals along with a digestive hormone called CCK PZ, both of which reduce the desire for more food. Some fat can even stimulate a desire to overeat.

There could be any number of nutritionally based reasons for cravings. Instead of being overly concerned about missing nutrients, a whole foods approach, and in some cases the temporary addition of a multivitamin-mineral food-based supplement, can help to balance nutritional factors.

2. Acid/Alkaline Balance

Opposites attract. This also applies to acid and alkaline foods.

As mentioned previously, the overall effect of excess acidity, of which Western diets have in plentiful amounts, is the leeching of minerals from bone, digestive fluid, and blood sources. If your diet tends to be more acid based, you might find the thought of reducing certain foods (meats, salts, mineral supplements) uncomfortable. However, limiting these high-acid foods and eating some low-alkaline source foods (vegetables, sea vegetables, some small amounts of sea salt cooked into foods, or miso, tamari) can quickly reduce cravings for foods that many people have difficulty resisting.

One theory suggests fat has a unique buffering effect and makes a comfortable middle-ground food choice to neutralize either extreme. Fats have the ability to buffer acids or acidify weak alkalis. Some dairy (salted and nonsalted cheese, unpasteurized milk, butter, yogurt, ghee) and soybean products (tofu) fall into this category.

3. Blood Sugar

Carbohydrates are broken into simpler units of sugar through digestion. This sugar can then enter the blood in order to nourish the cell. A number of hormonal mechanisms help to regulate this process. Ideally, for enduring energy and maximized emotional stability, you want a stable blood sugar level. Naturally, it will fluctuate, elevating and descending according to the kind of diet and activity you have.

If the sugar volume is excessive, the blood sugar will soar. When the blood sugar becomes too high, this is known as hyperinsulinism. Extremely high blood sugar can make you want to vacuum your entire house twice; you feel suddenly energetic, giddy, and talkative. However, it can also send you into a coma. To protect you, the body has an automatic insulin release that comes from the pancreas. Insulin bonds to the sugar as a carrier and transports it out of the blood and into the liver, where it can be stored.

However, if the sugar is really excessive and the liver storage warehouse is completely booked (storage capacity is approximately 60 to 90 grams), it'll be turned into a fat and stored in tissue, usually the less active tissues of buttocks and thighs—but you may already know this annoying fact.

As it happens, the amount of insulin released is unregulated—it just keeps on pouring in until sugar levels are lowered and nonthreatening. The problem with this function is that it frequently results in an opposite condition, called hypoglycemia (*hypo* = low; *glycemia* = sugar).

With low blood sugar, fatigue increases as the muscles have lessened sugar supply for energy. You might also feel negative and irritable—like most people just before entering a bar at Happy Hour. But within ten minutes, imbibing customers go from uptight, tired, and quiet workers to uninhibited Karaoke superstars belting out Top 40 lyrics with gusto. Having a distillation of sugar (alcohol) after a full afternoon of work, office stress, and growing hunger makes Happy Hour an appealing ritual.

Sometimes, a low blood sugar condition is initially mistaken for hypothyroidism because of slowed reaction times and sleepiness.

CONTROLLING BLOOD SUGAR LEVELS

Simply speaking, whole grains, vegetables, beans, and fibrous fruits will keep blood sugar at a more manageable level. When blood sugar soars, you're likely to crave salted foods or animal protein. With low blood sugar, you typically crave sweet foods. I've observed that the two most common physical reasons for sweet cravings and overeating tend to be skipped meals or long periods between meals. Long periods without eating lower blood sugar, giving way to ravenous sweet appetites. Sometimes, eating fat in place of sweet is an unconscious strategy that pacifies the sweet tooth, since fats take nearly three hours to leave the stomach. You feel satisfied with the feeling of fullness that comes from the slow digestion time of fats or from the possible acid/alkaline buffering effect of fat on blood chemistry. Pay attention to blood sugar. It's one of the most common ways to sabotage good eating habits.

4. Emotional

Eating can be a nurturing activity. Sometimes, when we feel emotionally deprived, we may automatically turn to eating for this nurturance. It can be a conscious or an unconscious attempt to get our needs met. Learning to identify and express emotions is the first step toward stopping this self-destructive cycle.

Psychologically, self-esteem and social value are frequently connected to physical appearance. The modern concept of beauty, perpetuated by Hollywood images, women's magazines, and men's action heroes, suggests that a uniformly thin (or muscular), hard-bodied, smooth-skinned, young and vital ideal is the ultimate goal. Considering that less than 1 percent of the population probably fits this ideal, it's not surprising that many young people become dissatisfied with their bodies. The popular media and its unrealistic portrayal of beauty and chic seduces them with unattainable ideals. Inability to meet these ideals can lead to developing lowered self-esteem and often result in self-punishing behaviors.

For some, eating is not a nurturing fuel or a pleasure ritual. It becomes a convenient drug of choice; a friend, a companion, a comfort and a distraction from the frustrating, unfulfilling experiences of daily life. Eating then becomes a way to medicate

---

WHAT CAUSES COMPULSIVE OVEREATING?

More serious compulsive overeating is characterized by an inability to cease eating when one's physical hunger has been satisfied. The most common factors that drive compulsive overeaters are the following:

- High levels of anxiety and/or shame
- The preoccupation with and fear of becoming fat
- Negative body image and lack of acceptance of a "normal" body
- Extreme dieting; alternating restrictive periods with binge eating
- Sensitivity or allergy to specific foods or food groups

pain. Unfortunately, the association between eating and easing emotions gets reinforced on a daily basis. Loneliness, stress, and fear, experienced regularly, are common eating triggers.

Some therapists recommend ten-minute journaling when the urge to eat, not arising from actual hunger, occurs. Questions to be addressed at this time on paper might be the following:

- How am I really feeling presently?
- Has anything happened that has made me feel upset, sad, or fearful?
- When I feel these feelings, what do I really need?
- What is familiar about these feelings?
- When have I felt this way in the past?
- When is the first time that I can remember feeling this way?
- What can make me feel better other than eating?
- Where do I feel discomfort in my body? Shoulders? Jaw? Chest? Abdomen?
- If I do eat, how will I feel?
- What will I feel if I wait until the next meal?

Recommendations for combatting emotional eating include the following:

1. Give up restrictive dieting and eat well-balanced meals.
2. Develop a healthy self-image by focusing on positive aspects of yourself and others. Think about people that you admire. Why do you admire them? Realize that physical appearance is a very small part of a person's attractiveness.
3. Get involved in interesting hobbies, creative pursuits, or activities that challenge you and inspire good feelings.
4. Increase your physical activity and focus on the pleasure of movement instead of weight loss, heart threshold levels, or calorie burning.

5. Encourage the healthy expression of your emotions. Learn better ways to articulate how you feel, simply and directly.

Emotional eating is frequently a symptom of deeper issues, which can also be fueled by physical factors, such as blood sugar instability, poor nutrition, or inactivity. However, emotional components cannot be overlooked. "Mind and body are not separate," goes an old Chinese saying. Make your efforts unifying. For some, a therapist who has experience with emotional eaters can help to bring deeper awareness and resolve underlying traumas to strengthen coping ability and regain a deeper sense of accountability for the choices we make in nourishment.

The healthiest physical perspective is to view dietary change not as a futile exercise in deprival, but as a "temporary experiment" you've chosen to conduct in order to test its personal value. This makes your efforts more of an independent challenge and not just someone else's rule. Changes you exert and the discipline to carry them out with the commitment of self-discovery, quickly prove their positive worth and continually inspire you to remain committed.

Here's an example: If you begin to stabilize blood sugar levels and find that you can resist eating late at night, you'll happily discover the following day that you have more energy, enjoy deeper sleep, and feel restored hope. Your noticeable positive changes sustain your will to continue. You connect cause and effect. This is the power of an informed choice.

5. Genetics

True or false: Cravings are your parents' fault. Dad ate sugar by the wheelbarrow, and so what else is a chip-off-the-old-block supposed to do? Mom was a compulsive eater, so naturally it's in your "genes."

The answer is false—with a bit of true. Most people seem to believe that heredity is the prime factor for many of their ills, addictions, and habits. In reference to disease, while there might be valid genetic components, what is inherited is a susceptibility to develop disease and not the disease itself. It is immeasurably difficult to separate the effects of genetics from the influence of the upbringing lessons, which occurred in the home with mom and dad, our first teachers and role models. This is referred to as the familial factor. Our eating habits and mannerisms were originally influenced and absorbed by the example of our family members.

Sometimes, certain cravings you experience may remind you of similar cravings indulged by your parents, or for foods you shared with the cherished celebrations of childhood. Usually, such cravings have little to do with biochemical inheritance, but more with the search for sentimental re-connecting to the past through familiar comfort foods.

6. Allergy Response

In 1906, scientist C. E. Pirquet coined the word *allergie* from Greek *allos* (meaning "other" or "different") and *ergon* (meaning "work" or related to English energy). The derivation can be translated as *altered reaction*. However, many modern allergists are divided between a definition that considers "allergy" specifically as reactions between antigens and antibodies and a broader definition that encompasses more than a reaction to just pollen, molds, dust, and dander.

Allergic reactions occur when different offenders (food, pollen dust) interact with our immune system and produce harmful responses. While allergists devote much of their attention to respiratory problems, food-allergy specialists focus on the relationship between our immune function and food reactions. Two approaches can be used to deal with allergy reaction:

1. Determine the offender and eliminate your intake of it or exposure to it.
2. Strengthen your immune system to create greater resistance to the foods or substances that produce reactions.

Among the many symptoms of food allergy, fatigue and sleeplessness are the most common. Other symptoms are wide ranging and commonly include weakness, headaches, mucous congestion, irritability, poor concentration, memory problems, and depression.

Food allergies are distinct from other allergies in that many food allergies can foster addiction for the very foods that create debilitating symptoms. The analogy allergists frequently use is one that relates to drug addiction; a heroin addict must use continuously to avoid painful withdrawal symptoms. The risk of "cold turkey" withdrawal can be a prolonged ordeal of varied pain. A continuous dose of the drug, in whatever volume available, keeps the addict symptom free. Food can produce similar reactions. However, the principal difference between food and drug addiction is the degree of severity. I have heard clients say they're "climbing the walls" for chocolate, but this is more figurative, whereas with ordeal of heroin withdrawal, it's not uncommon literally to climb walls.

Because a person may be constantly including an addictive food within the general mix of the daily diet, it can easily go unrecognized. The worst food addictions are to caffeine, alcohol, dairy products, sugar, and chocolate. In most cases, your favorite treat can be your most allergic.

Generally, if you find yourself obsessing about a particular food, have it stashed around your house, and constantly find yourself yo-yo dieting and experiencing strong cravings for it,

---

EVERYDAY FOODS CAN CAUSE ALLERGIES

Some of the most common foods that cause allergic reactions are the following:

apples	chocolate	peanuts
beef	eggs	pork
cane sugar	green beans	potatoes
carrots	lettuce	soy products
chicken	dairy products	tomatoes
coffee	oats	wheat
corn	oranges	yeast

these may be indicators that you have food allergies. It might also be easy to confuse low blood sugar or sugar cravings from acid/alkaline imbalance with allergy symptoms. The best test is to abstain completely from "suspect" foods, and to watch for withdrawal symptoms.

7. Elimination/Detoxification

Elimination cravings can arise when you are in a cleansing process and have begun to change your diet. Theoretically, as we cleanse our bodies from toxins and foods that are not health supportive, stored toxins from fat tissue dissolve and release these toxins back into the blood for elimination through the liver, kidneys, lungs, and skin. During this time, it's not unusual to crave foods that originate from this storage. While this theory, also known as detoxification, belongs to some of the cultural folk medicine models and the natural hygiene schools of early twentieth century Western Europe, I've seen this occur in clients often enough to recognize that it does have relevance despite the lack of so-called scientific merit.

Some years ago, I read about a group of businessmen who were undergoing a sauna cleansing process. They spent abnormally long periods in saunas, with 10-minute breaks every hour, and constantly hydrated themselves with bottled water. Many of these men had been marijuana users in their hippie heydays but had long abandoned all drugs and had since embraced more conservative living.

After a number of hours, many of them began talking about their marijuana days. Those of them that had been heavy users found that they experienced a craving for marijuana. Still, several of the men claimed they could even taste it in their saliva.

The author of the article theorized that the potent THC resins from the cannabis plant had been long stored in their fat tissues. As it was dissolving, due to the prolonged heat exposure of the sauna, the resins reentered the blood and while recirculating through their systems, passed into the blood/brain barrier, triggering the marijuana memory and cravings. Several also remarked that they felt slightly stoned.

Most elimination cravings should not be overwhelming and will usually disappear after several hours. If the craving lingers, it might be wise to satisfy it in small quantities as part of your growing respect for the body's innate wisdom.

8. Expansion/Contraction

This last craving category is based on identical concepts that appear throughout cultural medicines, from Asian medicine to Ayurveda to Central American forms of folk medicine. It's a concept based on looking at things in terms of opposites and the natural laws between them.

If we can look at the world with an unprejudiced view, we can see that all phenomena exist in opposition and support each other: light and dark; strong and weak; hot and cold; centrifugal force and centripetal force; short wave and long wave; sodium and potassium; animal and vegetable; male and female, etc. Numerous cultures categorized these differences under specific terminology. In the Orient, for example, *yin* and *yang* were used to describe these opposite forces. For the sake of simplicity, I refer to these extremes as expansion and contraction.

Overeating produces distension, swelling, and bloating. It can be physically described as a state of expansion. The opposite of overeating is fasting—a state of gradual contraction. Eliminating food constricts the intestines. Eating an excess of salt has the same contractive reaction. It can create a strong attraction for sugar or alcohol. Tobacco users can find giving up the habit easier if they eliminate some of the factors that make

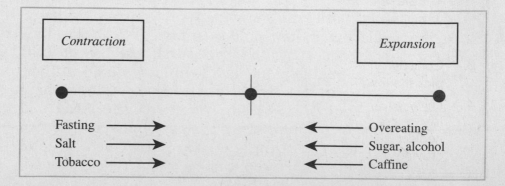

tobacco so much more physically desirable—namely, caffeine, alcohol, overeating, and/or sugar.

The physical effects of certain foods on tissue can be contractive or expansive. When we feel tense, we crave foods that have a relaxing or expansive effect. Watch a man enter a bar, tight-lipped and tense. Twenty minutes and several drinks later, he's gesturing broadly, is all smiles, and has little inhibition about serenading the entire bar. Aside from sociocultural factors, the influence of environment, psychological development, and biochemistry, all relevant and important influences, an excessively tense condition will seek foods or substances to relax, loosen, or simply chill. The reverse also applies.

FOUR KEYS TO HANDLING YOUR CRAVINGS

Here are four factors to consider when you have strong cravings, so that you can understand the basis behind them and determine the most satisfying and safe way to handle them.

1. Recall what you had in previous meals. This might be a key to why you are craving certain foods. For example, if you had a salty breakfast, you might be craving something sweet by afternoon. If you had pancakes with lots of syrup in the morning, you might crave something with animal protein or salted food several hours later. Opposites attract. Cravings work in the same way. If you don't eat for long periods, you'll want to overeat; if you take excess salt, you'll crave sugar.

2. Get specific about what is most appealing about the food you are craving:
   - *Taste:* Sweet, salty, bitter, pungent, sour
   - *Texture:* Crunchy, creamy, dry, liquid
   - *Temperature:* Hot, cold

3. Consider your options, plan your purchase or preparation, and pick the lesser of the evils, so to speak.

4. Enjoy yourself. If you're beating yourself up with guilt as you satisfy a craving, particularly for some kind of food treat, you neglect to enjoy an important part of the whole "satisfying-your-craving" equation—psychological pleasure.

Chocolate Romance in Aisle 10: A Sad Tale of Love Gone Wrong

I remember when I first changed my diet. I was dreaming about this package of chocolate wafers I used to buy that contained about a ton of sugar. (I would practically devour the bag before I reached the cash register. Mmmm, they were good.) After a year of diet change—and no chocolate wafers—I suddenly began thinking about them … a little too much. Actually, I was *dreaming* about them. I decided the only worthwhile solution would be an experimental session of "chocolate wafer treat therapy." A little bit won't kill me, I rationalized. I've been "good," but now it's time to be "bad." I call this rational *junk-dessert schizophrenia*, where you think of foods only in terms of good and bad and give unhealthy treats "reward" status.

With growing excitement, I left for the market. On the way, I enjoyed some chocolate wafer foreplay—I visualized sinking my teeth into that luscious rich chocolate, savoring that unique wafer crunch as its delicious filling melts over my tongue. The thought drove me into sensorial realms of bliss for the expected pleasures to come. My excitement grew. Why had I deprived myself for so long? No matter. It was time. I was ready.

If this seems to have sexual undertones, just ask any indulger to describe their favorite treat and you'll get an earful that sounds unquestionably like an intimacy encounter. Perhaps it's displaced passion. Who knows? Who cares? Now, about those wafers …

In the market, at aisle 10, I found my treat. It was neatly packaged in pretty foil with hot red lettering. It lay there, alone on the shelf in that vast, sterile, and cold market, eagerly awaiting my gentle, warm touch to grab it and make it mine. But, this was not going to be an ordinary affair. For that tortuous year of sacrifice I endured, our reunion demanded the respect of ritual. After all, we hadn't been with each other for more than a year. No, this had to be special. I was going to go home, light some candles, make some exotic drip grain coffee, put my wafers on a plate, and chew, in timeless moments of rapture, to my heart's content, reliving the fond remembrance of sweet times past.

Well, I did all of that—and it was a colossal disappointment; a bust; an *un*-event. The wafers were disgusting! Yeech! and Blah! of the highest order. Their artificial taste lingered in my mouth. The wafer felt like I was chewing air and the chocolate had this stale milky, bitter, chemical taste. I didn't remember them tasting like this! In my profound self-absorbed mourning, I began to laugh. A realization came clear: My taste buds had gotten used to whole food, fresh food, natural food that had real sweetness as it was chewed and felt good going down, staying down and leaving me with a feeling of true satisfaction and nourishment. This stuff I used to consider a treat from heaven now seemed like the wasted money dessert from hell. I felt a mixture of disappointment and elation at the same time. Disappointment for an expectation unrealized and elation for my new freedom; free from the longing, free from deprivation, free from the addictive bondage of chocolate-wafer-itis. Free, at last.

CRAVING SUBSTITUTIONS

With all the seminars, courses, and private instruction I had involved myself as a student, I've yet to find really practical and specific solutions for cravings. The subject is not something that's really "taught." Most so-called craving information entirely blames nutritional deficiencies and recommends plentiful supplements as a solution.

I had to learn through the trial and error of personal experimenting, from peers who developed similar strategies, and from the feedback of many thoughtful and diligent clients who made no bones about telling me what worked and didn't work.

So the following is some general substitution information about certain foods and food groups followed by more detail for specific cravings. Remember that the idea is not to feel you can never have your favorite goodies again. Rather, it's about no longer having to depend on them. You no longer have to compromise your health for a "treat" because you'll learn what to avoid that *drives* the craving. You might also discover, as I did, that your tastes change; what you once thought was delicious and something you could never live without or depend on soon becomes something you no longer desire, enjoy or depend on.

Food Craved	Substitution Strategy
• Sugar	Fruit, fruit-juice-sweetened desserts, grain-based sweeteners such as barley malt and rice syrup. Include more sweet vegetables in the daily diet, such as corn, onions, squash, and carrots.
• Animal Protein	If you do not want to give up animal protein use white meats, such as chicken and clean varieties (deep water) in small 3- to 5-ounce servings with abundant servings of vegetables.
	Choosing a vegetarian path is easier if you include a variety of protein-rich beans and bean products such as soybean burgers (tempeh), tofu, beans, and miso. Including a small amount (1–3 teaspoons) of olive, sesame, or flax oil with these dishes makes it easier to feel satisfied without animal protein.
• Dairy	Dairy cravings can often be satisfied with foods that supply some fat, protein and mineral content. Having ample portions of leafy dark greens, sea vegetables, and beans and bean products, and using small amounts of added oils and roasted seeds or nuts as condiments, helps to reduce or eliminate these cravings. For milk cravings, try some of the soy or rice milks and dilute them with water to use in cereals or recipes. For ice cream cravings, try any number of the frozen soy ice creams to avoid offending dairy-based proteins. There are also some pure fruit sorbets that are equally satisfying.
• Bread	Often, a lack of complex carbohydrates can inspire cravings for bread and flour products. Another reason for eating bread lies in its convenience—it's easy to make an instant sandwich or a quick snack. In this case, meal planning is crucial. However, one of the most common reasons for bread cravings has to do with the craving for hard, chewy textures, especially if your meals contain predominantly soft textures (like pasta

and sauce, or soup). A variety of textures will make a meal feel more balanced.

- Caffeine

For some people, this represents the most difficult challenge. Some of the factors that can create caffeine cravings are foods or practices that create fatigue, overeating, too much exercise, eating excessive dietary fat, mineral deficiency, and, as strange as it sounds, caffeine itself, since it sets up an addictive pattern. The two methods to stop are complete elimination or gradual reduction, replacing it with any of the many cereal grain, coffee-like hot drinks available at most natural foods stores (Roma, Pero, Cafix, Barley Brew, Dandelion Root Tea, Inka). Beware, caffeine can appear in many over-the-counter medications as well as soft drinks. One to two weeks after getting off caffeine, you'll pleasantly find that you have more energy of enduring quality. I would sometimes drink coffee when I was writing, telling myself that I felt more creative and energetic if I did. What I eventually realized was that while I did have greater bursts of energy, my thinking tended to be more fragmented and my endurance suffered. I also got impatient more easily and my rest quality was poor.

- Alcohol

Some factors behind the craving for alcohol have to do with high dietary sodium, excessive animal protein, and lack of fermented foods, aside from the obvious factors of addictive personalities, genetic predisposition, or psychological issues. Reduce animal protein by abstaining from red meat and chicken. Eat fish, if desired, one to three times weekly. Do not overeat; eat more frequently and less in volume. Reduce salt to very low, incidental amounts. Do aerobic walking or biking five times weekly to promote good circulation and oxygen increase. Try to include a little bit of fermented food, such as vinegar on salads, a small piece of pickle with your main meal, and some miso soup (approx.: $1/2$ to $3/4$ level tsp. miso paste in vegetable soup broth).

Ten Strategies to Eliminate Sugar Cravings

Read each of the following suggestions and notice how they apply to your eating patterns or lifestyle. Reducing your desire or addiction for sugar should not require Herculean will power. Becoming conscious of the physiological and lifestyle factors that stimulate sugar cravings should make taming your sweet tooth a piece of cake—so to speak.

1. Reduce Salt Consumption

The need for dietary salt is dependent on several factors: a lack of salt can cause fatigue, stimulate a desire to overeat, and often result in a craving for animal protein. However, with the availability of good-quality sea salt, miso paste, tamari soy sauce, and natural pickles, it's quite easy to overdose. Thirst, irritability, and a craving for sweet foods are reliable indicators of excess dietary salt.

2. Reduce Animal Protein

The standard four-basic-food-group propaganda was force-fed to the American public along with the myth that animal protein should be a dietary staple. This meat-and-potatoes mentality has to be rethought, since established research now demonstrates that excess animal protein can lead to colon and prostate cancer. If this applies to you, eat less in volume (2- to 4-ounce servings) and limit it to three to four times per week (maximum) as opposed to daily. You might want to experiment with abstaining completely from animal protein for a while, if your sugar habit feels out of control.

3. Reduce Food Volume

Overeating leads to fatigue and sluggishness. This makes a stimulant like sugar (or coffee) tremendously appealing. Eating more frequently (see suggestion 4) will allow you to reduce overeating with a minimum of effort.

4. Eat More Frequently Throughout the Day

Going for long periods between meals is one of the most common reasons for sugar cravings—especially at night. By skipping meals or waiting long periods, you stop supplying your blood with glucose—muscle fuel. Your blood sugar drops, and by the time you finally get around to eating, you're going nuts for something very sweet. You're also likely to end up overeating or craving something fatty as a compensation for sugar. Initially, don't wait more than 3½ to 4 hours between meals.

5. Avoid Eating Prior to Bed

If your body is digesting when it requires much needed rest, you'll later require more sleep, dream excessively, and find it difficult to awaken with alertness. Good deep sleep will result in wide-awake days. Eating too close to bedtime creates a groggy awakening and the morning craving for sugar (or caffeine). Eat a light evening dinner at least 2½ to 3 hours before retiring.

6. Avoid Sugar

This may sound obvious, but continuing to eat simple sugars results in a continuously low blood sugar state. This stimulates the need for more sugar, and the cycle continues. Even though fruit is a simple sugar, switching to fruit instead of refined or more concentrated forms of simple sugar is a good first step. Eat the skin of the fruit as well, for the value of its fiber.

7. Exercise Moderately, but Consistently

Daily aerobic exercise will increase circulation and strengthen will power. Brisk walking, biking, or light jogging naturally increase sensitivity to the effects of sugar. Try to get 20 to 30 minutes of some type of pleasurable exercise at least five times per week. Enjoy this. It should not be a chore.

8. Emphasize Whole Complex Carbohydrates

If your daily diet includes whole grains (brown rice, oats, millet, barley, buckwheat, etc.) and vegetables (roots, greens, and round vegetables such as squashes, cabbages) as a primary fuel, you'll find that you automatically crave less sugar. Emphasizing sweet vegetables such as carrots, cooked onions, corn, cabbage, parsnips, or squashes adds a natural and satisfying sweetness to meals. Try introducing some sea vegetables (a.k.a. "seaweed") for enhancing your minerals.

9. Don't Suppress Feelings

This doesn't mean you have to broadcast every feeling—only those that matter and to those who really matter to you. Food indulgence, especially with sweets, is a convenient way to anesthetize feelings. Sugar can consume you with sensory pleasure, temporarily providing mental relief from whatever might be stressful. Conversely, sweets can hinder energy levels and mental clarity, so in the long run your emotional coping ability becomes diminished.

10. Beware of Psychological Sugar Triggers

The many psychological associations we connect with food have a powerful influence. Consider the influence of family associations, movie rituals, familiar restaurants, and childhood habits.

SIX WAYS TO DEFEAT YOUR FAT TOOTH

Fat—in the form of french fries, deep-fried shrimp, tempura vegetables, pizza, and melted cheese on just about anything— has become America's dietary passion. Fat's slow digestion time accounts for that "stick-to-the-ribs" feeling after a rich meal. Here are six general reasons for fat cravings.

1. Carbohydrate Imbalance

A lack of complex carbohydrates and an excess of simple carbohydrates can create a strong desire for fat. Years of looking at client dietary records has convinced me that a substantial reason for craving fat is this very imbalance. Here's how it looks when diagramed:

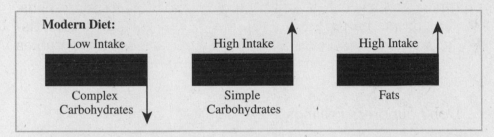

The lack of whole complex carbohydrates in the modern diet (particularly whole grains) triggers carbohydrate cravings. We eat refined sugars and concentrated simple sugars in an attempt to satisfy our carbohydrate needs. Due to their quick digestion, however, they create irregular blood sugar levels. As a result, we are attracted to fat to feel more satisfied, to regulate blood sugar, and to experience fat's natural ability to hold more flavor.

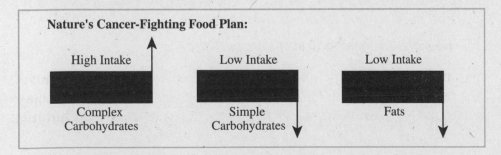

On *The Nature's Cancer-Fighting Food Plan,* the abundance of mineral- and vitamin-rich whole grains, beans and vegetables, and fruits, offers a more enduring fuel and more satisfying nourishment. Automatically, our desire for fat is reduced.

2. Excessive Bread and Flour Products

Eating too much bread can often trigger cravings for oil. Rarely does anyone eat bread dry. You dip your bread in olive oil, butter it, or spread nut butters on it. It only stands to reason that the more bread you eat, the more you'll want something, usually oil-based, to spread on it. I once had an Asian nutrition teacher who recommended that students steam their bread for about 30 to 45 seconds. I thought this had to be the most bizarre suggestion I'd ever heard. After trying it (it only works with real whole grain, unyeasted bread), I loved it! However, that's not always convenient or appealing for most people. Therefore, if you have a fat tooth, go easy on the breads and flour products.

3. Need for Fermentation

One of my teachers used to claim that fat cravings resulted from intestines that are weak or not accustomed to digesting whole foods. Some fermented products can help the intestines synthesize nutrients more effectively by adding breakdown enzymes and contributing to the growth of healthy bacteria. Miso soybean paste as a vegetable soup ingredient, small amounts of tamari soy sauce (naturally processed), tempeh, and even some natural sourdough nonyeasted breads are good forms of fermentation. As some of these products contain sea salt, be sure to use in minimum quantity.

4. Need for Protein

Another reason for fat cravings might be due to a need for more protein. Since fat usually accompanies protein, it is best to take daily small amounts of beans, bean or soy products, and occasional fish (optional) to satisfy this craving.

5. Stimulating Foods and Fat-Dissolving Foods

In observing different culinary combinations and from listening to client feedback, I began to see a dietary connection between specific foods that, in combination, were well suited to fat. It only made sense that if you began to restrict these foods, the desire for fat would diminish. I have found this strategy consistently effective with clients and in my personal life. The following are two categories of foods:

1. Foods that have a fat-dissolving effect. They emulsify— like the old kitchen pot-cleaning tip of adding a bit of salt to an oily skillet to dissolve the oil.
2. Foods that have a stimulating effect. These foods counter the fatiguing effects of excess fats and sharpen the senses.

Vegetables that are considered to be fat emulsifying are onions, scallions, leeks, watercress, parsley, white (daikon) and red radish, ginger, mushrooms, dandelion greens, burdock root, peppers, and tomatoes. If your previous diet has been high in fat and animal products, these vegetables are considered to have a detoxifying effect on fat storages in the body.

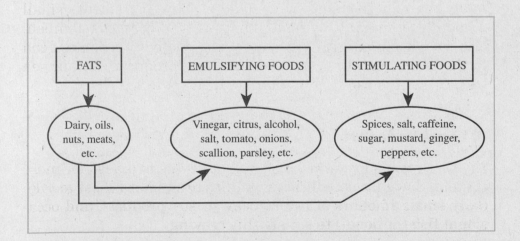

FOODS THAT BALANCE

Think about the following food combinations to see how they are often complementary:

- Wine and cheese
- Alcohol and salted nuts
- Tempura (Japanese deep-fried vegetables) and a soy sauce-ginger dip
- French fries and ketchup, or fries with vinegar and salt (British)
- Eggs and salt, pepper, or with a spicy hot pepper sauce
- Coffee with cream; toast with butter
- Meats with salt, onions, mustard, ketchup, or tomatoes
- Cheese enchiladas with spicy green or red sauce

Each of these combinations represents some kind of balance. When I've counseled people who had strong cravings for fats, applying this paradigm usually worked well. If the favorite emulsifying or stimulating food was reduced, fat cravings became minimized with less of an effort.

6. Need for "Comfort" Food

Fat is one of the macronutrients often considered a comfort food. Mother's milk has nearly four times more fat than protein. It has been theorized that this alone might be ample reason for the comforting effect of fats. Ice cream, cheese, butter, and warm milk are typical foods associated with comfort.

Fat with a sweet taste, as in ice cream, might provide some psychological refuge for us in times of stress. However, in the long run, it could compromise our emotional coping ability, instigating such symptoms as immune dysfunction from sugar excess or allergy response from poorly digested dairy-based proteins. If the attraction to fat does not seem to relate to any of the reasons previously mentioned, it might be a comfort craving or a craving based on certain psychological associations from your past. Sometimes, an occasional indulgence is therapeutic. The real concern is when we indulge in these foods often, or in large volume.

Au Revoir to Overeating—Six Keys for Handling Monster Appetites

For people in dietary transition, especially changing to a diet lower in fat and sugar, overeating is a common practice. The following are six key reasons for overeating.

1. Emotionality

There are many emotional factors that are the basis for overeating or binge eating. If you feel that this is a component to your overeating, first, remove the dietary imbalance factors mentioned in this section that may be pushing you in this direction. Second, accept that your overeating may be emotionally based and either seek support or do some research to get a better perspective on what some of these emotional factors might be.

2. Excessive Animal Protein/Excessive Salt

I've seen the craving to overeat occur in people who begin eating miso and soy sauce and pickles—some of the traditional, salt-based products recommended for their alkaline properties and enzyme nourishment. This may be the fault of a previously high-acid diet that stimulates a continued craving for salt products when people first begin to sample these traditional foods. They end up craving large amounts of food. I suspect this is mainly because they're trying to avoid what they're really craving: sugar. So, overeating then becomes a compensatory act. This can also occur with excessive intake of animal protein.

3. Irregular Blood Sugar

Waiting long periods between meals can make you ravenous! This is one of most common reasons for overeating. If you suspect this might be a cause of your overeating, plan more carefully, and eat more frequently throughout the day—not one continuous meal, but perhaps four to five smaller meals. You're less likely to have a late-night appetite if you do so.

4. Inactive Lifestyle

Becoming more physically active on a daily basis can make you more sensitive to the subtle, and not-so-subtle, negative effects of overeating. If you know you're going to take a bike ride or long walk, the last thing you'll want to have is a belly full of food to accompany you. Changing your evening ritual can help as well. If you normally watch television and snack late at night, consider watching earlier programming and do some gentle stretching, or several yoga postures, or slow sustained stretching prior to bed. You'll have a more relaxed and deeper sleep instead of digesting while you toss and turn, as a panorama of nonstop dreaming keeps you in a superficial and dissatisfying sleep.

5. Poor Nutrient Assimilation

Poor absorption could be another reason at the root of frequent overeating. We're not satisfied and so we'll eat to capacity. The solution to overeating as a result of poor assimilation is dietary experimenting; not just the random popping of pills, but the elimination of foods that threaten your vitamin and mineral status, such as frequent sugars, or excessive fat. We can experiment with adjunctive foods, such as herbs and even supplements, as part of a more detailed inquiry into our needs. In more serious cases, a blood panel or stool sample may reveal more chronic conditions, such as anemia, or parasites, which could sometimes be the root cause of chronic overeating. Consistent, good nutrition, daily activity, rest, and a wide variety of foods and cooking styles can help restore intestinal strength fairly quickly.

6. Insufficient Chewing

I used to have a teacher who claimed overeating was due to a lack of chewing. Period. That was his theory. Based on what I've observed around me, sometimes I think he was right.

> ### FOOD KILLS!
>
> I once heard a news brief, from The National Safety Council, that the sixth major cause of accidental death in this country, ranking ahead of airplane crashes, is choking on food. Nearly 3500 people die yearly from what is technically called "food inhalation." This term sounds appropriate for some of the meals I've witnessed people consuming in public. The brief claimed that some of these people who choked had tried to swallow pieces of meat the size of a cigarette package!

When all is said and done, good digestion begins with the simple act of thorough chewing. Fat and protein do not digest in the mouth. They begin their digestion in the stomach and in the following stage, the duodenum. If our diets are high in these factors, we're less likely to chew.

Whole foods have the distinction of beginning their digestion in the mouth. Their taste becomes naturally sweet and fills you up, without filling you "out." Most people shovel a tremendous amount of food into their mouths. It's difficult to chew a large volume of food because you become so overwhelmed with saliva and the impulse to swallow is automatic. So, I suggest small volumes, chewed thoroughly.

Hopefully, these lists of generalized recommendations will help you to recognize what factors might pertain to you. Sometimes, as Mark Twain said, "eat what you want and let the food battle it out inside" might be good advice. However, when you need tools to aid a desired, healthy diet change, you'll find that many of these factors will be of enormous support.

7

THE BEST KEPT SECRET OF THE ORIENT: THE SOUP THAT HEALS

A HEALING FOOD STEEPED IN CULTURE

Over 1000 years ago, Chinese Buddhist monks traveled to Japan, bringing with them a vegetarian religion as well as their traditional Chinese recipes for fermented soybean products. Two of these enduring products are a thick paste made from salt-fermented soybean and grain called miso, (mee-so) and the dark liquid run-off from this process commonly called soy sauce, but traditionally known as tamari (made without wheat), or shoyu (made with wheat). These vegetarian staple foods were eventually assimilated into the Japanese diet, using native Japanese grains, soybeans, and vegetable molds. Today, a small number of rural families throughout Japan still make their own miso from products they've personally cultivated.

While it is well known that soybeans provide a wealth of good-quality protein and many other nutrients, only a small amount of these nutrients can be made available to the body when the whole beans have been cooked by boiling, baking, or roasting. However, when fermented, the complex proteins, carbohydrate, and fat molecules of soybeans are converted into digestible amino acids, simple sugars, and fatty acids. The unique fermentation process also unravels a full panoply of aroma, flavor, and texture.

Simply speaking, miso is a thick paste made by combining soybeans, whole grain (usually rice or barley), a vegetable-based enzyme starter (koji, yeast mold), natural sea salt, and water. It has a sweet, rich flavor and contains living enzymes that aid digestion, strengthen the blood, and provide a nutritious balance of complex carbohydrates, essential oils, protein, vitamins, and minerals. According to Asian folk legends, miso was a gift from the gods to ensure humanity's health, longevity, and happiness.

Miso can be made with many different ingredients. In addition to barley and rice miso, an infinite number of co-starring ingredients can be added. On the commercial natural foods market, chickpea miso, plain soybean miso, leek miso, and sweet rice miso are currently available.

The mixture of ingredients is cooked and then allowed to age from three months to three years, depending on the strength of miso desired and grain, or added bean. According to Asian folk medicine, miso aged for more than 3 years contains more powerful healing qualities. The liquid run-off from this fermented mash is how natural soy sauce was originally created, while the paste, at the bottom of the vat, became miso. This savory and versatile paste is then packaged and sold as a seasoning to be diluted with water and added to vegetable soups, sauces, gravies, salad dressings, dips, marinades, pickles, and assorted pates.

Unfortunately, in modern Japan, miso quality has considerably declined. Most of the commercial miso available today is made with refined grain, contains numerous chemicals, MSG, sugar additives, and is artificially aged. Fortunately, a number of American natural food companies now manufacture traditionally aged miso made with unrefined organic ingredients and packaged in small plastic tubs. It is available at most natural foods stores in refrigerated sections.

The flavor of this unique and healthy seasoning characterizes the essence of Japanese cooking. Most Japanese begin their day with a fortifying broth of miso soup. Consider it the traditional equivalent of a morning coffee, and when used for sickness, a replacement for the traditional chicken-soup remedy. To Americanize this cultural product, I usually call it "vegetarian beef bouillon paste"—its hearty and full-bodied flavor being somewhat reminiscent of beef broth.

MISO'S NUTRITIONAL WAREHOUSE

Containing all essential amino acids, miso offers rich vegetable quality protein. In fact, miso has been a traditional key source of protein in the Japanese diet and accounts for up to 25 percent of the island's inland, rural protein consumption. The Japanese national individual miso consumption is approximately 16 pounds per year.

More than an ordinary seasoning, miso has been considered an essential part of the East Asian grain-based diet. Due to its abundance of amino acids, which many foods lack, combining miso with other foods acts as a protein booster, increasing protein by as much as 30 to 40 percent.

Protein amounts in miso can very from 9 to 18 percent. The protein chains are broken down during the fermentation process into seventeen different amino acids, making for superior nutrition and easy digestion.

Japanese researchers have discovered trace amounts of vitamin B_{12} in certain types of traditionally produced miso. B-vitamins riboflavin, niacin, and B_{12} are each increased by microorganic synthesis during the fermentation of the miso mash. The fungi and bacteria within the fermenting mash manufacture the B_{12}. Whether or not these micronutrients are passed on to humans is still in question. However, it is interesting to note that for centuries, Japanese Buddhist monks, notorious strict vegetarians, ate generous amounts of fermented vegetable foods such as tempeh soybean mash, tofu, seaweeds, natural soy sauce, and miso and were renowned for their good health, vigor, and longevity.

Miso, due to its salt content, has an alkalizing effect on the blood; therefore, it has the ability to neutralize mild acids. Miso soup is frequently used in Japan in the same way Westerners might use Alka-Seltzer or Milk of Magnesia to settle an upset stomach, reduce the effects of a hangover, or remedy indigestion.

THE FUNGUS AMONG US—YEAST, MOLDS, AND ASSORTED MICROFLORA

The organisms found in the miso fermentation comprise hundreds of species and can be generally classified as molds, yeasts, and bacteria. Molds are fungi, related to mushrooms, and can be delightfully discovered growing abundantly on the foods we've forgotten about in the back of the refrigerator. The blue, black, and green dust covering advanced cultures are molds that have been reproduced by spores.

Molds, matter in a decomposing state, contain enzymes that help transfer complex compounds into simple ones. Yeasts, similar to molds, are also fungi, but typically reproduce by budding instead of by spores. There are many types of yeasts that are partially responsible for miso, natural soy sauces, certain fermented diary products, and pickled vegetables. In these products the alcohol produced is not only responsible for the aromatic bouquet, but has a preserving ability in the lactic acid content, which is produced by a specific type of bacteria present in the fermenting food.

An Intestinal Voyage

The microscopic world of human intestinal bacteria is a complex sort of ecosystem with over 400 species residing just within the last 5 feet of intestine. Consider the colon a virtual microbial factory. Coexisting with assorted yeasts and fungus species, our colon contains trillions of microscopic bacteria, known as gut microflora. Intestinal flora allow our intestines to assimilate nutrients and eliminate waste more efficiently. On the typical American diet, one-third of the dry weight of the feces is composed of bacteria. On a healthier whole-foods diet, this bacteria count is diluted by the fiber content.

The functions of intestinal microflora include

1. Helping to further digest food through fermentation
2. Synthesizing water-soluble vitamins
3. Protecting our body from disease-causing bacteria
4. Enhancing our immunity

Indigestible complex carbohydrates, dietary fiber and plant-derived sugars, provide the bulk of the food for these bacteria. In a *Journal of Nutrition* study, it was noted that individuals following a vegetarian diet have higher counts of aerobic bacteria than meat eaters. Aerobic bacteria (the "good" twin) can only live in the presence of oxygen, whereas anaerobic bacteria (the "evil" twin) are not oxygen dependent. Anaerobic bacteria are considered "unfriendly" bacteria and health compromising.

The health of our gut microflora can be negatively influenced by the following factors:

*   Temperature
*   Illness
*   Antibiotics/drug treatments
*   Dietary changes

THE MICROFLORA SOLUTION—MISO!

Miso is prized for its ability to aid in the digestion and assimilation of different foods. At least four digestive agents are contained in all nonpasteurized forms of miso:

1. Natural digestive enzymes
2. Lactic-acid forming bacteria (a.k.a. *Lactobacillus*)
3. Salt-resistant yeasts
4. Mold and other microorganisms (present in the starter, koji)

WHAT'S GOOD FOR THE FLORA

A whole foods diet of unrefined grains, vegetables, and beans appears to support the healthiest mix of bacteria in the intestinal flora. This mix can be diminished by a refined-foods diet high in simple sugars and by frequent use of broad-spectrum antibiotics. To regenerate this bacteria, many health practitioners recommend eating a number of unpasteurized fermented foods, particularly yogurt, acidolophilous milk, and miso. The premise for this recommendation is that the lactic acid bacteria available from these foods will help, once it arrives in the colon, to recolonize healthy bacteria. However, three requirements are frequently overlooked:

- For the bacteria to adapt to the severe elements it encounters as it travels from the mouth to the intestines, and tolerate the environment of harsh intestinal conditions, it should be a species that is naturally part of the gut flora. The bacteria must also be able to coexist with organisms already residing in the gut.

- The bacteria species must also be able to implant itself within the gut and not bond with bowel matter that will be discharged and lost.

In some cases yogurt has been found to aid intestinal health, but this is thought to be more of a result of natural antibodies than the introduction of lactic acid bacteria. The problem with dairy-quality bacteria is that they are not of the species normally found within the gut. It has not been conclusively demonstrated that bacteria species derived from yogurt can effectively colonize within the human intestine.

Additionally, yogurt has many of the negative qualities of dairy products:

- It is often high in fat and cholesterol.
- It contains allergy-producing proteins.
- It is frequently infected with potentially harmful viruses and bacteria and chemicals.

It takes a hearty variety of enzyme to survive the severe ritual of several years' fermentation in a mild brine solution. This ability empowers the microorganisms to continue the work of nutrient breakdown in the human intestines, where proteins, carbohydrates, and fats are reduced to simpler and more easily digested molecules.

Enzymes (digestion-promoting catalysts) are destroyed at temperatures above 104°F. Lactic acid is also heat fragile and can be destroyed within minutes of a simmering heat. For this reason, unpasteurized miso is recommended to foster a living digestive culture within the intestine.

Numerous laboratory tests have checked for the existence of mycotoxins and especially aflatoxins (toxins caused by harmful molds) in miso. All reports have been negative, indicating no findings of any toxins.

MISO'S SALT CONTENT

Miso's salt content varies from 8–12 percent. Natural unpasteurized miso is made with natural, trace-mineral-rich sea salt. It does not contain aluminum, sugar, iodine, or any other chemicals generally added to common (mine-source) salt. Natural sea salt's many trace elements are essential for our metabolic balance. Recent experiments show that the fermentation process actually changes the effect of salt on the human body; rats demonstrated a higher salt tolerance when the source was miso instead of common table salt.

Miso's salinity is four times greater than seawater. That may sound quite salty; however, miso's amino acid and natural oil mellow it. When made properly with a vegetable base, miso soup should not taste salty. Miso is best used as a soup addition and not a flavoring. A general recommendation is use $3/4$ to one level teaspoon of miso per large bowl of soup containing vegetables.

I once had a client call and complain, "Boy, that miso is pretty salty stuff." I asked how much he was using. "Not more than two tablespoons," he said. "That's way too much," I replied. "Two tablespoons means you're using six teaspoons of miso paste!"

"Well," he said with defeat in his voice, "I thought it was supposed to be good for you."

My client thought that if a little was nutritious, then loading up would be doubly nutritious. Unfortunately, it doesn't work like that. More is not always better—especially in regard to foods with substantial salt content.

STRONGER THAN STRONTIUM?

A survivor of the Nagasaki bomb blast one mile from its epicenter, Dr. Shinichiro Akizuki, was convinced that his resistance to radiation was due to his daily habit of taking miso soup. In 1972, stimulated by Dr. Akizuki's writings, a number of prominent Japanese scientists doing agricultural research discovered that miso contained dipicolinic acid (*zybicolin* in Japanese). Produced by miso microorganisms, it is an alkaloid that chelates (bonds) to heavy metals such as radioactive strontium and discharges them from the body. This discovery received front-page coverage in Japan's major newspapers.

MISO'S ROLE IN FIGHTING CANCER

You would be well advised to add miso to your diet for the general health benefits it promotes, But miso can also be an active participant in cancer prevention.

- "Friendly" bacteria within the intestine can protect us from cancer in several ways. They can bind and arrest cancer-causing substances in the food we eat. Lactobacillus, living or dead, can absorb cancer causing chemicals known as pyrolysates, which are produced by cooking meat at high temperatures. These chemicals are deactivated when absorbed into the cell walls of lactobacillus bacteria—the kind of bacteria found in miso.

- The friendly bacteria in miso also have the ability to neutralize cancer-causing substances such as, *N*-nitrosamines. Another type of friendly bacteria called *Bifidobacteria* produces antitumor substances that cause our white blood cells to engulf and destroy tumor cells.

- An Alabama study showed that a diet supplemented with miso reduced the incidence and delayed the appearance of mammary adenocarcinomas in female rats. The miso-supplemented diet group showed a trend toward a lower number of cancers per animal, a trend toward a higher number of benign tumors per animal, and a trend toward a lower growth rate of cancers compared with controls.

- A Japanese medical school reported the following: "Japanese soybean paste miso, which has reported to prevent gastric and mammary cancer and chronic nephritis, was demonstrated by electron spin resonance spectrometry as a scavenger of free radicals." The report showed that miso acts as an "antioxidant by scavenging free radicals."

HOW TO USE MISO

Miso is a tremendously versatile food. Its uses in food preparation seem unlimited. Most frequently it is diluted into soup or used as a salt/soy sauce substitute. As a broth ingredient it imparts body and offers a savory, hearty taste that is both nourishing and satisfying.

When buying miso, it is best to experiment by purchasing small quantities of different varieties. This will enable you to become familiar with its unique flavors, colors, textures, and aromas. Naturally-aged miso is available at most natural food stores and usually stored in plastic tubs. It should say "unpasteurized" on the label. Miso is best stored in a cool, dark place. Sweet varieties of miso, which are aged for shorter lengths of time, require refrigeration.

Keep in mind that natural miso is a living food containing many beneficial microoogranisms that are easily destroyed by prolonged cooking. It is best to add the miso to soups, or other dishes, just before they are removed from the heating element of your stove.

I'm fond of making a lentil, barley, carrot, onion, and celery soup. It's a simple soup that can act as a one-bowl lunch. I might make a general amount and store it in the refrigerator. After I warm up the amount I intend to use for one serving, I'll then add a level teaspoon of miso (diluted in several tablespoons of water) immediately after I've turned off the element.

When traveling, I take along dry instant miso soup packets. They can be diluted into a cup or a bowl of hot water. I've even used a small amount of dry instant miso as a condiment mixed into hot oatmeal. Frankly, fresh miso can spoil your taste for the instant version, but in a pinch it does well.

In Chapter 12 there are directions for several delicious recipes that use miso. A wonderful and thorough reference is William Shurtleff and Akiko Aoyagi's *The Book of Miso*. It offers 400 recipes and even offers miso-making details for the ultra-ambitious.

8
HARVESTING THE GOOD EARTH—MEDICINAL HERBS AND MUSHROOMS

HERBALLY HOPELESS OR HERBALLY HELPFUL?

There was an uncomfortable silence after the patient, a youthful woman of 43, was diagnosed with a reoccurrence of breast cancer. In considering additional rounds of chemotherapy, she feared the possibility of responding poorly, experiencing those same nasty and debilitating symptoms despite advances in drip-and-cocktail developments. She asked about alternatives. The doctor shook his head. "There's very little out there that seems of any merit," he said flatly.

"What about herbs? I had a friend who took some Chinese herbs and she responded really well—"

"There's very little research to support that," he interrupted.

It has become increasingly clear that the concept of a magic bullet for curing cancer does not lie in one formula, one food, or one particular practice. A healthy diet, lifestyle, positive disposition, and will to live still constitute the main elements for healing. In this regard, herbal therapies should not be overlooked as they may present strong adjunctive support as a healing catalyst.

Since there are only a handful of clinical trials to show that plants can prevent or treat cancer, the scientific community still considers herbal recommendations as only a "theoretical possibility." Despite the fact that herbs have been used for thousands of years and quite effectively by other cultures, the evaluative final word is still documented scientific study. Considering the calvacade of "cures" claimed in various herbal advertisements bolstered with dramatic anecdotal testimonies, skeptical attitudes are understandable.

Herbs are nature's botanic gift of an extremely vast and powerful pharmacopoeia. Over the centuries, numerous cultures have developed extensive medicines from native plants in the form of tinctures, tonics, powders, salves, and external applications. About 300 years ago, thousands of plant species were the primary source of drugs for the world's population. Herbal remedies were routinely prescribed until the late 1800s, when the American Medical Association (AMA) used its enormous wealth and political clout to control or eliminate alternative forms of treatment.

Ironically, many of our most potent and qualified modern drugs are derived from herbs and other plants. The origin of penicillin is from a mold and, in this regard, is herbal or plant based. Numerous antibiotics are based on substances produced by fungi. A number of prominent drugs originate from herbal plants. For example:

- Digitalis is an extract from the dried leaves of foxglove, which contains various substances, including digitoxin and digocin, that stimulate heart muscle. Used to treat heart failure, it is given orally or, in emergency, through injection.

- Atropine is a drug that is extracted from the "deadly nightshade" plant belladonna. Atropine relaxes smooth muscle and is used to treat biliary and renal colic and also reduces secretions of the bronchial tubes, salivary glands, stomach, and intestines, and is used before general anesthesia.

In China, the government has funded an intensive study of traditional Chinese herbal medicine, called Fu Zhen therapy, which plays a featured role in the Chinese health care system.

Backed by centuries of empirical experience, China's huge pharmacopoeia contains thousands of substances of plant, animal, or mineral origin, most of them herbs. According to a National Academy of Sciences study of 796 Chinese herbal and animal remedies, at least half of the remedies have scientific basis for their reputed claims. Yet many an uninformed Western physician will raise an eyebrow and claim that there exists little proof that herbs are beneficial, that they are dangerous or even a waste of money.

INTELLIGENCE IN THE ABSENCE OF WISDOM

One reason for this attitude is due to modern medicine's approach of isolating active ingredients from various plants to assess the value of using them in concentrated form, a process known as standardizing. This unbalanced approach often diminishes the potency of the herb. In whole form, nature's herbal gifts are composed of multiple chemicals in moderate proportions which synergistically work together. As concentrated carriers of sunlight and vitality, herbs have a unique, natural healing energy absent from synthetic drugs.

The distinguishing difference between herbs and synthetics is that herbs work harmoniously with the body's natural ability to regenerate, bolstering immunity as opposed to suppressing it, a negative result of many drugs. From the perspective of traditional herbal medicine, the linear method of focusing on only one ingredient, while successfully interfering with the disease process, ignores the rich matrix of existing chemical proportions that herbs naturally contain, maximizing healing while minimizing toxicity.

In trying to isolate the most potent of the chemicals, we run the risk of losing or diminishing the synergy of the natural chemical matrix contained in the herbs. Often, an ingredient considered "inert" ends up being essential to the entire matrix, perhaps enhancing absorption or as a toxicity reducer of the active phytochemical. In the words of author and physician David Simon, "we have extracted the intelligence, but discarded the wisdom of the herb."

DRUG COMPANIES AND HERBAL PRODUCTS

A number of pharmaceutical companies today have done this very thing: they have developed herbal products based on the standardization of a single active ingredient. By isolating this bioactive substance and made molecular modifications, the resulting synthetic product can become proprietary, an exclusive product, which they are then entitled to patent. This is how the pharmaceutical giants can recoup the $125 million it costs to test a new drug and bring it to market.

Commenting on this pharmaceutical practice, Richard Walters suggests the following:

> If you and I could simply pick some weeds or herbs, brew them into a tea, drink the tea, and avoid or reverse a terrible disease, drug companies and doctors would watch their enormous profits evaporate. This is why the parameters of drug-industry science are totally regulated. We are told that the medical monopoly's restrictive regulations are necessary for two reasons: safety and efficacy. But substantial evidence for the effectiveness of some herbal cancer treatments (and other nontoxic alternative therapies) belies this rationale.

Despite the appearance of financial motive, there are some medical benefits to this process of standardization. Several chemotherapy drugs are derived from ordinary plants. The most recent newsmaker has been taxol, which comes from the Pacific yew tree. On the plus side, taxol has been used successfully in women with ovarian cancer. On the minus side, it suppresses the bone marrow and causes nausea. Etoposide comes from the mayapple plant and is used to treat lung and testicular tumors. From the periwinkle plant we get the vinca alkaloids, vincristine and vinvlastine, two of the most widely used agents to inhibit tumor growth, which are used in the treatment of lympohmas. These plant-derived vinca alkaloid drugs are used aggressively for fast-growing cancers. However, with less aggressive cancers, the danger of "curing the disease, but killing the patient" might outweigh the potential benefits of these cyotoxic agents.

Herbs can be very powerful restoratives, but they should not be used based solely on the say-so of self-help books. A commitment to using herbs as an adjunctive therapy should include formal and individualized recommendations by a qualified, experienced practitioner. A truly qualified practitioner will recommend formulas, in specific dosages, for an experimental time only after evaluating a patient's condition. This will include an assessment of the patient's appearance, medical history, current diet, allergy potential, and general lifestyle. A number of common herbs can also be toxic and should be avoided during pregnancy, or with certain medications, such as those for high blood pressure and kidney problems.

This chapter will offer a general outline of the possibilities herbal support can offer. It is not meant to be a specific directive, as individual sensitivities are highly unique. The subject is vast and continually growing as more research and public awareness develops. Please refer to this book's bibliography for references, herb sources, and practitioner organizations for more detailed and individualized support.

HERBAL CANCER PREVENTION

From epidemiological studies that indicate the risk of various cancers and the long-term consumption of particular herbs, we have learned that there are literally thousands of plant-derived products which are associated with a lower risk for most types of cancer.

For instance, herbs that contain plant sterols can help with breast cancer by filling the estrogen receptor sites in the body and preventing an individual's estrogen from "feeding" the cancer. Other herbs that have undergone research in this area are red clover, evening primrose, soy, and alfalfa.

Perhaps it may be our "medicine mentality" that can relate only to taking pills or even herbal formulas as "medicine," yet fails to regard food with equal importance. The individual who

SEVEN WAYS THAT HERBS HELP HEAL

While it may be dangerously naive to think of herbal treatments as magic bullets for combating cancer, some herbs can offer crucial support for cancer prevention treatment, reducing the damaging effects of chemotherapy and radiation. Here are seven ways by which herbs can assist the healing process:

- Strengthening the body's natural detox systems to aid liver and kidney function
- Stimulating immune response to galvanize the body's natural healing ability
- Preventing further cellular mutation characteristic of cancer development
- Soothing inflamed tissue from drug therapy side effects
- Stimulating digestion for better assimilation and elimination
- Providing antioxidant protection to fight free radicals.
- Promoting emotional and physical calmness without sacrificing health

invests time, money, and hope in herbal or supplemental support, but neglects to eat and live in a way that supports healing, compromises the effectiveness of his or her herbal therapy. Moving three steps forward with herbs, but four steps backward with poor diet and erratic lifestyle, because a self-sabotaging effort. This tendency may also account for some of the "official" statistics which judge herbal or vitamin supplements as "ineffective." The healing possibilities of many natural medicines, from acupuncture to herbal medicine to vitamin supplementation, can be minimized, if not undermined, by daily diet, stress levels, and bottled-up emotions.

1. Detoxification

Detoxification, an area generally overlooked by conventional medicine, can take place at three levels:

A. *Within Cellular Structures*. Herbs described as blood purifiers and lymphatics work at this level. Every cell goes through its process of absorption and discharge. Cells discharge their waste products into the lymph and blood systems.

Some examples of herbs that have detoxifying action are oils of lemon and orange; cumin; poppy seed; basil; thuja; turkey corn; poke; extracts of rosemary, peppermint, and spearmint; sulfur compounds from onions, garlic, cruciferous vegetables (cabbage, broccoli, brussel sprouts, various greens); and many of the common flavonoids, such as carotenoids as well as organic acids found in fruits and vegetables.

B. *Liver Cleansing*. A healthy liver is essential for cancer prevention and treatment. Many of the toxins that we are exposed to on a daily basis are filtered through the liver. Many of these toxins can cause mutations of our genetic material, specifically DNA. Some toxins can promote the growth of cancer once it develops. Detoxification, according to nutrition author C. Leigh Broadhurst, occurs as a series of biochemical reactions in the liver, intestines, and kidneys, changing harmful chemicals into relatively nontoxic chemicals for the body to excrete.

Some phytochemicals have been shown to protect against cancer by aiding detoxification reactions, indicating a high intake of plant foods as a good hedge against cancer. Some herbs that assist the liver, as well as other eliminative organs, are the hepatic bitter herbs, such as dandelion, burdock, and celandine, all of which have shown to be tumor fighters. Instead of cursing dandelion's wild prolific growth on our lawns, we might consider actually eating it!

Milk thistle is another herb with tremendous cleansing abilities. An extract of the seeds of milk thistle has been shown to be conclusively liver protective even against one of the most virulent liver toxins known, the death cap mushroom. Pretreatment of animals with milk thistle demonstrated 100 percent protection against this poison. Milk thistle has also been shown to help regenerate liver tissue and increase the production of glutathione, which is essential for the cell to protect itself from hydrogen peroxide production.

Since the liver is the body's main detoxifying organ, it becomes directly involved in the internal cancer battle. A cancer that has spread to the liver makes cancer treatment more complicated.

C. *Excretion Organs.* The major organs of elimination in the body are the kidneys, intestines, lungs, and skin. In addition to previously mentioned herbs, the following can be added: nettles, horsetail, butternut, pectin, elder, yarrow, and boneset.

2. Immune Response

Our immune system recognizes and destroys anything foreign to the body, including cells like bacteria, microbes, foreign particles, and toxic compounds. Immune cells circulating within the blood and lymphatic systems primarily do this. The immune system is a very complicated system with parts scattered throughout our bodies. These parts range from our skin, which is the largest component, to the cellular level of white blood cells.

Through advances in cancer research, scientists believe there are more than 100 million immune cells whose response is governed by several different types of white blood cells. Normally, foreign substances (pathogens) such as viruses, bacteria, fungi, and protozoa activate the white blood cells to seek out and destroy them.

There is a class of herbs called adaptogens which can help the body better adapt to its environment, whether that environment is one of harmful chemicals or simply one of rapid change.

Research has shown that adaptogens work by the following:

- Supporting adrenal function to counter adverse effects of stress
- Enabling the body's cells to have access to more energy
- Helping cells to eliminate toxic byproducts of metabolism
- Providing an anabolic (building-up) effect—as in the use of adaptogens by body builders

- Helping the body to utilize oxygen more efficiently
- Enhancing and speeding the proper regulation of biorhythms

Common herbal adaptogens are echinacea, golden seal, schizandra (magnolia vine), ashwaganda, gotu-kola, wild oats, bupleurum, astragalus, fo-ti (or Ho Shou Wu), burdock, suma, and the mushroom varieties of reishi, shiitake, and maitake.

3. Preventing Cell Mutations

The dominant initial cause of cancer is the mutation of our genetic material, or DNA. Many reactive and toxic chemical compounds bond directly to DNA, damaging and altering its structure. As a cancerous cell divides, the altered DNA replicates itself, causing continuous reproduction of this "mutation error.

According to Donald R. Yance, author and clinical herbalist, "There are herbs that either increase the innate immunity and cytotoxicity of one's immune system or have direct antitumor/antineoplastic activity. The most common antitumor active principals found in plants are terpenes and alkaloids." Yance explains:

> Gene repairing is a mechanism in which plant compounds genetically alter cancerous cells to revert back to normal cells, possibly by inhibiting cell division through means of a DNA repair mechanism or by extinguishing the malignant information that can eventually kill the cancerous cell.

Such mutations can happen to the body thousands of times in the normal course of a day. Usually, the immune system of a healthy body will send its troops to destroy these mutations before they can amount to any threat. The beginning of cancer is when these mutated cells survive and are permitted to continually replicate and grow out of control. One known mechanism by which plants can genetically affect cell proliferation of preneoplastic cells is by inhibiting certain enzymes (namely, tyrosine kinase and ornithine decarboxylase) that promote cancer growth.

If your work exposes you to potential mutation agents such as solvents, dyes, pesticides, or industrial chemicals, a number of antimutagenic herbs may help reduce DNA damage. Some mutation-fighting and tumor-inhibiting herbs and vegetables are aloe vera, sundew, mistletoe, garlic, Asian/Siberian ginseng, licorice, cumin, tumeric, thyme, cruciferous vegetables (cabbage, broccoli, brussel sprouts), citrus, cloves, black pepper, green and black teas, olives, isatis, ginko biloba, eucalyptus, and onions.

4. Soothing Inflamed Tissues

The side effects of drugs and radiation can often leave tissues irritated and inflamed. Known as mucositis, this can make nutritional absorption difficult, increase infection tendency, and create general discomfort, which increases internal stress.

Here are some of the choices generally recommended for relieving irritated tissues: sage, goldenseal, raspberry leaf, slippery elm, marshmallow, Solomon's seal and licorice.

These herbs can be prepared for gargling. Make an infusion by adding several tablespoons of these soothing herbs to a cup or a cup and a half of boiling water and allowing it to cool.

In addition, author, David Simon recommends the Ayurvedic herb Neem; it is "one of the most powerful cooling herbs in the Ayruvedic pharmacy which also helps to fight infections."

5. Herbs for Digestion and Elimination

"Are you regular?" is one of the first questions an informed physician will ask regarding your bowel condition. Good appetite, even digestion, and daily elimination are traditional hallmarks of good health. Two types of herbs can offer digestive support to reestablish regularity and digestion. Bitter and pungent tastes have been used to improve digestion for thousands of years in China and India. The bitter taste stimulates saliva and triggers stomach acid to secrete. A classic bitter tonic derived from roots and underground stems of several related plants is gentian. This bitter herb is a basic ingredient for some of the alcohol bitters traditionally used to stimulate the appetite before meals. Other bitter herbs reputed to improve appetite and digestion are the following: quinine, goldenseal, neem, and aloe vera. Fresh ginger root is a pungent herb that may also benefit digestion.

Some of the aromatic herbs that can reduce nausea, in addition to ginger root, are cloves, cinnamon, and peppermint. Cinnamon or whole cloves can be sucked on to reduce nausea. These herbs are also known for their ability to dispel lethargy, congestion, and mucus.

6. Antioxidant Protection

Free radicals are highly reactive molecules that can damage cell structures by oxidizing existing polyunsaturated fats within cell membranes. This makes us more prone to liver dysfuntion and DNA mutations. The following plants are known to assist detoxification function and promote antioxidant activity: ginko, ginseng, grapeseed, hyssop, licorice, reishi, pine bark extract, schizandra, tumeric, green and black teas, mint family (peppermint, spearmint, oregano, thyme), rosemary, and garlic.

7. Calming Herbs

Some herbs which provide natural sedative qualities to take the edge off tension or mental agitation and are referred to as nervines in Western herbology. Of these herbs, valerian has historical merit along with skullcap, chamomile, hops, and passionflower.

Within the common herbs of Western herbology, Chinese herbal medicine, American Native plants, and Ayurvedic medicine, there exists an entire world of health support that is both effective and relatively economical. Plant medicine, in whole form, as opposed to standardized form, is rapidly gaining recognition as a useful adjunct to dietary and conventional therapies. However, herbal medicine, from any source, should not be a substitute for qualified medical care from your practitioner of choice.

THE ESSIAC PROMISE

From informational books to volumes of anecdotal case histories and numerous Web sites promoting the "Herbal Indian Miracle Cure," Essiac has become a cottage industry with numerous companies battling for their market share with "new," "improved," or "original" versions.

The colorful story of Essiac began in 1922, when Rene Caisse (pronounced "Reen Case"), a surgical nurse working in The Sisters of Providence Hospital in Haileybury, Ontario, came across an elderly patient with a scarred, deformed breast. The woman had come thirty years earlier from England to join her husband prospecting in northern Ontario. Sometime after her arrival, she discovered a hardened mass in her breast. An Ojibwa Indian from the area "diagnosed" her as having breast cancer and recommended a "holy drink that would purify her body and place it back in balance with the great spirit."

The woman and husband dismissed the Indian's advice as "superstition" and left for a conventional medical diagnosis in Toronto. There, she was diagnosed as having a malignancy. The physician recommendation was complete breast removal (mastectomy). Feeling frightened and short of funds for the procedure, the woman returned to northern Ontario and reconsidered the Ojibwa's offer. She was given a pleasant-tasting herbal brew, the formula, and preparation instructions. The Ojibwa instructed her to drink the concoction twice daily.

According to the woman, the breast tumors gradually dissolved. She never had a reoccurrence and was 80 years old at the time of her meeting with Rene Caisse.

Caisse asked for the recipe, thinking, "If I should ever develop cancer, I would use it."

In 1924, Caisse's aunt, Mireza Potvin, was diagnosed with advanced cancer of the stomach and was told she had six months to live. Remembering the Indian brew, Caisse asked her aunt's physician, Dr. R. O. Fisher of Toronto, for permission to try it on her dying relative. With Dr. Fisher's consent, she gathered the herbs and brewed the tea. After two months of twice daily brewings, Mireza Potvin recovered and lived for 21 more years with no reoccurrence.

Until Caisse's death at 90 in 1978, she had treated thousands of cancer patients, refusing payment for her services and accepting only voluntary contributions. She brought remissions to hundreds of documented cases, many abandoned as "hopeless" or "terminal" by conventional medicine, and aided countless others in prolonging life and relieving pain. Her results were obtained against a variety of cancers, treating patients orally or through hypodermic injection.

Considering that herbs contain many proteins and impurities that can easily cause fatal allergic reactions if injected, Caisse was hesitant to use this method. She and Dr. Fisher worked for nearly two years to discover what ingredients could be given hypodermically without adverse reaction.

WHAT'S IN ESSIAC?

Caisse named the basic herbal healing tea Essiac—her last name in reverse.

The principal herbs in Essiac are burdock root, turkey rhubarb root (Indian rhubarb), sheep sorrel, and slipperly elm bark. Many of these ingredients today have been documented as having strong antitumor activity as well as immune-stimulating effects.

Caisse theorized that one of the herbs in Essiac reduced tumor growth while other herbs acted as blood purifiers, carrying away destroyed tissue as well as infections related to the malignancy. She also speculated that Essiac strengthened the body's innate defense mechanisms, enabling normal cells to destroy abnormal ones as "nature intended."

Essiac came within three votes of being legalized as an adjunctive cancer treatment by the Canadian parliament in 1938. Throughout the years, Caisse was in and out of court, being challenged on the legitimacy of her claims. People rallied to her cause, petitions with 17,000 names were presented to support her, and a dramatic political struggle developed that divided numerous medical professionals, organizations, and provincial governments.

Today, Essiac is widely available as a powdered tea or in herbal brewing packages from most natural food retail outlets.

HARRY HOXSEY'S SECRET

Single-handedly, Harry Hoxsey, a larger-than-life character with a fast-talking penchant for flamboyant self-promotion, initiated one of the most controversial cancer battles of the twentieth century, fiercely defending his family's herbal formula as a cure for cancer.

For over thirty-five years, Harry Hoxsey, high-school dropout, ex-coal miner with no medical training whatsoever, treated cancer patients, including the "terminally ill," with herbal-mineral formulas, which he claimed had been passed down through his family from his great grandfather. By the 1950s, the Hoxsey Cancer Clinic in Dallas was the world's largest private cancer center with branches in seventeen states that treated thousands of individuals with cancer.

Throughout his later life, Hoxsey faced relentless opposition and harassment from a hostile medical establishment. Despite this, two federal courts upheld the "therapeutic value" of Hoxsey's herbal-mineral tonic. Hoxsey's herbal formula changed slightly over the years; however, its base of red clover, cascara, poke, and burdock remained the same. Here is the current version of the Hoxsey formula:

Licorice root, red clover blossoms, cascara bark, burkdock root, barberry root, fresh poke root, and fresh stillingia root.

Note: The Hoxsey formula should only be used under an experienced physician's direction.

There are many versions of the Hoxsey formula available throughout the world along with his salves. Some of the formula's ingredients have shown to have antitumor characteristics and immune-stimulating qualities.

Hoxsey's protocols are still practiced at the Bio-Medical Center of Tijuana, located across the San Diego border in Baja California, Mexico.

HEALING UNDER THE MISTLETOE

Mistletoe (viscum album, or *Mistel* in German) is a semi-parasitic plant that was held sacred by Germanic tribes, Druid priests, and the Celts. It has been used medicinally for several hundred years. An extract of European mistletoe was first extracted in 1920 and is called Iscador.

Famed intellectual figure and founder of Anthroposophy, a spiritual philosophy and movement, Rudolf Steiner (1861–1925) first proposed mistletoe as a cancer "remedy"—basing his hunch on an analysis of the plant's unusual characteristics. He suggested mistletoe as a treatment for uterine and breast cancer prior to World War I. In 1917, he encouraged Zurich medical doctor Dr. Ita Wegman (1876–1943) to investigate mistletoe as a treatment for cancer.

MAGICAL MISTLETOE

According to legend, the Druids considered the mistletoe to be a sacred plant, believing it contained miraculous regenerative properties that could cure illness, serve as an antidote against poisons, ensure fertility, and protect against the negative effects of witchcraft. Whenever enemies met under the mistletoe in the forest, they had to lay down their arms and observe a truce until the next day. From this came the ancient custom of hanging a branch of mistletoe from archways to ensure reconciliation, represent good will, serve as an act of atonement, serve as a mystical ornament that could cause two people to fall in love, or bless their union.

After Steiner's death in 1925, Dr. Wegman published *Fundamentals of Therapy,* her book based on their work together. From her collaboration with famed Zurich pharmacist A. Hauser, and later with additional refinement by N. Kaelin and Drs. Alexandre Leroi and his wife, Rita, the first commercial preparation of mistletoe was created and called Iscador.

Numerous studies have demonstrated that mistletoe extract stimulates immune cells to inhibit tumor growth. Mistletoe stimulates the thymus, the body's main immune cell regulator, causing an increase in the scavenger white blood cells that consume invading foreign matter, which destroys other cells. Iscador has also been shown to increase the number of immune cells, activating the natural killer cells that specifically destroy tumor cells.

Extracts of mistletoe contain biologically active proteins called lectins and other substances that have demonstrated forceful antitumor activity in animal and cell-culture experiments. Iscador therapy is usually used as an adjunctive cancer therapy in tandem with conventional therapy, as well as by itself. It has shown to slow tumor growth, occasionally regress tumors, and in some cases cause remission.

Since its early use, Iscador has proven to be generally free of side effects, save for temporary fevers, headaches, chills, and, in some cases, mild inflammation at the injection site. Cancer patients under Iscador treatment have shown reduced pain, fatigue, and depression with improved sleep, appetite, and weight gain. Some patients have shown an increase of hemoglobin and red-blood cell levels. While Iscador has not resulted in dramatic remission, it has demonstrated an improvement in quality of life and a capacity to extend life.

According to Dr. Rita Leroi, a supervisor for many years at the Lukas Klinik in Switzerland, the best responders to Iscador are carcinomas of the bladder, genitals, and digestive tract, and also melanomas. At the Lukas Klinik, Iscador is an integral part of the recovery program, which also includes diet, herbs, and art, music, and movement therapies.

When Iscador is used with chemotherapy, hormone therapy, or radiation, it has relieved common undesirable side effects.

ANTICIPATING AN HERBAL BREAKTHROUGH

There are dozens of herbs known to increase immunity, inhibit tumor growth, and improve overall vitality that warrant continued scientific research. While much of this research occurs in Europe or Asia, it is still considered "fringe" by most American scientists. The positive attributes of phytomedicine present an exciting host of possibilities as adjunctive therapy, and in some cases, as possible solo therapies. Eventually, research will bear this out.

The growth of bone metastases is often decelerated with Iscador. It has also been used to treat cancers of the bone marrow, connective tissue, and blood-forming organs, specifically lymphomas, sarcomas, and leukemias, although it is less effective with these cancers than with solid carcinomas. Leukemia does not usually respond well to mistletoe therapy.

A study in 1990 found that in human cell cultures, mistletoe lectins increased the production of tumor necrosis factor-alpha, a hormone secreted by immune cells that destroys cancer tissue. This lectin also increased interleukin-1 and interlukin-6, both essential mediators of immune response.

Mistletoe can be extremely toxic; the American Herbal Products Association recommends a number of restrictions on its use. It is contraindicated in protein hypersensitivity and in advanced progressive infections such as AIDS and tuberculosis.

Despite the lack of toxic symptoms from many taking mistletoe tea, a standard textbook recommendation advises against self-administering. To avoid microbial contamination, Iscador is carefully filtered and processed to eliminate bacteria. The Swiss International Office for Drug Control routinely conducts testing of all Iscador products.

MEDICINAL MUSHROOMS—"THINGS GO BETTER WITH FUNGUS"

The first antibiotics were extracted and synthesized from fungi (mushrooms), molds, and yeasts. Penicillin, tetracyclene, and aureomycin, all derived from molds, were hailed as wonder drugs for communicable diseases and infections.

The word *antibiotic* is a compound of *anti* (against) and *bios* (life). Literally, it means "against life." This definition is appropriate since antibiotics are substances that interfere with the life cycle of invading bacteria. Unfortunately, antibiotics equally eliminates some of the "good" bacteria that reside in our body. This is one of many reasons why nutritional research is seeking more effective ways to fortify and stimulate the body's natural immunity as a disease-combating mechanism.

In 1928, Sir Alexander Fleming discovered that an accidental contaminant was killing off a culture of microorganisms. The contaminant was named *Penicillium notatum*. Remaining a lab oddity until the early 1940s, it was the pressures of World War II that reminded researchers of this incident. As a result of further investigation and experimentation, penicillin, as a medicine, was born.

It was hardly a new concept that molds could be used to combat infection. A number of traditional folk medicines utilized moldy bread, fermented soybean paste, and other materials applied to wounds that could potentially become infected.

While Western conventional and modern Asian medicine both continue developing antibiotics, Asian medicine, due to its unifying philosophy of relating to disease as a condition of physical and energetic imbalance, attempts to remedy imbalance through natural means. It has excelled in developing natural medicines to stimulate human immune function.

Mushrooms have a long history in traditional Chinese medicine. Their legendary positive effects on health promotion have been well documented by recent studies. The studies similarly conclude that mushrooms are probiotic—they help the body increase its resistance to disease. Many of the compounds within their cell structures have been classified as host defenses potentiators (HDPs). This is a primary reason for their use as adjunctive cancer treatments throughout the Orient, especially for counteracting the toxic effects of radiation and chemotherapy.

Naturally containing a high percentage of a difficult-to-digest polysaccharide called chitin, mushrooms must be cooked

POLYSACCHARIDES TO THE RESCUE

Polysaccharides (*poly* = many, *saccharides* = sugar) are the natural complex sugars of plant origin that have proved therapeutic on human immunity. While they are found extensively in grains, beans, vegetables, and many herbs, such as astragalus and echinacea, high levels of polysaccharides have also been discovered in many medicinal mushrooms. In China, Japan, Russia, and America, several unique polysaccharide antitumor agents have been developed from the fruiting body, myucelia, and culture medium of different medicinal mushrooms. It has been suggested that because polysaccharides are similar in size and weight to bacteria, they can stimulate an immune response. Some of their natural properties include the following:

- Antibiotic action
- Antiviral quality
- Lowering of blood pressure
- High blood fat reduction
- Antitumor activity

The anticancer properties of fungi polysaccharides are due to

- Inhibiting cancer growth
- T-cell stimulation and natural killer cells
- Increasing interleukin-1 production (a lymphocyte activator)
- Increasing immune ability of white blood cells

Because of these factors, mushrooms have been used successfully in the treatment of infections, flu, diabetes, heart conditions, and immune-related problems.

in order for the cell walls to release their nutrients. Another reason for cooking Shiitake (as well as common white mushrooms) is a chemical substance called agaritin, which may be carcinogenic unless neutralized through cooking.

The many compounds found in the varieties of Shiitake, Reishi, PSK, and Maitake are classified as HDP. Some of these compounds include hemicellulose, polysaccharide-peptides, nucleosides, triterpeniods, complex starches, and other metabolites. It has been shown that combinations of these products target the human immunity, while additionally aiding in neuron transmission, metabolism, hormonal balance, and the vital transport of oxygen and nutrients. Through a host-mediated (T-cell) immune mechanism, they help the body regulate lymphoid stem cell development and other important defense responses.

It is estimated that more than 100,000 species of fungi exist. While they are considered plants, their common characteristic is an absence of chlorophyll.

An extensive mushroom directory in Japan lists up to 1500 mushroom varieties, of which 700 are considered culinary. The "poisonous" varieties only amount to 50 species. Additionally, over 50 species are confirmed to have medicinal health-promoting properties.

This section will briefly detail four popular medicinal mushrooms: Shiitake, Reishi, PSK, and Maitake.

Shiitake—The Forest Mushroom

The Shiitake (pronounced she-tah-key) mushroom (*Lentinus endoles*), one of the most widely cultivated specialty species in the world, is both a prized medicine as well as a culinary favorite. Currently, Shiitake mushrooms are one of the most popular protein sources in Japan, as well as a major staple in China and throughout the Pacific Rim. Annual production of Shiitake is well over 200,000 tons, just second to America's favored white mushroom species. Shiitake is identified as a broad, dark-brown mushroom commonly grown on a number of trees that include the beech, chestnut, Japanese alder, maple, and walnut. Shiitake mushrooms are usually cultivated in the United States and not found in wild clusters.

Shiitake is a valuable source of carbohydrates (67 percent) and numerous fatty acids, particularly linoleic acid. Shiitake contains many enzymes and vitamins that do not appear in plants. It contains all eight essential amino acids in better proportions than soy beans, meat, milk, or eggs, Shiitake is a healthy source of vitamins B_1, B_2, B_{12}, niacin, pantothenic acid, and vitamin D, as well as calcium. Its cap contains higher amounts of nutrients than its stem.

The most active chemical component of Shiitake is lentinan. Lentinan, approved as a drug in Japan, is generally administered by injection to prolong survival of patients in conventional cancer therapy as well as in AIDS research. Lentinan is not only useful for cancer treatment, but is thought to prevent the increase of chromosomal damage resulting from anticancer drugs. Analysis has determined that lentinan, the principle active component of the shiitake, is a complex immunopotentiating polysaccharide referred to as beta 1,3-glucan, found in other medicinal mushrooms as well.

Lentinan's antitumor effects were first isolated and studied by the National Cancer Institute in Japan in 1969. Since that time, many studies have not only confirmed antitumor benefits, but a wide range of protective factors, such as improved host resistance to bacterial, viral, and parasitic infections, immune-regulating effects, liver-protective benefits, and positive cardiovascular effects.

Lentinan also inhibits metastasis, prevents chemical and viral oncogenesis (tumor growth), and has minimal side effects. The antiviral effects of Shiitake are attributed to its ability to

SHIITAKE VERSUS CHOLESTEROL

Japanese researchers have reported that consumption of Shiitake mushrooms lower blood cholesterol by as much as 45 percent. The active component responsible was found to be eritadenine, an alkaloid with extremely low toxicity, which lowered not only serum cholesterol but also phospholipids and triglycerides. However, the most dramatic results occurred when high-cholesterol foods were eaten simultaneously with Shiitake. In two human studies, cholesterol dropped 6 to 15 percent when the amount of Shiitake consumed was 9 grams per day, or approximately 10 dried medium-sized mushrooms.

Shiitake has a unique taste that goes well with soup, in any fat-containing dish (stir-fry, animal protein preparation), or with vegetables. A popular dish to increase fat-dissolving potential is to combine shiitake with onions. See the recipe section (Chapter 12) for some delicious and healthy shiitake sauces and soups.

produce interferon. It has also been shown to inhibit sarcoma growth in mice. Additionally, follow-up studies on patients with advanced and recurrent stomach and colon/rectal cancers have shown excellent results in using lentinan as a part of combination therapy.

Reishi—"Elixir of Immortality"

Reshi (pronounced "re-she") was introduced into diet and medicine by Asian herbal practitioners over 2000 years ago. In China, it is known as *ling chic,* or *ling qi*. Emperor Shih Huang To (259–210 B.C.), known for his Great Wall, is reputed to have dispatched an entire fleet of ships manned by 3000 young people to search for a mushroom called the "Elixir of Immortality." That mushroom was thought to be Reishi (*Ganoderma lucidum*).

Listed as a superior medicine in Japanese medical text *Shinnoh Honsohkyo,* Reishi is considered to be one of "God's herbs." Its special chemical make-up was considered a tonic for longevity or eternal life.

Reishi mushrooms are of polypore variety. Much like the apple is the fruit of an apple tree, mushrooms are the fruit body and reproductive structure of a higher-order fungus organism. The actual mushroom "tree" is a fine threadlike network called mycelium. For the most part, this mycelium is subterranean, living in soil, logs, and other forms of organic liter. Where green plants produce most of their own nutrients by photosynthesis, mushrooms get their primary nutrition from dead organic matter, or soil. Mushrooms and their mycelium are nature's original recyclers. Without them, the planet surface would be piled high with dead, decaying material.

From the mycelium, when the proper nutrients are absorbed and necessary environmental conditions are present, mushrooms blossom. At maturity, they release spores that the wind spreads. The spores land and the cycle begins over again.

In traditional Chinese medicine, Reishi is considered to be the highest class of tonics. Along with Shiitake mushroom, Reishi is one of the most widely consumed therapeutic mushrooms in the world. Within the Reishi family, six different varieties have been discovered. Each has unique medicinal characteristics and benefits, depending on the color of its cap—blue, red, yellow, white, black, or purple. Among the six types, red-colored Reishi is usually regarded as the most potent for medicinal purposes.

Due to their woody and hard texture, Reishi mushrooms are typically blended into a tea or tincture. In the West, Reishi can be found growing on oak trees, whereas in Japan, most Reishi are found on older Japanese plum trees.

The Reishi mushroom has traditionally been used in Chinese medicine for asthenia-type syndromes, characterized by a deficiency of vital energy and functions of the lower body. It is considered the perfect antidote for the typical American overwhelmed by constant stress. It has also been used successfully to minimize the toxicities of chemotherapy.

Reishi enhances white blood cell count (immune cells), platelets, hemoglobin, and various tumor-fighting cells. The potency of Reishi is partially based on its level of triterpenopids, which can be estimated by taste—increased bitterness means a higher level of triterpenoids. In general, Chinese medicine recommends that the average dose be from 3 to 5 grams daily.

Other applications for Reishi include skin beautification (attributed to its hormone-potentiating effects); as an ingredient in hair-loss formulas; for treating a form of arthritis known as lupus, allergies (by inhibiting the release of histamines), and coronary heart disease; and for regulating blood pressure.

A study at Cornell Medical College found that Reishi reduced side-effects during chemotherapy, prolonged survival, and minimized metastasis, while improving quality of life and in some cases preventing recurrence. Antitumor activity has been demonstrated in vitro as well as in tumor systems in animals. There is abundant in vitro and indirect clinical evidence to support its supplemental use in cancer.

Reishi also has a high germanium content, which some studies suggest contain antitumor activity. Germanium is said to neutralize pain during the final stages of cancer.

CHAPTER 8

THE NUMEROUS BENEFITS OF REISHI

Reishi's featured organic compounds of several ganodermic acids, classified as triterpenopids and a number of polysaccharides, are thought to be responsible for its benefits. Current studies have indicated that Reishi contains beneficial components that can work in a wide variety of ways:

* Antihypertensive
* Antiplatelet coagulation
* Antioxidant benefits
* Increases interleukin-1 and -2
* Liver detoxification/protection
* Analgesic
* Antiallergy
* Antibacterial
* Cardiotonic
* Increases white blood cells/hematoglobin
* Enhances natural killer cell activity
* Reduces caffeine effects by relaxing muscles

* Antitumor
* Anti-inflammatory
* Immunopotentiation
* Antiviral
* Antiulcer
* Expectorant
* Improves adrenal function
* Bronchitis preventive
* Enhances bone marrow
* Protects against ionizing radiation
* Anti-HIV

Christopher Hobbs, third generation herbalist and prolific author, recommends a traditional strengthening soup made from Reishi for one to two weeks or a period of up to six months.

* *Wei Chi (Protective vitality) Soup*
  Simmer for 30 minutes in 6 quarts of water:
  1 ounce of dried Reishi
  3 ounces of fresh Shiitake (or 1 oz. dried)
  1 ounce of Astragalus (optional)

  Add:
  ¼ cup of organic barley and a variety of slices or chopped organic vegetables (carrots, onions, and cabbage). Simmer for another 30 minutes, adding a quarter cup of sea vegetables (*wakame*) or to taste.

William H. Lee and Joan A. Friedrich recommend the following Reishi tea:

- *Popular Reishi Tea*
  1 teaspoon chopped reishi mushrooms
  5–10 thin slices fresh ginger root
  1 cup water
  Combine all ingredients in a saucepan and bring to a boil. Simmer for approximately 10 minutes. Makes one cup. Strain and drink at warm temperature. Good tea for multihealth purposes.

PSK—"Cloud Fungus"

PSK (*coriolus versicolor*), also known as "Turkey Tail," is an approved Japanese anticancer drug with 20 years of research behind it. In Japan, PSK accounts for hundreds of millions of dollars worth of sales each year. Based on Japanese sales alone, it is the number-one selling anticancer agent in the world.

There have been nearly 400 studies done on the safety and effectiveness of PSK. Some show increased survival rates and improved quality of life without toxic side effects from conventional therapies.

PSK shows great promise for other diseases, including herpes, hepatitis, systemic lupus, AIDS, rheumatoid arthritis, and many other viral, fungal, and bacterial conditions. It is also noted that PSK causes smooth muscle relaxation, making it especially helpful for treating chronic coughs, asthma, and other bronchial conditions.

PSK is the subject of several large, randomized, double-blind clinical trials with hundreds of patients running as long as seven years and showing up to two- to threefold survival benefits versus controls. For example, PSK plus radiation yielded 22 percent 5-year survival for stage III non-small-cell lung cancer versus 5 percent 5-year survival for those patients receiving radiation alone. In another phase III study, oral ingestion of PSK after complete surgery for colon cancer yielded a 30 percent disease-free survival versus 10 percent for the control group.

PSK stimulates both T-killer lymphocytes and macrophages, which are the primary white blood cells responsible for dissolving tumors. It stimulates not only the number of macrophages, but the motility of macrophages to the tumor, at the same time inhibiting the tumor cell's motility.

PSK has also been used successfully with chemotherapy to produce remissions and extend survival time in cases of leukemia. The vast majority of *Coriolus* (approximately 70 percent) is excreted through the lungs, which makes it very effective when kidney or liver function is impaired.

Both PSK and lentinan (Shiitake mushroom derivative) have demonstrated benefit to colon and cancer patients in controlled clinical trials; however, PSK has the strong advantage in that it may be taken orally, while lentinan is normally given via injection.

As an arsenal against cancer, PSK is frequently combined with other mushroom extracts, such as Maitake D-fraction. PSK does not seem to have enjoyed the "hype" associated with other alternative therapies, but it does have one very strong advantage to its credibility—the extensive documented results published in mainstream medical journals.

PSK is generally available in tea or capsules.

Maitake—"The Dancing Mushroom"

"We have been involved in research on medicinal properties of edible mushrooms for the last 15 years and have reported that, of all medicinal mushrooms studied, Maitake mushroom (Grifola frondosa) has the strongest antitumor activity in tumor growth inhibition both when administered orally and intraperitoneally. In fact, most of the other mushroom extracts are reported ineffective when given orally."

—Department of Microbial Chemistry, Kobe, Japan Pharmaceutical University

WHAT'S IN A NAME?

Maitake (pronounced my-tah-key) comes from the common name of a fungus found in Italy. The name refers to a mythical beast, which is half-lion and half-eagle. Maitake has come to be known as "the dancing mushroom." There are several possible reasons for this nickname.

Some say the name is associated with Maitake's shape, which resembles a "dancing nymph." Others say it is so named because of its rippling form with no caps and its bent for growing in clusters, presenting the image of a dancing butterfly. Traditionally, another reason is given for this name: In ancient times people who found the mushroom danced with joy since its prized worth would allow the finder to exchange its weight for silver.

Maitake, also known as "hen of the woods," has a colorful history—collectors in Japan traditionally guarded their hunting grounds with hatch marks on trees bordering the trove and keeping others, often by forcible means, out of the marked areas. Maitake hunters have been known to forage alone and rarely divulge the location of their treasure—even to their own family. Until cultivation techniques were developed in 1979, Maitake was only available as a wild harvested mushroom.

In 1990, Japanese cultivators produced nearly 8000 tons of Maitake, and since then production and worldwide distribution have increased tremendously as awareness of its healing potential becomes known. When matured, the Maitake mushroom can weigh as much as 20 pounds, offering a visual feast, with its flower-shaped clusters often growing to the size of a basketball. Its large and fleshy clusters are dark gray-brown and lighter gray and often yellowish as it ages.

In Chinese medicine, Maitake is called "Keisho." Shen Nong's scripture of herbal medicine (*Shen Nong Ben Cao Jine*) states that Maitake has been used for improving spleen, pancreas, and stomach aliments, calming nerves and relaxing the mind, and treating hemorrhoids.

MUSHROOMS AND IMMUNITY

The following chart illustrates immunity benefits from the four types of mushrooms discussed in this section.

Mushroom Variety	Compound	Compound Type	Immune Effects
• Shiitake	Lentinan Beta-glucans	Polysaccharide Stranded DNA Triterpenes	Stimulates T-helper cells, natural killer-cells, and macrophages, antitumor, adaptogenic
• Reishi	Ganodermic Beta-glucans	Triterpenes Ganoderma polysaccharide (GPS) Triterpenes	Antitumor, immuno-stimulant, adaptogenic
• Cloud Fungus	PSK Beta-glucans	Polysaccharides Triterpenes	Immune enhancer, antioxidant, antiviral, antitumor, adaptogenic
• Maitake	Beta-glucans	Polysaccdarides Triterpenes	Antitumor, adaptogenic, immunostimulant

Although Maitake is a relatively "new kid on the block" and may not have thousands of years of medicinal folklore experience behind it, as Reishi and Shiitake do, a rapidly growing body of scientific research supports its effectiveness as an immune system enhancer. It is also reported to have anticancer properties and has proven effective in treating diabetes, high blood pressure, bacterial and yeast infections, and HIV/AIDS.

Fresh Maitake (fruiting body) at harvest contains 91 percent moisture, 3.4 unsaturated fatty acids, a valuable source of vegetable protein, organic acids (including 47–50 percent malic acid) polysaccharides, niacin, phospholipids, vitamins B_1 and B_2, and ergosterol—provitamin D). It has neither vitamin A nor C and small quantities of minerals.

Chemically, Maitake also contains powerful active polysaccharides, especially the immuno-enhancing beta-D-glucans. Recent studies have documented that a particular Maitake extraction process called D-fraction provided increased immune protection by

- Triggering cellular immunity
- Stopping normal cells from carcinogenesis
- Inhibiting tumor growth
- Preventing metastasis of tumor cells
- Reducing side effects when administered with chemo-therapy

Maitake's extract does not directly kill cancer cells, but activates the individual's immunity to increase the body's self-healing power. In animal observational studies, it was noted that D-fraction alone demonstrated superior tumor-growth inhibition to that of mitomycin (MMC), a popular antibiotic drug used in cancer treatments in Japan and the United States. When D-fraction and MMC were given together, with each dose cut in half, tumor inhibition was further enhanced by

HEALTH BENEFITS OF MUSHROOMS

Here's a quick look at the health benefits of each of the four mushroom types discussed in this section.

Mushroom Uses	Shiitake	Reishi	PSK	Maitake
Antiviral	*	*	*	
Antitumor	*	*	*	*
Immune enhancer	*	*	*	*
Anti-inflammatory		*		
Blood pressure	*	*	*	*
Cardiovascular	*	*	*	
Cholesterol lowering	*	*	*	
Libido enhancing	*		*	
Kidney tonic		*	*	
Asthma-bronchial		*	*	
Stress reduction		*	*	
Diabetes				*
Liver; hepatitis	*	*	*	*
Chitin	*	*	*	*

nearly 98 percent. Maitake's anti-HIV activity was also confirmed by both the Japan National Institute of Health and the U.S. National Cancer Institute in 1992.

Maitake is said to be the tastiest of mushrooms and a Japanese favorite. Numerous cooking styles suit Maitake's uniqueness. It can be roasted, served with radish or vinegar, included in soups (popularly, miso soup), and made into sauces, stews, and fried dishes.

Currently, extensive clinical trials of Maitake's effectiveness in cancer treatment are being conducted at various cancer treatment institutes in the United States.

A representative I spoke with from one of Maitake's distributors suggests that individuals seeking maximum immune enhancement take the D-fraction powder form in capsule as well as the D-fraction extract together on a daily basis.

9
HEALTH SUPPORTIVE SUPPLEMENT STRATEGIES

OF CAPSULES, PILLS, AND POTIONS

Pick up any general-interest newsstand magazine and you'll see numerous advertisements hyping miracle potions that promise everything from reversing cancer to restoring hair growth and improving intelligence. Since 1994, when Congress deregulated the Food and Drug Administration's control of nutritional supplements claims, there's been a virtual explosion of "health-enhancing" megavitamins, magic pills, and cure-all potions guaranteed to relieve pain, deepen sleep, and boost virility.

The supplement industry, a $6+ billion-dollar-a-year business, is sustained by over 25 percent of the American population, who confidently take supplements. While a small percentage rely on daily usage of supplements, seventy percent of this amount use nutritional supplements on an "occasional" basis, while one in three people with chronic disease rely on herbal remedies for help.

Do we need supplements? Can they really work as promised? Are they safe?

The answers to these questions are widely debated and not always precise. Even within medical circles, as pro and con research is reported almost daily, there are very clear divisions between supporters and detractors.

Despite the growing evidence of the benefits of supplements, very little has filtered down to the rank and file. The average physician still regards food and nutritional supplements with suspicion and doubt, or considers the supplement issue merely as adjunctive therapy to the "fundamental" or "real" treatment—drugs and surgery. However, new research has opened the door a bit wider, and many physicians now concede that pregnant women need folic acid, which has been proven to prevent spina bifida. Still, few obstetricians have made the necessary connection that nutritional supplements may prevent many other birth defects as well.

This chapter will address new research and examine conventional, alternative, and traditional folk medicine perspectives on supplements. Basic recommendations will be offered and, in the second half of this chapter, a supplement-repairing protocol will be detailed for minimizing the negative effects of chemotherapy and radiation therapy. Before undertaking a supplement regime, it is imperative that you check with a qualified health practitioner regarding possible harmful drug–supplement interactions and with a qualified nutritionist for supplement updates, brands, and dosages tailored to your own particular condition.

VITAMIN ORIGINS

As far back as 3500 years ago, ancient Egyptians recognized that night blindness (attributed to a lack of vitamin A) could be treated with specific foods. The folk medicines of many cultures often included herbs and food combinations as remedies for certain ailments.

During the late nineteenth century, it was discovered that the substitution of unpolished for polished rice, in a rice-based diet, could prevent a disease called beriberi.

In 1906, the British biochemist Frederick Hopkins, discovered that foods naturally contained what he called "necessary accessory factors" in addition to the macronutrients of carbohydrates, fats, and protein, along with minerals and water. In 1911, Polish chemist, Casimir Funk discovered that the anti-beriberi substance in unpolished rice was an amine (a nitrogen-containing compound). Funk named it vitamine—for "vital amine." Soon, this term was applied to all accessory nutritional factors. When it was later discovered that many vitamins do not have nitrogen-containing amines, the final letter *e* was dropped.

By 1912, scientists Hopkins and Funk advanced their theory of vitamin deficiency, explaining that physical deficiencies of certain vitamins were connected to specific diseases. This was a major finding, prompting industrious animal experiments

PUTTING THE LIME IN LIMEYS

In 1747, a major milestone occurred in nutritional medicine when the Scottish naval surgeon James Lind, discovered that an unknown nutrient in citrus foods prevented a common disease called scurvy, whose symptoms included spontaneous bleeding, loose teeth, pain, brittle bones, and fatigue. Scurvy was often deadly and claimed more British sailors than war casualties. Lind's experiment, one of the first controlled nutritional studies involving human subjects, provided unprecedented evidence of the curative value of oranges and lemons.

Scurvy, recognized from ancient times as a serious disease, was often a deadly problem when fresh fruits and vegetables were unavailable during harsh winters or during long ocean voyages. Sailors were especially vulnerable to this wasting illness which afflicted them because the only food given them on these long voyages was hardtack biscuits and salted meats.

The disease is characterized by frequent hemorrhaging of capillaries in the skin to produce blood spots and structural weakness of cartilage and bone. In the mid-eighteenth century it became clear that simple additions of vegetables and fresh fruit, particularly limes and oranges, would prevent scurvy. This was the reason that British sailors were nicknamed "limeys." It took until 1928, when chemistry had become more advanced, for a researcher to identify the "scurvy-curing" substance as vitamin C.

throughout the early 1900s in which scientists succeeded in isolating and identifying many of the numerous vitamins recognized today.

In 1939, Nobel laureate Albert Szent-Gyorgyi, M.D., Ph.D., who had discovered vitamin C and the flavinoids, gave a series of lectures at Vanderbilt University Medical School. He claimed that it would be impossible to predict how many more vitamins would be discovered and proposed that there be a minimum and optimum dose for different nutrients.

Around the same time, Dr. Evan Shute, along with colleagues, began using large optimal doses of vitamin E to treat patients with a variety of cardiovascular diseases. Dr. Frederick R. Klenner began to successfully treat several different viral diseases (including polio) with large doses of vitamin C. By 1952, Dr. Abram Hoffer had begun treating schizophrenics with vitamins C and B_3. This was the start of an exciting new perspective and attitude about the use of vitamins in supporting health and preventing sickness.

During 1945, Linus Pauling, Ph.D., developed the concept of "molecular disease" and established a new basis for modern molecular biology. Pauling observed that aging occurs within the 60 trillion cells of the body due to functional breakdown, resulting in subsequent disease development.

The coup de grace occurred in 1954 when Denham Harman, M.D., Ph.D., conceived the free radical theory of aging, an idea that medicine is just now beginning to embrace. Harman's idea was clear and uncomplicated: Molecules with an unbalanced pair of electrons (free radicals) can damage DNA structure and other cell components, stimulating the aging process. Harman also discovered that antioxidant nutrients, such as vitamins C and E, had the power to neutralize free radical factors.

Nearly two years later, Roger Williams, Ph.D, published his theory of biochemical and nutritional individuality, which was based on extensive biochemical data and generic research. William's primary argument was that individuals varied widely in their nutritional needs. He felt that the minimum daily requirement (MDR) and recommended dietary allowance (RDA) were vain attempts to create unrealistic statistical norms. Williams proposed striving for "optimal nutrition" values—nutrient dosages far above the RDA recommendations.

Today, nutritional medicine is divided in its position concerning human nutrient requirements. It is plainly evident that free radicals damage DNA and that this can lead to premature aging and diseases such as cancer, heart disease, arthritis, and Alzheimer's. Research has shown that vitamins can protect against DNA damage and that amino acids and B vitamins are necessary for the repair and synthesis of DNA. However, while one side proposes optimal nutrition, the other claims that adequate nutrition is available from "a balanced diet." Exactly what constitutes a balanced diet is still a hotly debated issue.

While many researchers claim that supplements offer much needed insurance against deficient soil quality, poor diet, and modern everyday stresses, another fraction claims whole foods from organic sources can prevent and treat deficiencies. As the industry's advertising cry of "nutritional deficiency" rallies substantial weight for the supplement argument, the true problem might be more a matter of excess: an *excess* of macronutrients (too much simple carbohydrate, fats, and protein); an *excess* of overall dietary acidity; an *excess* of inactivity; and an *excess* of stress, both physical and emotional.

Clearly, good health first requires dietary and lifestyle restructuring. Supplements, by their very name, should supplement our health without creating dependency and be used in an alternating manner, as opposed to every day. Go vitamin-free on weekends, or take supplements for on-off periods of 10 days on, 5 days off. This keeps the body in a state of change and free from dependence on supplements.

From a more traditional perspective, macrobiotic educator Michio Kushi suggests that supplement use be examined in a more sociological light, explaining that if "true health is universal it should be available to all and not only those who can afford expensive preparations and formulas." Kushi suggests that this be accomplished with particular detail to food percentages, believing that carefully balanced, consistent eating of complex carbohydrates (grains, vegetables, sea vegetables and beans), chiefly derived from plant sources, are best suited for the design of our digestive systems and our good health.

However, until that ideal time when we can reestablish health and energy by eating in a balanced way, moderate use of supplements to support our diets—especially for conditions where individuals are physically challenged by sickness or weakness—may be a valid interim solution.

WHO CAN BENEFIT FROM SUPPLEMENTS?

People falling into the following categories may require supplementation to maximize health and disease prevention:

- **The Elderly**

  With a population of more than 25 million and continuously growing, individuals over 65 may need supplement support for their diets. Nutritional problems affecting this group may be due to reduced caloric intake, inadequate absorption, poor dentition, medication/nutrient interactions, lack of exercise or physical handicap, loneliness, or any combination of these factors. Deficiencies identified for this group include calcium, the B group (vitamin B_6, thiamine, folate, riboflavin, niacin), vitamin C, and vitamin D.

- **Chronic Illness**

  In the United States approximately 32 million people are chronically ill, a position where inadequate nutrition puts them at risk for further debilitation. Equally alarming is that over one million new patients develop some type of cancer each year. Diseases of the liver, gall bladder, intestine, or pancreas or previous digestive surgery may interfere with digestion and nutrient absorption. Problems of assimilation or malnutrition can impair immune function.

- **Surgery: Pre- and Postoperative Care**

  For the 24 million patients undergoing surgery annually, it is well known that operative trauma compromises nutrition. Operations may also interfere with digestion, ingestion, and food absorption. Taking specific nutrients (exceeding the RDA) prior to and after surgery ensures stronger immunity, faster recovery, and a better mineral profile, often diminshed by the use of medication at the time of surgery.

- **During Weight Loss Regimes**

  An estimated 40–50 million Americans go on and off dieting regimes at any given time. Strict weight-loss regimes of less than 1400 calories a day, make meeting adequate vitamin and mineral requirements more difficult. Vitamin needs remain the same despite changing caloric intake, even during periods of total fasting. Another risk factor may be the continued use of high-protein diets, which for prolonged periods can create an excess of the various acids that compromise mineral balance.

- **Pregnancy and Nursing**

  The diet of many American women, when examined, reveals only marginal intakes of vitamin A, vitamin C, vitamin B6, calcium, iron, and magnesium. Pregnant and lactating women usually require nutritional support beyond the standard RDA. In even normal pregnancies, during the time of delivery, 25 percent of mothers were observed to have had a deficiency in at least one essential element.

- **Smoking**

  There are over 55 million tobacco smokers in the United States. Studies have confirmed that the vitamin C plasma level in heavy smokers can be almost 40 percent lower than in nonsmokers. Additionally, other antioxidants, such as beta-carotene, vitamin E, and vitamin B6, have been recorded at low levels in heavy smokers.

- **Alcohol Consumers**

  Over 90 million Americans drink alcoholic beverages. More than ten million of us are estimated to be alcoholic. The effects of increased alcohol consumption include decreased levels of beta-carotene, folic acid, thiamine, riboflavin, niacin, vitamin C, vitamin B6, vitamin B12, magnesium, and zinc. Deficiencies of these nutrients begin to appear when three or more drinks are consumed on a regular weekly basis.

- **Medication Users / Oral Contraception Users**

  Millions of people who rely on therapeutic drugs are at risk for nutritional deficiency. Common drugs available over the counter such as laxatives and mineral oil can deplete your body of fat-soluble vitamins; and oral contraceptives deplete your body of vitamins B_6, B_{12}, C, folic acid, and beta-carotene.

THE HARDEST WORKING NUTRIENTS IN THE BUSINESS

In the miraculous composition of our body, proteins, carbohydrates, and fats combine with other substances to create energy and construct tissues. In the right amounts, they provide normal growth, digestion, mental clarity, and immune function. Essentially, vitamins and minerals are substances required in small amounts to promote fundamental biochemical reactions in our cells. However, since we don't "burn" vitamins, we don't derive direct energy (calories) from them.

Together, vitamins and minerals are called micronutrients. A prolonged lack of a micronutrient can lead to a specific disease or condition, which can often be reversed when the micronutrient is again provided.

Vitamins are divided into two categories: (1) water-soluble vitamins (B vitamins and vitamin C), and (2) fat-soluble vitamins (A, D, E, and K).

At this point in nutritional history, there are 13 known vitamins, which our body strives to keep at constant and optimal levels as they circulate within the bloodstream. The four fat-soluble vitamins (A, D, E, and K) are stored within your body's fat tissue. The nine water-soluble vitamins (C, and eight B vitamins) are not stored in significant amounts in your body's tissues. The eight B vitamins are B_1 (thiamine), B_2 (riboflavin), niacin, B_6, pantothenic acid, B_{12}, biotin, and folic acid (folate).

Surplus water-soluble vitamins are excreted in urine, while surplus fat-soluble vitamins are stored in body tissues. Since fat-soluble vitamins (A and D) are stored in tissues, they can accumulate to toxic levels.

Your body also needs 16 minerals to help regulate cellular functioning and provide structure for cells. These minerals include phosphorous, calcium, and magnesium. In lesser amounts, your body also needs copper, iron, iodine, chromium, molybdenum, selenium, zinc, chloride, potassium, and sodium.

- **Vegetarians**

  Vegetarians who have eliminated all animal products from their diets may need additional vitamin B_{12}. There is some debate about the bioavailability of B_{12} in the frequently cited sources of sea vegetables, tempeh, miso, and brine pickles. This is still somewhat controversial. A reliable source of B_{12} is nutritional yeast, which differs from brewer's yeast or torula yeast and can be used by those sensitive to other yeasts.

As long as we depend on foods that are chemically sprayed, processed, refined, canned, frozen, stored, hormonally fed, overcooked, artificially chemicalized, genetically modified, and laden with sugar and excessive salt, we run the serious risk of deficiency and increased malabsorption. In this way of eating, a supplement regime is akin to the ice pack analogy: "Allow me to batter you with a 2×4 plank, but worry not; I'll give you an ice pack soon afterward."

THE CANCER-PROTECTION SUPPLEMENT PLAN

Antioxidant and nutrient supplements have demonstrated an ability to bolster and reinforce the body's ability to counteract the effects of free radicals (substances that promote tumor growth) and enhance immunity. There are also other micronutrients and nutritional factors that can help prevent cancer and are essential with any cancer therapy.

The following antioxidants are generally recommended for cancer prevention:

- **Beta-Carotene**

  The precursor of Vitamin A, beta-carotene is a plant pigment found naturally in various vegetables and fruits. It has repeatedly proved helpful for immune enhancement of natural killer cells and other immune cells against tumors. However, the vegetables containing beta-carotene (carrots, sweet potatoes, and most green leafy vegetables) may have even more protective effects. One study from Dartmouth Medical School in New Hampshire showed that vegetables are better than supplements in lowering the risks of developing colon cancer. Beta carotene has shown particular importance for women as a cervical cancer deterrent and for lung protection from smoking and smog exposure.

- **Vitamin E**

  As one of the body's key micronutrients for protecting cell membranes and supporting the immune system's ability to fight cancer and infection, between 400 and 800 units of vitamin E daily is generally recommended. According to Lawrence Taylor, M.D., vitamin E also increases the effectiveness and specific toxicity of chemotherapy agents against tumors and helps to protect against radiation treatment-toxicity. E vitamins can be found in dark green vegetables, eggs, wheat germ, unrefined vegetable oils, liver, and some herbs. Researchers claim that a mixture of several vitamin E sources (natural d-alpha tocopherol succinate) may prevent cancer more efficiently than other forms.

- **Coenzyme Q10**

  Also known as ubiquinone, CoQ10 is a general antioxidant that energetically supports cellular function and has an ability to enhance immunity and protect the heart. It is one of a family of brightly colored substances, called quinones, that appear abundantly in nature and are essential for generating energy in living things that depend on oxygen. While the body produces small quantities of CoQ10, it diminishes with aging. CoQ10 is naturally found in high concentrations in fish (particularly sardines), soybean and grapeseed oils, sesame seeds, pistachios, walnuts, and spinach. General amounts recommended are 200 to 300 milligrams daily. CoQ10 is best absorbed with a small amount of dietary fat.

- **Inositol (IP6)**

  Inositol (IP6) is an unofficial phytochemical and powerful antioxidant member of the B vitamin family derived

THE DIFFERENCE BETWEEN NATURAL AND ARTIFICIAL

Are we getting more than we bargained for in commercial supplements? There are a variety of ingredients used in the manufacturing of vitamin supplements. Some of these compounds known as excipients, are typically used to make tablets and may be classified as fillers, binders, lubricants, preservatives, dyes, disintegrators, coatings, drying agents and sweeteners. Many of these ingredients are thought to be potentially harmful and could compromise the benefits of the supplement.

Noted vitamin authority and author, Earl Mindell, PhD., advises to "look for an all natural formula that does not use any artificial colors, dyes, preservatives."

Here is a brief explanation of ingredients that may be hiding in your supplements:

- *Dilutents or fillers*—gives bulk to the tablet.

- *Binders*—added to bond ingredients together. Fillers and binders such as cellulose and gum arabic or calcium stearate also get absorbed through digestion and can negatively affect the rate of absorption.

- *Colors, flavors, and sweeteners*—added to synthetic formulas to give a uniform appearance.

- *Drying agents*—prevents moisture water materials from picking up moisture during the processing stages.

- *Lubricants*—these keep the supplement ingredients from sticking to the machines that punch the tablets out.

- *Natural coatings*—helps keep moisture from penetrating the tablet.

- *Disintegrators*—this is to make certain that the tablet effectively disintegrates when swallowed.

- *Preservatives*—added to maintain market shelf-life. Avoid supplements with polysorbate 80 or polyethylene glycol. These preservatives can cause allergic reactions.

from high-fiber foods containing phytic acid (legumes, cereal grains, and citrus fruits). Inositol is found in nearly all body cells and aids the liver in removing excess fat from its tissues, which prevents fat and bile asccumulation in the liver. Inositol plays an essential role in transferring signals between cells and the environment. In 1989, Drs. A.M. Shamsuddin and Asad Ullah reported in the journal *Carcinogenesis* that IP6 prevented large intestinal cancer. IP6 worked even after exposure to a carcinogen. In 1995, Dr. Shamsuddin showed that IP6 inhibits growth of prostate cells, commenting in a publication of the American Institute of Nutrition that the "substance is instantaneously taken up by malignant cells."

The following nutrients are generally recommended for cancer prevention:

- **Vitamin B Complex**
  This group of vitamins is comprised of B_1, B_2, B_3 (niacin), B_6, folic acid, and pantothenic acid. Together, they act as a biochemical support system to accelerate chemical reactions as catalysts, regulate overall energy metabolism, and help regulate proper nervous system functioning. B vitamin deficiencies can inhibit the immune system's natural ability to destroy cancer cells. It has been observed that pantothenic acid and vitamin B_6 inhibit tumor growth. Folic acid has also been shown to inhibit development of chemically-induced tumors. Growing evidence indicates that B_3 (also known as niacin or nicotinic acid) can increase the efficacy of cancer treatment. Food sources of B vitamins are dark green leafy vegetables, brewer's yeast, wheat germ, whole grains and grain products, and various animal meats.

- **Vitamin C**
  Vitamin C has proved foundational for a healthy immune system. Vitamin C limits free-radical damage to DNA that may lead to cancer. The natural killer (NK)

cells of the immune system are only active when they contain large amounts of vitamin C. However, patients with leukemia should be cautious about taking large doses of vitamin C. General recommendations vary from 500 to 2000 milligrams daily in two or three doses. Vitamin C can be found in green leafy vegetables, broccoli, green peppers, and numerous other vegetables and fruits.

- **Vitamin D**

  Classified as a hormone, vitamin D has shown antitumor qualities. It has been shown to increase the number of vitamin A receptors on cells, stimulate the reversal of cancer cells back into normalized cells, and induce "cell suicide" (apoptosis) in cancer cells. Some Australian research has indicated that vitamin D could offer prostate cancer protection. Suggested dosage varies from 400 to 800 international units (IU) daily.

- **Selenium**

  Considered important for its strong syngergistic effects with vitamin E, enhancing its cancer-fighting potential, the recommended dosage is 100 micrograms per day. According to biochemist Gerhard Schrauzer, Ph.D., selenium is often deficient in cancer patients. Selenium supplements have been shown to impede the reappearance of tumors in animals whose tumors regressed following ovariectomy. This trace mineral is found in vegetables, fruits, and some nuts.

- **Calcium**

  Essential for bone and tooth development, blood clotting, and cellular metabolism, calcium offers protection against colon cancer. Calcium can be sufficiently obtained from dark green vegetables and sea vegetables, as well as from nuts, seeds, sardines, and salmon.

- **Magnesium**

  Helping to maintain balanced blood pH and the synthesis of RNA and DNA, magnesium offers solid cancer protection and can be found in various fish, green vegetables, whole grain and grain products (particularly brown rice), legumes, and most nuts.

- **Iodine**

  Iodine has been shown to offer protection against breast cancer and is required for cellular energy metabolism and the growth and repair of all tissues. It is found abundantly in seafood and sea vegetables such as kombu, nori, wakame, hiziki, arame, and kelp.

- **Zinc**

  Zinc, known for its prostate-cancer protection, is a necessary factor in RNA and DNA formation and for enhanced immune function. Good sources of zinc include whole grains, various seafoods, beans (notably soybeans), sunflower seeds, pumpkin seeds, eggs, and onions.

- **Omega-3 Fatty Acids**

  Some studies have shown that essential fatty acids can inhibit breast cancer. Good sources of omega-3 fatty acids include fish such as salmon, mackerel, haddock, cod, and sardines, and flaxseed and flaxseed oil. A 20-million-dollar study underwritten by the National Cancer Institute (NCI) in 1990 found that flaxseed oil reduced the growth of breast cancers and metastases in laboratory animals when compared with cancerous growth in animals receiving corn oil. While this study was not completed, it was determined that strong anticancer factors in flaxseed due to flaxseeds' high lignan content. Flaxseed oil contains up to 100 times more lignans than any other plant food. Researchers have discovered that lignans can bind to estrogen receptors in the body and diminish the cancer-stimulating effects of estrogen on breast tissue. The recommended amount of flaxseed oil varies from 1 to 2 tablespoons per day.

- **Germanium**

  Germanium is an unusual trace element that increases oxygen to both healthy and cancer cells. It has been established that cancer cells cannot live under oxygen-rich conditions. Germanium sesquioxide blocks or slows tumor growth and has been shown to lengthen survival times in laboratory animals. Highly esteemed Japanese cancer physician and researcher Keiichi Morishita, M.D., suggests Korean ginseng, a particularly rich source of germanium, to patients at his Ochanomizu Clinic in Tokyo, Japan. Morishita claims that germanium from this source improves liver function and strengthens the blood-cleansing ability of the body.

- **Green Tea**

  In 1997, researchers at the University of Ohio published a report in the journal *Nature*, which showed that green tea inhibits the protein urokinase, a protein central to the growth and spread of cancer cells. Additional studies over the years have shown that green tea offers breast cancer protection. Researchers found that increased consumption of the tea was closely associated with decreased numbers of axillary lymph node metastases among pre-menopausal patients with stage I and II breast cancer.

  Suggested amounts are from 2 to 4 cups daily. For those people who might be caffeine sensitive (30–40 milligrams per cup), decaffeinated versions are available.

WHEN MORE IS NOT BETTER—A WORD OF CAUTION

Vitamins cannot replace food. In fact, vitamins cannot be assimilated without ingesting food. This is the reason for taking most vitamins with or shortly after a meal. Vitamins help to regulate metabolism, convert fat and carbohydrates into energy, and assist in forming bone and tissue. However, vitamin-mineral supplements should not be used as substitutes for a healthful diet. High doses do not usually offer extra protection, instead increase the risk of encountering toxic side effects. For example, taking large amounts of vitamin D can indirectly cause kidney damage, while large amounts of vitamin A can cause liver damage. Even modest increases in some minerals can lead to imbalances that limit your body's ability to use other minerals. Supplements of iron, zinc, chromium, and selenium can be toxic at just five times the RDA. Virtually all nutrient toxicities stem from high-dose supplements.

Supplement tolerance and the individual needs for specific conditions is still a very young science. Isolating key nutrients, as in standardization processes, often leaves out the natural matrix of many assisting trace nutrients that synergistically aid in assimilation and cellular use. Also in question is whether or not it is necessary to take supplements continuously on a

SOME DANGERS OF VITAMIN EXCESSES

Here are some miscellaneous facts about vitamin excesses and the imbalances they can cause:

- High amounts of calcium inhibit absorption of iron and other trace elements.

- Folic acid excess can mask hematologic signs of vitamin B_{12} deficiency, which, if untreated can result in irreversible neuroligic damage.

- High dosages of zinc supplementation can reduce copper status, impair immune responses, and decrease high-density lipoprotein cholesterol levels.

- An excess of vitamin E can interfere with vitamin K action and enhance the effect of coumadin anticoagulant drugs. Over 25,000 IU per day can cause headaches, dry skin, hair loss, fatigue, bone problems, and liver damage.

- A study of 22,748 pregnant women found that women taking more than 10,000 IU of vitamin A had a greater risk of giving birth to babies with cranial neural crest defects.

- Iron supplements intended for adult household members are the most common cause of pediatric poisoning deaths in the United States.

- Excessive zinc and vitamin C has an antagonistic effect on the body's copper levels.

daily basis, as opposed to irregular consumption (example: four days on, three days off) as an attempt to keep nutrient dependency at a minimum. At best, an on-and-off regimen might offer a greater understanding of what works for the individual and what doesn't. Ultimately, the answer is not in research but results. This is best determined through additional study, personal experimenting, and self-evaluation.

MINIMIZING CHEMOTHERAPY TOXICITY

Chemotherapy is the systemic use of anticancer drugs and still is a standard treatment for many cancers. While its effectiveness with some cancers has been shown to be useful (acute lymnphocytic leukemia, Hodgskin's disease, testicular cancer, ovarian cancer, and a small number of rare tumors), justification of chemotherapy as an across-the-board therapy for the majority of cancers, particularly advanced carcinomas, is still highly debatable. Often, the actual "benefits" might amount to weeks or months of "remission" but not to years. Unfortunately, the trade-offs for this extended time are life-threatening side effects and a serious decrease in a patient's quality of life.

An often-overlooked point worthy of consideration made by author Ralph Moss in *Questioning Chemotherapy* (Equinox Press) is that chemotherapy "reduces the likelihood of benefiting from other promising nontoxic, nutritional, or immunological treatments." This can occur by damaging bone marrow and other organ structures, which diminishes a patient's chance of benefiting from promising treatment that may offer stronger immunity and better constitutional health.

Anyone considering chemotherapy would be better informed by diligent research of chemotherapy's effectiveness, pertinent to their own special cancer, before considering it as an automatic choice. For instance, how many cases of this kind of cancer have been helped or cured? May you speak to a patient with your type of cancer about his or her experience with chemotherapy? These are important questions worth discussing with your physician.

Most of the following suggestions have not been evaluated with the rigorous attention of randomized clinical trials. Fortunately, they do not have the kind of serious side effects attributed to chemotherapy. Therefore, they cannot threaten health, but can hopefully stimulate immunity, trigger the body's internal cleansing function, and enhance nutrition. These recommendations and dosages for use during chemotherapy should be thoroughly discussed with your nutritionally oriented physician:

Malabsorption Problems: A multiple vitamin and mineral supplement is highly recommended to counteract the negative effect of chemotherapy on nutrient absorption.

Nausea: Some research has shown the *N*-acetytl cysteine (aka NAC), an amino acid-like supplement that has demonstrated strong antioxidant activity, may reduce nausea and vomiting caused by chemotherapy. Recommended dosage is 1600 milligrams per day.

Mouth Sores: Known as mucositis, chemotherapy often leaves patients with painful mouth sores. The topical application of 400 IU of vitamin E, according to double-bind research, has proved helpful.

Enhancing the Effect of Chemotherapy: Antioxidants, such as vitamin A, vitamin E, and vitamin C, are known to increase the effectiveness of chemotherapy.

Folic Acid Warning: The chemotherapy drug Methotrexate interferes with folic acid (B vitamin) metabolism. Cancer patients taking methotrexate should not supplement with folic acid beyond the recommended 400 micrograms usually found in a daily multivitamin without first discussing this with their oncologists. Typically, oncologists will recommend leucovorin (a form of folic acid) after methotrexate is used, to counter any side effects.

Heart Damage: Some chemotherapy drugs (adriamycin, also known as doxorubicin) may damage heart tissue. A number of antioxidants are capable of reducing this toxicity. In particular, CoQ10 has been found successful in recommendations of 90 to 120 milligrams. In animals, vitamin C has been shown to give enough heart protection for dosages of several grams per day. Vitamin B_2 supplementation may also protect the heart from damage when taking adriamycin.

ANTIOXIDANT PHOBIA?

Some physicians fear that supplements could negate the effectiveness of chemotherapy. The basis for this concern was from a 1999 paper by a naturopath, Dan Labriola, and oncologist Robert Livingston in the journal *Oncology*.

Well known and respected researcher and author, Ralph Moss, Ph.D, addresses this issue in his, *Antioxidants Against Cancer*:

"I don't agree with this. The actual data (which I present throughout this book) overwhelmingly contradicts the idea that antioxidants cancel the effects of toxic treatments. Quite the opposite: almost every experiment on the topic supports the idea that there is synergy, that is, increased benefits when antioxidants and toxic treatments are used together. Another reason to take supplements is that toxic treatments routinely rob patients of key nutrients. Almost every vitamin, from A to K, has been found to be lacking in some cancer patients after they receive chemotherapy. Plus, cancer itself can sometimes cause deficiencies and malnutrition . . . The same holds true for radiation therapy. The decline in antioxidants after radiation can be subtle, but long-lasting. Many oncologists believe that antioxidants spring back after radiation. Not so . . . Scientists in Tubingen, Germany, have looked at the levels of vitamins C and E, beta-carotene, etc., before, during, and after high-dose chemotherapy. The drug etopside significantly increased free radical damage to fats. Beta-carotene levels fell by 50 percent and vitamin E (alpha-tocopherol) levels by 20 percent . . . Antioxidant supplements can play a role in restoring a cancer patient's nutritional status to normal. So taking supplements is a logical way of returning what was lost due to conventional treatments and disease."

If you have chosen to undergo chemotherapy, share your desire to take antioxidants as a part of your overall treatment plan, with your medical specialist. It might be worthy to point out that there exists a preponderance of data to support the use of antioxidants with chemotherapy.

Hair Loss: There is some anecdotal material that claims hair loss as a result of adriamycin, can be reduced by taking elevated amounts of vitamin E—usually up to 1600 IU per day. Nutritionally oriented physicians generally recommend at least 800 IU of vitamin E to patients taking adriamycin.

Magnesium Loss: The chemotherapy drug Cisplatin frequently leads to depletion of magnesium. Magnesium levels should be checked for this reason. Cisplatin toxicity can also be reduced by taking glutathione; however, this must be administered intravenously by a physician. Taking an excess of magnesium can result in diarrhea, which can occur with a dose as low as 350 to 500 milligrams per day. Additionally, people with kidney disease should not take magnesium supplements without consulting a nutritionally oriented physician.

Palm and Sole Pain: The drug Flurouracil can sometimes cause pain on the skin of the palms and soles. It has been suggested that vitamin B6 can eliminate this pain.

A CHEMOTHERAPY SUPPLEMENT PROTOCOL

Here is a sample supplement recommendation for your consideration and further research, to take during and after chemotherapy. Supplements should be taken 15 to 25 minutes after meals. There is not ample evidence to justify megadoses of vitamins and minerals, but there is strong evidence demonstrating that modest amounts of major vitamins and minerals are protective against most major illnesses, including cancer. Use this list below as a reference when checking multi-vitamin/mineral labels for contents and amounts.

VITAMINS AND MINERALS	PREVENTION/THERAPEUTIC
Vitamin A	5000 international units
Vitamin D	400 international units
Vitamin E	200–400 international units
Vitamin B1	100 milligrams
Vitamin B2	50 milligrams

Vitamin B6	25 milligrams
Vitamin B12	500 micrograms
Vitamin C	500–1000 milligrams
Niacin	10 milligrams
Niacinamide	150 milligrams
Pantothenic acid	500 milligrams
Choline	100 milligrams
Inositol	100 milligrams
Para-amino benzoic acid (PABA)	50 milligrams
Bioflavanoids	100 milligrams
Calcium	500 milligrams
Magnesium	500 milligrams
Potassium	99 milligrams
Maganese (aspartate)	10 milligrams
Copper (gluconate)	2 milligrams
Boron (chelate)	1 milligrams
Zinc*	20 milligrams
Folic acid	400 micrograms
Biotin	300 micrograms
Iodine	100 micrograms
Molybendum (chelate)	100 micrograms
Selenium	100–200 micrograms
Vanadium	25 micrograms

Note: Calcium may interfere with zinc absorption as well as the phytates in grains and beans. This is one nutrient that should be taken separately.

ANTIOXIDANTS	PREVENTION SUGGESTION	THERAPEUTIC SUGGESTION
• Beta-carotene*	15 milligrams	45 milligrams
• Bioflavonoids	2 grams	8 grams
• Co-enzyme Q10**	30 milligrams	100 milligrams
• Pycnogenol	25 milligrams	100 milligrams
• Lipoic acid	30 milligrams	100 milligrams
• N-acetyl-cysteine (NAC)	300 milligrams	600 milligrams

Note: Beta-carotene is best obtained from food sources.

**Note:* Should be taken with a meal containing some fat for better absorption.

AMINO ACIDS	PREVENTION SUGGESTION	THERAPEUTIC SUGGESTION
• L-glutamine	500 milligrams	1000 milligrams

MUSHROOMS	PREVENTION SUGGESTION	THERAPEUTIC SUGGESTION
• Maitake D-Fraction	320 milligrams (2 capsules)	480 milligrams (3 capsules)

CHEMOTHERAPY HERBAL SUPPORT

Certain herbal preparations, taken after chemotherapy treatment, can help boost bone marrow white blood cell production and increase immunity. Three herbs have shown the most consistently successful following chemotherapy.

1. *Astragalus:* 2–3 500-milligram capsules, 3 × daily. Astragalus is usually combined with another Chinese herb: ligustrum (Ligustrum Lucidum).
2. *Eleuthero* (Siberian ginseng): 2–3 grams of dried root or 300–400 milligrams daily of solid extract standardized on eleutherosides B and E).
3. *Asian ginseng:* 100–200 milligrams daily of standardized herbal extract.

Additionally, schisandra, shiitake, reishi, and maitake have proved helpful for immunity enhancement.

> **Note:** Ginseng should not be used with uncontrolled high-blood-pressure conditions. Ginseng could also cause insomnia and gastrointestinal upset when taken with caffeine. Long-term use of ginseng may cause menstrual abnormalities and breast tenderness in some women. Ginseng is not recommended for pregnant or lactating women.

In *Herbal Medicine, Healing & Cancer,* numerous herbs are recommended to combat side effects from chemotherapy and radiation. The following herbs for minimizing chemotherapy and radiation damage are mentioned as inspiration for further research:

- Ligustrum (one of the "main herbs used in China to offset toxicity from chemotherapy and radiation. It is usually combined with schizandra, reishi, ginseng, and astragalus)
- Wild Geranium (inflammation)
- Aloe Vera (antiviral and immune boosting)
- Ashwagandha (antitumor, immune boosting and for radiation after-effects)
- Atractylodes (immunity)
- Bitter Melon (antioxidant, especially for leukemias and prostate cancer)
- Boswellan (antiinflammatory, for weight gain and immunity)
- Butterbur (tumor pain)
- Chapparral (antitumor agent, antiviral, antifungal)
- Dandelion (liver detoxification, diuretic, replenishes potassium, used with breast cancer)
- Echinacea (immunity boosting, wound healing, inflammation)
- Eclipta (liver regeneration, chemo detox)
- Goldenseal (breast, stomach cancers, antitumor, particularly against brain tumors)
- Ho Shou Wu (graying of hair, bowel irregularity, chills, fevers, high cholesterol)
- Jaborandi (dry mouth induced by radiation, fever— usually combined with echinacea, prickly ash, and kava for use as a mouth spray)
- Lotus Seed (to stop diarrhea and promote lymph health)
- Milk Thistle (exceptional herb for liver detox)

- Nettles (anti-inflammatory, anemia, poor lymph function)
- Nux Vomica (essential plant for low vitality, weak nervous system—can be toxic if taken in single concentrated form. For maximum effectiveness it is usually combined with other herbs in extract form)
- Rabdosia (sore throats, anticancer activity)
- Yellow Dock (glandular swelling, laxative)

The decision to begin or remain on chemotherapy is an individual one. Nobody can make that for you. Often, a client will tell me, "They want to put me on chemotherapy." I'll ask, "What do you want? Is that your choice?" They'll usually shrug their shoulders in an unsure manner. I encourage them to become more of an activist in their pursuit for healing, to ask questions and not be intimidated, in certain cases, by the brusque, fleeting manner of their physician, who will usually assume control with patients who feel overwhelmed and unsure.

10
NATURE'S CANCER-FIGHTING FOOD PLAN

SO MANY THEORIES, SO LITTLE TIME

The late comedian George Burns, once said, "Too bad all the people who know how to run the country are busy driving taxis and cutting hair." This equally applies to nutrition; everybody seems to have their own theories and everybody seems to have passionate and dogmatic convictions supporting them.

Obviously, there are many dietary paths that can lead to a healthy destination. Thirty years of personal and professional experience have convinced me that there exists no one dietary solution for all of our ills. Practically speaking, our needs are far more complex and often require a flexible, individualized approach.

There are impressive case histories of people using a raw foods approach, just as there are for those adopting a more cultural macrobiotic approach, where a majority of the food is cooked. Some people do not fare well with a strict vegetarian approach and respond better with regular, but small quantities of animal protein. The factors that determine a healthy dietary approach have to do with a person's genetic make-up, upbringing, lifestyle, former diet, and current health condition. A successful dietary plan, one from which you quickly experience noticeable benefit and can feel comfortably committed to following consistently, might be difficult to maintain without considering these factors.

Why do so many theories seem to contradict each other? What's the secret of creating a balanced food plan? Can someone else advise you about what's right for your body?

It's a fact that we're all biochemically unique. We may have similar organic functions and needs, but our strengths, weaknesses, nutritional profiles, and habits, distinctively vary. A body builder, an office worker, a messenger, an athlete, and a homemaker might each require different and varying percentages of nutrients or food groups (fats, simple and complex-carbohydrates, protein).

The presumption that one theory can serve all is naively simplistic. A generic approach to nourishment definitely has convenience appeal and might sound good theoretically, but in the real world nutritional needs have to be individualized for consistent success.

HOW TO ASSESS A DIETARY PLAN

Let's take a closer look at the important considerations (see *Seven Key Questions*) for evaluating a food plan:

SEVEN KEY QUESTIONS

Here are seven questions to consider when evaluating a food plan:

1. What are the short- and long-term benefits?
2. Is there a sound principle behind the theory?
3. Does the food plan have a successful track record?
4. Can the dietary benefits be supported by science?
5. Does the plan offer good nutrition?
6. Is the plan affordable?
7. Is it a plan you can enjoy or grow to enjoy?

Short-Term Versus Long-Term Benefits

With our increasingly fast pace of living, a premium on time, and a modern hunger for short-term solutions, it's difficult not to be influenced by popular diet-of-the-month "best-seller" food plans promising rapid weight loss, instant cures, and dynamic health.

Does the diet plan you're currently considering lure you with the promise of a quick fix? What are its long-term benefits? Liquid diets, as a more extreme example, fit this point— short-term rapid loss, long-term inevitable gain.

Comparing short term to long term prevents dietary self-sabotage. Our blood chemistry is immediately influenced by the daily food we consume. After two to three weeks we should be able to notice positive signs that the path we're following is a positive one. Our sleep quality, bowel movements, energy levels, cravings, and general nutritional satisfaction all reveal the validity of the approach we follow. This is one of your best barometers.

Principle Behind the Theory

What is the theory based on? Is it a generic plan for all of humanity for all time? Does it change with your own evolving condition? With the seasons? Is it physically compatible with what the human body is designed to eat? What signs, physically or otherwise, indicate you might need to make dietary adjustment?

Track Record

Is it a "new, breakthrough" food plan? Has it been used and tested successfully? Does it have the basic ingredients found in healthy cultural diets practiced for thousands of years?

Scientific Support

Does the program have some scientific merit? Can its claims be verified? Is there any potential of jeopardizing your health?

Natural Quality

Are we talking about genetically engineered food? Irradiation? Artificial additives? Ingredients you cannot pronounce or understand? Is it a whole food or a refined variety? Is it naturally grown or waxed and cultivated with chemicals?

Nutritional Balance

Does the program contain a good variety of foods, textures, colors, and cooking styles for a sense of variety? Is there flexibility for situations where the recommended foods might be unavailable? Does the program offer satisfying nutrition?

Economics

Is the program affordable? Practical? Are the ingredients only available at specialized and exotic stores? Can anyone follow such a program? Ingredients that constitute a healthy diet should be available to everyone and not just those who can afford exclusive preparations. While certain natural medicines and supplements may enhance health, there should be a way of nourishing the body that can accomplish the same result without depending on rare items that are difficult to obtain, or that come with high price tags. If used, they should be adjunctive as opposed to staple parts of the diet.

Enjoyment

Finally, is the program pleasurable? Of course, every mouthful doesn't have to be an experience of rapture, but does it taste good? Does it *feel* nourishing? Can you grow to enjoy it? Are you satisfied after the meal? Meals that are designed exclusively for taste might be highly pleasurable while being consumed, but afterward, as you're searching for that antacid, it's another story.

You have to appreciate the food you're eating. It shouldn't be something you have to "put up with." I've seen clients, reportedly on "healing diets," who approach their meal preparation as if it were gum surgery. This attitude can make a simple meal a stressful event—hardly conducive toward good digestion, healing or long-term commitment.

These considerations can help to sort out the idealistic from the practical while helping you to distinguish between the hazardous and the safe. Ultimately, the best test will be your own experience, not studies, theories, or blind loyalty to a program. You must determine whether or not you can maintain the program guidelines.

Having the flexibility of different programs to shift between according to circumstances, changing needs, or a sudden desire for variety prevents the compulsion to do "all or nothing." *The Power to Fight Cancer Program* is the opportunity to positively transform your health.

THE *NATURE'S* CANCER FIGHTING FOOD PLAN

The focus of my program is to introduce whole foods in a gradual way that you will find inspiring, healthy, and healing. Depending on your previous way of eating and individual needs, *The Nature's Cancer Fighting Food Plan* offers two dietary plans.

1. Transition Plan
2. Prevention/Therapeutic Plan

Here is an outline of each program:

- The Transition Plan offers a gradual change for increasing cancer-fighting agents by adding new, healthy, whole foods and decreasing foods that are not health supportive. This introductory plan is best suited to someone who is not familiar with many of the foods recommended since it permits greater dietary flexibility.

- The Prevention/Therapeutic Plan greatly increases cancer-suppressing foods with a higher percentage of wholesome healthy foods and higher reductions of foods that are not health supportive. It can yield quicker results for general health that can be noticed within weeks.

- The Therapeutic Plan increases cancer-fighting foods and offers the highest level of anti-cancer protection. It minimizes, or eliminates, animal protein, permits only the lowest level or total elimination of dairy products, and raises the percentage of whole grain, vegetables, beans, bean products, and fruits in the daily diet. This is a more demanding approach, however, it can be interchanged with the transition plan.

WHOLE GRAINS: THE STARTING POINT

Every great culture cultivated corn, rice, wheat, barley, oats, rye, or buckwheat. Frequently, these plants were worshipped as the sacred source of life.

In Will Durant's historical books, the dietary habits of different societal groups are outlined with fascinating similarity:

- The Babylonian civilization, established thousands of years prior to the birth of Christ, produced a healthy variety of grains, peas, beans, fruits, and nuts. Meat was rarely used; however, fish, being more affordable and available, was eaten occasionally. Small quantities of goat products along with grapes and olives supplemented their diet.

- North of this civilization lived the near-vegetarian Assyrians, whose fields were ripe with wheat, barley, millet, and sesame. Meat eating was limited to the aristocracy; however, an occasional fish was taken from the Tigris River.

- Throughout India, rice, peas, lentils, millet, vegetables, and fruits were cultivated and considered staples, limiting meats to be consumed by the wealthy or social outcasts. In the south, the cuisine was predominantly made more elaborate by the addition of numerous spices.

- Dominating the vast terrain throughout China were fields of millet, barley, wheat, and soybeans, as well as paddies of numerous rice varieties.

- The Japanese, limited in land space, cultivated varieties of rice, buckwheat, small beans (aduki), soybeans and seaweeds in dried and fresh form.

- Despite harsh mountainous terrain, the ancient Greeks were a hearty population whose staple grain was barley, from which they made porridge, flat breads, and cakes, typically mixed with honey. Olive oil, goat products, beans, peas, cruciferous vegetables, lentils, onions, garlic, figs, grapes, and wine were regularly consumed along with their staples.

- The Roman diet shared similarity with Greek dietary traditions until their empire declined. Meals then became legendary rituals of prolonged feasting with richer foods and higher percentages of animal protein.

- For the past five thousand years, the chief crops of Mexico have been corn, or maize, and rice. Along with a variety of beans, tomatoes, onions, peppers, and small amounts of meats, Mexicans enjoyed a wide array of vegetables, fruits, berries, and coffees. The cow was unknown prior to the advent of the Spaniards. Until then, the largest animal consumed was a guinea pig. Lard, used extensively today, is a recent addition as well as the increasingly common use of cheese, which you'll find in virtually every bean dish. As food refinement increased, fats became more prominent.

The common thread obviously apparent in most of these traditional societies was the regular consumption of whole grains, beans, and vegetables as primary carbohydrates and protein sources. Unfortunately, when grain polishing was introduced, valuable fiber, minerals, and vitamins were stripped. This initiated a pattern of inadequate food preparation that continues to this day. It has been pointed out that many of the subsequent

THE WHOLE TRUTH ABOUT CEREAL

For most people, hearing the term *cereal* usually brings to mind a visual of boxed breakfast cereal, the kind you soak in milk and typically topped with fruit. Not so. These common breakfast cereals are merely grain products. The once whole grain has been through unnatural processing that has made cereals into a grain product.

Cereal grains go through different styles of processing. While whole grains are preferable, cut and rolled grains are also acceptable. However, powdered forms (flour) are recommended only as a minimum percentage of grain products, if desired. They are less satisfying and in some individuals can elevate blood sugar since they're quicker to be absorbed.

Here's what I call the Oat Story:

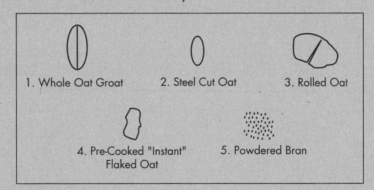

1. Whole Oat Groat   2. Steel Cut Oat   3. Rolled Oat

4. Pre-Cooked "Instant" Flaked Oat   5. Powdered Bran

A whole oat groat (1) may take an hour and a half to cook. If it's cut with a steel-tooth machine it becomes a steel-cut oat, (2) that cooks in approximately 20 to 30 minutes. If it is rolled flat from its whole form, for quicker cooking purposes, it now becomes a rolled oat (3). This style of oats usually cooks in 10 to 15 minutes. If the grower decides to cook it for the consumer and then dry it, you now have instant, one-minute oats (4). But it doesn't stop here. As an additional product, companies will remove the layers of bran and powder it to make oat bran (5), which requires no or little cooking and is suggested to be added to foods as a topping or mix.

Since the word *meal* literally means "grain," any form of the above can be called oatmeal. Generally, I'll recommend whole, steel-cut, or naturally rolled oats (1, 2, 3) and save the instant for an "in-a-pinch fiber-source" situation, such as when traveling.

food additions (increased dairy, fat, and protein) to these once traditional diets are the result of a compensatory attempt to make meals more filling and nutritionally satisfying.

H₂O FACTOR

Have you had your eight glasses of water today? Did you have to force it down or were you genuinely thirsty? Contrary to popular thought, it's really not necessary to drink large volumes of fluid throughout the day—unless you're eating in a way that requires it. Our kidney systems are much more complex mechanisms than dual toilets that simply "flush."

Traditional wisdom regarding fluid intake was simply to drink when thirsty. However, the notion of "the daily eight" might actually be based on acquired need. Considering heavy salt use, abundant meat proteins, high fat, plenty of flour products, and frequent sugar, combined with the lack of soups, whole grains (high water content), vegetables, and fruits in our diets, drinking "plenty of liquids" is necessary.

Our modern diets are laden with fat. Fats thicken the blood. When our fat intake becomes excessive, the red blood cells aggregate in the narrow capillaries. Since they carry oxygen, this clumping partially traps much needed oxygen and prevents it from entering tissues. Meanwhile, our overconsumption of animal protein breaks down into harmful by products of sulfur, ammonia, and purine wastes, including uric acid.

Now, include meat hormones, pesticide residues, assorted bacterial strains, food industry chemicals, and a gross volume of refined sugar, and you're left with a highly carcinogenic mixture that's supposed to nourish and sustain our health.

Such dietary habits might be the reason we're always trying to "replace" fluids. If you're on a typical Western diet, drinking a lot of fluids, or "washing down your meals," is probably a necessity. One theory suggests that water, in this case, may dilute the effects of this carcinogenic mixture to thin the blood and keep the kidneys in continuous eliminative mode. Drinking more to "flush toxins," in this regard, obviously makes good sense. However, this advice might be better phrased as, "eat toxins less and reduce the need to feel like you have to constantly irrigate your body."

A Chinese doctor I once interviewed told me that he thought the American diet created so much internal "heat" that Americans *needed* to drink in order to put out their "fire." This is exactly what we do; from fruit juice, coffee, ice water, tea, cola, carbonated beverages, alcohol to milk—and we're still thirsty. Somehow, we went from 12-ounce soda cans to "32-ounce, Big Gulp® specials" along with designer water bags to tote that omnipresent plastic water bottle that inspired comedian, George Carlin to remark, ". . . Will you tell me when we suddenly became so thirsty? . . ."

On a whole foods diet, you'll find your thirst at a minimum and the need for fluids far less than during your previous diet. The idea is not to *restrict* your fluids, but to *reduce*. Big difference. A difference determined by your changing needs. A difference based on your individual condition, exercise profile, daily diet, and sensitivity.

Most people will find that once they are on *The Nature's Cancer-Fighting Food Plan,* their liquid needs lessen. Generally, between the high liquid content of the program's foods, soups, a cup or two of tea after meals, and water as a

---

BOOSTING THE NEED FOR LIQUIDS

Here are five other reasons for liquid needs:

1. *Stress*—Although this can vary from individual to individual, as stress levels rise, our need for liquid frequently increases.
2. *Supplements*—Excessive supplement intake usually requires increased liquid consumption.
3. *Exercise*—Strenuous exercise demands more liquid than you'd normally consume.
4. *Pregnancy/Lactating*—Pregnancy needs require increased liquid throughout the pregnancy and into lactation months.
5. *Conventional Cancer Therapy*—For chemotherapy protocols, the need for liquid is essential in order to make chemical intake less toxic.

thirst quencher, little more is rarely needed. Use your own intuition and craving symptoms as a guide, not mechanical rules that are based on generalities. Drinking with meals can dilute nutritional elements from your meals and result in poor chewing. Liquids and meals should be separate, preferably, after your meal of moderate temperature and sipped slowly.

Cold liquids, frequently brought to the table before meals in most restaurants, may inhibit digestion for up to 30 minutes. Become more sensitive to your liquid needs. If you have to attack a pitcher full of water immediately after eating, this is a telltale sign that your meal has not been balanced; the culprit could be excessive salt, sugar, spice, or an excess of dry textures. Satisfy your thirst and be more conscious of meal preparation for the next meal.

FOOD CATEGORIES AND LISTING

The following are lists of foods within the guidelines of *The Power to Fight Cancer Program*. Later, guidelines for each program will be outlined in detail.

Whole Grains

- Whole oats
- Millet
- Amaranth
- Buckwheat
- Wheat, spelt, or kamut
- Brown rice (short, medium, long grain)
- Sweet brown rice
- Barley
- Quinona ("Keen-wa")
- Teff
- Rye

Cracked, Ground, or Rolled Grains

- Bulgur wheat
- Cracked wheat
- Rolled oats
- Oat groats
- Wild rice (seed)
- Corn grits
- Polenta

Whole Grain Products

- Popcorn
- Rice cakes
- Chapatis/tortillas
- Rye flakes
- Natural breakfast cereals

- Pasta
- Crackers/flat breads
- Mochi (sweet rice product)
- Flours
- Yeasted/unyeasted bread

Minimize/Avoid

- Refined grains and flours
- Sweetened flours with oils, artificial coloring, perservatives, conditioners, etc.

VEGETABLES

Leafy Greens and Cruciferous

- Broccoli
- Chinese broccoli
- Collard Greens
- Green cabbage
- Turnip greens
- Endive
- Spinach
- Butterhead lettuce

- Bok choy
- Daikon greens
- Parsley
- Red cabbage
- Brussel sprouts
- Swiss chard
- Mustard greens
- Dandelion greens

- Cauliflower
- Watercress
- Chinese cabbage
- Arugula
- Kale
- Escarole
- Romaine lettuce

Root, Round, and Ground Vegetables

- Onion
- Parsnip
- Lotus root
- Leeks

- Turnip
- Red radish
- Beets
- Acorn squash

- Carrot
- Burdock
- Scallions
- White radish (daikon)

- Summer squash
- Corn
- Celery

- Kabocha squash
- Rutabaga
- Cucumber

- Zucchini
- Patty pan squash

Miscellaneous Vegetables

- Sweet potato
- Snap beans
- Green beans
- Garlic
- Celery root
- Mushrooms
- Fennel

- Yams
- Snap pea
- Green peas
- Artichoke
- Kohlrabi
- Plantain
- Shiitake mushroom

- Chives
- Wax beans
- Sprouts
- Ferns
- Shepherd's purse
- Salsify

"Sweet" Vegetables

- Butternut squash
- Onion
- Daikon

- Kabocha squash
- Corn
- Parsnip

- Carrot
- Cabbage

The Sweet Vegetable category is made up of vegetables that become naturally sweet with cooking. They are used to combine with whole grains or make delicious additions/bases for soups.

"Nightshade" Vegetables

- Green/red peppers
- Potato

- Tomato
- Eggplant

The Nightshade Vegetables category is made up of vegetables that tend to be more acid producing. Although clinically unproven, nightshade vegetables may trigger arthritic symptoms in susceptible individuals.

Minimize/Avoid

- Vegetable Juices—These are fine to enjoy as a vegetable supplement, but not as a substitute for vegetables.

BEANS

Beans

- Great white Northern beans
- Anasazi beans
- Lentils (green, brown, red)
- Navy
- Black turtle beans
- Peas (whole/split, green, yellow)
- Lima
- Fava
- Chick peas
- Aduki
- Kidney
- Black-eyed peas
- Mung
- Soy beans
- Pinto

Bean Products

- Fresh tofu
- Vegetarian burgers
- Tempeh burgers
- Dried tofu
- Soy milk
- Tempeh
- Soy yogurt

Minimize/Avoid

- Canned beans with sugar, coloring, artificial perservatives, added meats, oils, etc.

SEA VEGETABLES

Sea Vegetables (a.k.a. Seaweeds)

- Nori
- Dulse
- Kombu
- Wakame
- Sea palm
- Kelp

- Sea cress
- Hiziki
- Ocean ribbons
- Agar agar
- Arame

Minimize/Avoid

- Most commercial seaweeds sold in Asian markets are either processed or colored. Check carefully before purchasing.

ORGANIC SEEDS/NUTS

SEEDS

- Pumpkin seeds
- Sunflower seeds
- Sesame seeds
- Other seeds
- Seed butters
- *Sesame butter*
- *Tahini butter*

NUTS

- Almonds
- Walnuts
- Hazelnuts
- Nut Butters
- *Peanut Butter*
- *Almond Butter*

- Chestnuts
- Peanuts
- Pine Nuts
- Pecans
- Other Nuts

ANIMAL PROTEIN—OPTIONAL/TRANSITIONAL DIET

Fish/Chicken/Red Meat

- Fish (white meat varieties): Sole, Halibut, Flounder, White/Orange Roughy, Perch, Haddock, Cod, Snapper, etc.)
- Salmon (preferably ocean-originated)
- Eggs (free range, naturally raised)—*Transitional Diet/ Preventive Diet* (Minimize)
- Poultry (free range, hormone free)—*Transitional/Preventive Diet* (Minimize)
- Red meat (grain fed, hormone free)—*Transitional Diet*

Minimize/Avoid

- Seafood high in cholesterol such as crab, shrimp, and lobster.
- Cured or processed meats for this transition diet stage.
- Whole eggs are recommended twice weekly, at a maximum, for the transitional food plan.

DAIRY—TRANSITIONAL DIET

Certified Raw, Organic Dairy Products

- Organic raw butter—*Transitional Diet* (Minimize)
- Ghee, clarified butter—*Transitional Diet* (Minimize)
- Kefir—*Transitional Diet* (Minimize)
- Raw goat milk—*Transitonal Diet* (Minimize)

Minimize/Avoid

- This category is suggested for transitional diets and in minimum amounts.
- Dairy-free cheeses—These products are usually highly processed and typically difficult to digest.
- Mayonnaise—There is tofu-based mayonnaise that might act as a good occasional substitute.

FRUITS

Seasonal Fruits

- Apples
- Peaches
- Cantaloupe
- Blackberries
- Strawberries
- Lemon
- Apricots
- Pears
- Cherries
- Blueberries
- Plums/Prunes
- Orange
- Nectarines
- Watermelon
- Raisins
- Raspberries
- Honeydew

Minimize/Avoid

- Tropical fruits—This category of fruit tends to be more concentrated in sugar. Best if used less frequently.
- Fruit juices—Juices are especially concentrated in sugar and are best minimized or diluted with water.
- Fruit syrups—are strong concentrates and best minimized.
- Fruits can be dried, cooked, or fresh. Be cautious of overeating dried fruit; a seemingly innocent handful might be equivalent to many fruits.

NATURAL SWEETENERS

- Barley malt
- Fruit juice
- Maple syrup
- Molasses
- Amasake
- Chestnuts

Minimize/Avoid

- Honey—Highly concentrated in sugar and and best minimized.
- Refined sugar (white, brown, Turbinado, Kleen-raw, etc.), corn syrup, saccharine, Nutrasweet, fructose, etc.

FERMENTED FOODS/PICKLES

FERMENTED FOODS

- Miso soy bean paste
- Natural soy sauce (tamari)
- Tempeh
- Sauerkraut

PICKLES

- Brine pickles
- Umeboshi (salt plums)
- Miso pickles
- Radish pickle

ORGANIC OILS

- Sesame oil
- Safflower oil
- Olive oil
- Sunflower oil

Minimize/Avoid

- Margarine, coconut oil, lard, shortening, palm-kernal oil, refined and chemically processed, non-organic vegetable oils.

BEVERAGES

Grain "Coffees" (No Caffeine)

- Instant grain coffees
  American brand names: Roma®, Cafix®, Pero®, Barley Brew®, Inka®, Dandelion Coffee

Teas

- Herbal teas (numerous)
- KuKicha Twig Tea
- Ashitaba Plant Tea
- Roasted barley tea
- Dandelion root tea

Other

- Purified spring water
- Soy milk
- Rice milk
- Spiced cider
- Fruit juice
- Natural (nonsugar) cola—*Transitional Diet*
- Mineral water—*Transitional Diet* (Minimize)
- Nonalcoholic beer—*Transitional Diet* (Minimize)
- Naturally brewed beer—*Transitional Diet* (Minimize)
- Wine/spirits—*Transitional Diet* (Minimize)

Minimize/Avoid

- Caffeinated beverages, sugared soft drinks, tap water, hard liquors, frozen drinks, fruit juice

FAMILIAR FOOD SUBSTITUTIONS

The following is a list of healthy alternatives to familiar, less healthy foods. These suggestions do not pose any long-term health risks and will eventually prove equally, if not more, satisfying to your health.

MODERN LOW-FIBER, REFINED DIET	NATURE'S CANCER-FIGHTING FOOD PLAN
• Red meats	Poultry > Fish > Vegan (optional)
• Dairy products	Natural cold-pressed oils, beans, nuts/seeds
• White breads, enriched flours	Whole grains, natural breads (Yeasted/unyeasted) & unrefined whole grain products
• Frozen, canned vegetables	Fresh vegetables (prefer organic)
• Sugar & sweetened desserts	Fruits, moderate amounts of fruit-juice-sweetened products. Soy and fruit purees can be used in place of sugared, dairy ice cream. For cola cravings, try fruit "spritzers."
• Shortening/lard/ butter	Cold-pressed vegetables oils, some nut/seed butters
• Mayonnaise	Soy varieties
• Coffee	Transition from caffeine with natural decaf varieties, then a final switch to grain coffees.
• Alcohol (Beer, wine, spirits)	Occasional natural beer or wine, nonalcoholic beers

1. THE TRANSITION PLAN

The Transition Plan introduces whole grain while decreasing the amount of refined grain products normally consumed. It increases the amount of daily vegetables, introduces beans, and decreases the amount of animal protein and dairy products consumed. The Transitional Foods wedge is for part of your previous diet, provided that you reduce the quantity and seek better quality. The circle diagram represents an approximate percentage volume of food consumed in the course of one day.

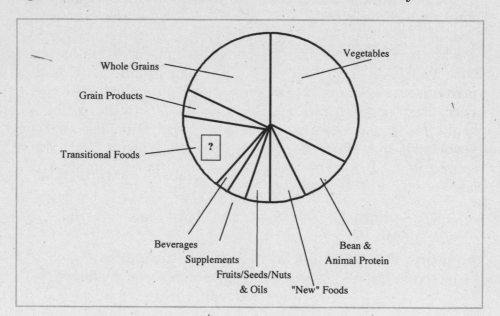

TRANSITION PLAN APPROXIMATE AMOUNTS FOR ONE DAY:

- **Whole Grains**—1 to 1½ cup (cooked)
- **Grain Products**—Bread, pasta, crackers, etc., 1–3 slices daily
- **Vegetables**—2–3 cups (variety of cooking styles, including raw)
- **Bean/Animal Protein**—Fish or chicken (meat, rarely) 3–4 times weekly. Have beans during vegetarian days.
- **"New" Foods**—Experiment with bean products/sea vegetables/ soy, etc.

- **Fruits**—2–3 times daily
- **Oils**—1–3 teaspoons daily (flax, olive, sesame)
- **Beverages**—After meals/in between meals
- **Supplements**—As per choice (see Chapter 9)
- **Transitional Foods**—Best quality of previous foods in smaller amounts

2. THE PREVENTION/THERAPEUTIC PLAN

The Prevention/Therapeutic Plan increases the amount of grains and vegetables while suggesting that three to four days weekly be vegetarian fare, replacing animal proteins (optional) with vegetable proteins (beans and bean products). This plan introduces sea vegetables and a section called the Swing Percentage—a percentage evenly divided between grain and vegetable or just emphasizing one category. This plan also suggests switching from fruit juices to whole fruit as a sweet source. *The circle diagram represents an approximate percentage volume of food consumed in the course of one day.*

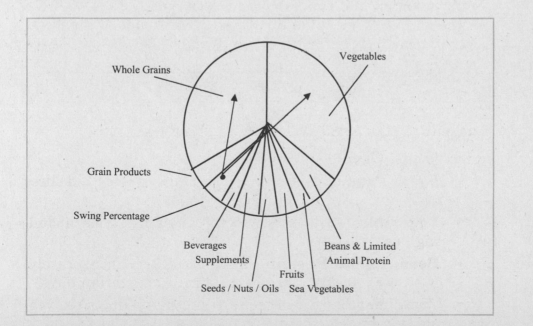

PREVENTION/THERAPEUTIC APPROXIMATE AMOUNTS FOR ONE DAY:

- **Whole Grains**—2–3 cups (cooked)
- **Grain Products**—Bread, pasta, crackers, etc., 1–2 slices daily
- **Vegetables**—3–4 cups (variety of cooking styles, including raw)
- **Bean/Animal Protein**—Fish or chicken (meat, rarely) 2–3 times weekly. Have beans during vegetarian days.
- **Sea Vegetables**—Condiments, side dishes, soup stocks
- **Fruits**—1–2 times daily
- **Oils**—1–2 teaspoons daily (flax, olive, sesame)
- **Beverages**—After meals/in between meals
- **Supplements**—As per choice (see Chapter 9)
- **Swing Percentage**—More of grain or more of vegetable, according to desire

THE BIG PICTURE—DAILY FOOD SERVINGS

Grams, calories, and ounces: three words synonymous with the word *diet*. Get an earful of television commercials or glance at cover titles of popular women's magazines and you'll be

THE ART OF CHEWING

"Drink your food, and chew your drink."
—Ghandi

The importance of thorough chewing cannot be overemphasized. Complex carbohydrates first begin digestion in the mouth. Alkaline enzymes found in saliva initiate carbohydrate breakdown. Chewing is how we expose the surface areas of food to these powerful enzymes. While you may notice an increase in appetite and an ability to tolerate more food, be wary of stuffing yourself; even good quality food, in excess, can result in hyperacidity, poor assimilation, and subsequent fatigue. Whole food becomes naturally sweeter the more it is chewed. Chewing helps us to distinguish the real from the artificial.

reminded about our national obsession with serving sizes, ounce and gram measurements, and calorie counting.

The dietary guidelines of *Nature's Cancer-Fighting Food Plan* makes these measurements unnecessary. Cup suggestions are given only as an approximation. The natural fiber content of the program's staple foods will fill you up without filling you out—so to speak. Another way to look at amounts is by visualizing the general percentages for an entire day's consumption, as illustrated by the divided-pie-plate suggestions. If you've been very active, you'll naturally crave more food.

Here are your daily dietary guidelines under *Nature's Cancer-Fighting Food Plan:*

- *Eat a good portion of whole grain.* This will help with bowel regularity, provide valuable B vitamins, regulate blood sugar, and naturally curb cravings for sugar and dietary fat. Sample whole grains: brown rice, oats, barley, millet, buckwheat, quinoa.

- *Eat a generous serving of dark leafy greens.* These can be selected from the previous food listings. Dark leafy greens are natural blood cleansers, high in valuable minerals with documented anticancer qualities. Sample leafy greens: broccoli, collards, mustard greens, turnip greens, bok choy, kale, Chinese and regular cabbage, brussel sprouts.

- *Eat a serving of root vegetables.* Containing concentrated minerals, root vegetables offer a very satisfying meal addition. Sample root vegetables: carrots, beets, celery root, red and white radish (daikon), parsnip, rutabaga, turnip, burdock, onion, leek, scallion.

- *Eat a serving of yellow-orange vegetables.* High in the cancer-fighting antioxidant beta-carotene, many of these vegetables offer a naturally sweet taste. Sample yellow-orange vegetables: squashes, carrots, yams, sweet potato, rutabagas.

- *Protein serving.* Vegetable-quality proteins: beans, tofu, tempeh, miso. Limit animal source proteins according to the plan you choose (from 1–3 times weekly and in 3- to 5-ounce portions).

- *Fruit serving.* Ideally, seasonal fruits with ample fiber, such as apple, pear, peach, apricot, melons, berries. Tropical fruits, more concentrated in sugar, should be limited. Fruit juice is not recommended as frequent fare because it is highly concentrated in simple sugars. Fruit is best enjoyed separately, between meals, but should be limited in cases of fatigue.

- *Oil serving.* A small portion of oil on a daily basis can make meals more satisfying and reduce cravings for dairy and meat products. Essential fatty acids can be obtained from the following oils: olive, sesame, flax, and borage. These can be added to cooking (except for flax) at the end of a water stir-fry, or used as a salad dressing addition. Choose organic oils stored in the refrigerated section of your natural foods outlet. Oils are best if kept cool and not directly heated on the skillet surface when cooking. If added to cooking, they are usually added at the very end stages when there is a slight bit of water at the bottom of the pan. This keeps the oil from getting too hot. In the course of one day, your combined fat intake of oils, nuts, seeds, and animal protein might be excessive, so be aware of your overall fat content. Generally, about 1 to 2 teaspoons of oil per day is all that is necessary. This can vary either way, but as a general rule, it should suffice.

MAKING A CHANGE

There seem to be two schools of thought when it comes to the idea of change:

- *A Gradual Transition Approach.* This plan is a progressive weaning from non-health-supporting foods while increasing natural whole foods and health-supportive lifestyle strategies.

- *The "Dive In" Approach.* This plan involves no testing of the water temperature. You immerse yourself completely and immediately stop all non-health-supportive foods and lifestyle practices at once.

Deciding which program to choose should be based on your health priorities; available time to plan, shop, and cook; and rest. It might also depend on your food habits or food addictions—in the mild sense of the word. For example, if you mechanically drink several cups of coffee every morning, to stop suddenly will only work if you can tolerate possible headaches and fatigue while combating cravings for stimulants.

If your daily work requires energy levels that caffeine has previously helped you to maintain, it might not be practical to cease immediately, as one of the withdrawal symptoms can be extreme fatigue. It might be less stressful to consider a gradual decrease over several days or weeks to avoid such withdrawal symptoms. However, I've found that both methods have their place, and choosing one over the other has to be a personal choice.

My own experience with coffee runs a little more to the extreme. Whenever I've begun to drink coffee and find myself with a renewed habit, withdrawal, for me, has rarely proven successful. I find that a morning half-cup becomes three-quarters and then justifies itself to a cup because I can rationalize: "Well, I was going to have a half-cup and then it became three-quarters—guess I might as well have a whole cup ..." and suddenly, I'm back to where I began. Being aware of my own addictive tendencies with coffee, I am most successful when I stop completely; cold turkey, no mas, finito, adios café.

If one method does not serve you successfully, try the other—a formidable challenge beckons!

11
FOOD PREPARATION AND COOKING FOR LIFETIME HEALTH BENEFITS

No Time to Cook?

The most common reaction I hear about cooking, or the familiar aphorism "slaving in the kitchen," is "I really don't have time to cook." Whenever I hear this, I'm always reminded of the cynical response to this statement I heard an 89-year-old naturopath from the Pacific Northwest give to his patients:

> *"That's all right. You should just wait ..."*
> *He'd pause after that sentence and wait for his client to respond.*
> *"Wait for what?" would be the reply.*
> *Then, with an uncharacteristic intensity, he'd lean forward and say:*
> *"Wait until you come out of the hospital after your tumor removal, or the bypass you're headed for, and as you recuperate—hopefully—you'll have plenty of time to cook and plan."*

I doubt most of his patients appreciated his humor, but his point was clear. Why wait until you get sick? Why wait until you become too sick to take care of your health? Choose to change now, instead of later being forced to change.

Many years ago, I was asked to consult with a very wealthy single businesswoman, in her early sixties, at her home. She pulled up in her chauffeured Bentley as I arrived and waited by the gate. She waved me in behind her car. She stepped out of the car and formally greeted me. We walked up her front stairs, past the marbled Roman columns to a large wooden door with strange carvings of animals, which was framed around a beautiful color montage of stained glass.

Her 22-room mansion had high-tech security, perfectly manicured landscapes, thick, natural fiber carpets, antique furniture, and magnificent art and sculpture throughout its main rooms. Five household employees greeted her at the door; one with the day's home telephone messages and numerous faxes, one whose sole function was to walk her many dogs and give a written daily dog report, a housecleaner, personal assistant, and a full time landscaper.

However, there was no cook. She was adamant about doing that herself. But she really didn't cook. "I *warm*," she told me flatly. "If it takes more than ten minutes, I'm not interested—don't even talk to me about it." She was consulting me because her friend found great relief from arthritic pain with my program and another friend's breast lumps had noticeably reduced within two months. I gave her all the details of my program, but with some quick rearranging in my head for her specific needs; I suggested boxed, canned, and frozen items that could all be prepared within her ten-minute limit. It was an ideological compromise for me, but, I rationalized, any change in the direction of my program would serve her better, maybe even inspire her to do more.

I explained that I was customizing this for her and if she found improvement, she might want to accelerate her progress by actually doing some cooking. With that statement, she peered at me from over the rim of her eyeglasses and succinctly said,

"Don't bet on it."

I dropped the matter and smiled understandingly.

Two weeks later, my telephone machine carried this message:

"Hello, this is Ms. _____ . I seem to be doing quite well, surprisingly, on this program of yours. And uh ..., well, ... if ... if I were going to actually cook, could you furnish some recipes?"

It was a definite triumph for her. A noticeable improvement in energy levels, sleep, bowel regularity, and sense of calm opened her mind to even greater possibilities. Suddenly, she had a new value for preparing food because of her conviction that the recent changes had come as a result of her new diet and lifestyle.

This is what it's about: redefining your relationship with your kitchen, from relating to cooking as a "chore" to instead thinking about your kitchen as the "Alchemical Center for Health Transformation." In fact, I once had a client who made a sign out of that title and hung it over the entrance to his kitchen as a daily reminder.

Another important perspective is that cooking, food preparation, and planning are simply another way we self-parent ourselves. We assume responsibility for controlling our health,

---

SHOPPING HINTS

Here are a few guidelines to help you purchase healthy, nutritionally sound foods:

- Buy local, seasonal, fresh, and organic whenever possible.
- Find out if your city has open street farmers' markets and get to know your growers.
- Buy in bulk whenever possible. This is usually less expensive but requires storage room.
- Read labels. Remember, "Natural" is just a marketing slogan. Sugars usually end in "-ose" (such as fructose, dextrose, etc.), and beware of corn syrup, evaporated cane juice, Sucanat ©, and brown sugar—all still highly concentrated forms of sugar.
- Consider the hidden sources of oil in baked goods, crackers, cookies, tofu, veggie and soy burgers, and tofu salads, etc., when attempting to lower fat intake.

to the best of our abilities and recognize that the first step begins with the commitment to care for yourself in a disciplined and consistent way. This begins with the food fundamentals of educating yourself, planning meals, creating new cooking rituals, and cultivating a willingness to adventure into self-experimentation. Eventually, you'll discover numerous short cuts that will save time without compromising the integrity of your efforts. That's the inspiring part.

Planning the next day's meal, having staples on hand, making sure you have leftovers for fast and easy dishes or roll-ups (tortilla, chapattis, pocket-bread [pita]) makes cooking more efficient, less stressful, and quicker.

VARIETY—THE NATURAL SPICE OF YOUR MEALS

The Western diet has an enormous amount of variety, from textures and colors to consistencies and tastes. Not being conscious of how to use these different elements can be a recipe for boredom. Here are some general techniques for achieving variety:

- *Food Selection*—You can choose from whole grains, cracked or rolled grains, grain products, vegetables, beans and bean products, sea vegetables, animal proteins, fruits, condiments and seasonings, herbs, natural pickles, and beverages.

- *Methods of Cooking*—Foods can be pot cooked, pressure cooked, made into soups and stews, steamed, boiled, stir fried with water or oil, pressed, dry roasted, marinated, served raw, pickled, baked, or grilled.

- *Cutting, Slicing, and Chopping*—Foods can also be prepared in different shapes and sizes to quicken cooking times, concentrate flavors, or inspire visual appetite.

- *Use of Water*—The amount or type of water used in cooking can also lend variety. A vegetable stock can be created for cooking soups or adding to vegetables.

- *Use of Seasonings and Condiments*—These can be herbal seasonings, sea salt, soy sauce, vinegar, miso, flaked sea vegetables, spices, or roasted nuts and seeds.

- *Length of Cooking Time*—Lengths of time usually vary according to the season. In temperate climates, we are usually inclined to cook less during the summer, whereas in winter, stews and porridges produce more desirable warmth.
- *Combinations*—The mixing of various dishes and different foods lends variety to the diet.

METHODS OF COOKING

There are many methods of cooking that are used to create variety, offer cooling or warming aspects to your meals, and enhance nutrition. Some methods are considered healthier than others. Ultimately, your intuition might be the best guide in choosing a cooking method.

Traditionally, foods were cooked over burning embers that had to be tended. According to natural food chef and author Rebecca Wood, "The more solid the fuel a food is cooked upon, the longer the food retains warmth, the more energy it imparts and the more delicious it tastes. How good is a marshmallow cooked over an electrical range or in the microwave?"

Wood and gas heat produce infrared radiation, which some nutritional educators claim energizes the food. Many upscale restaurants and ethnic eateries (Southwestern cuisine or East Indian, for example) advertise their natural wood ovens and mesquite grills for the unique flavoring and taste they produce.

Here's a rundown on the key sources of food-cooking energy:

- *Wood Cooking*—Unless you're living in the country and have the time (and the wood), this might be a bit impractical. The popularity of eating over a campfire or the ritual of the American cookout during outdoor gatherings or picnics contains a sensory appeal that stems from food being cooked over a wood-generated flame.
- *Natural Gas*—This is one of the healthiest options for everyday cooking. Many people claim that food cooked by natural gas tastes better than food cooked on electrical ranges. It is also easier to regulate heat and gauge tem-

perature. A potato cooked in a wood or gas oven differs in taste from one cooked electrically or in a microwave.

- *Electrical Cooking*—One of the disadvantages of electrical ranges is the limitation they impose on the cook's creativity, since the heat settings are limited to fixed heat temperatures. Electricity is the alternating charge between a positive and negative pole at 60 cycles per second. Its heat energy, unlike wood or gas, does not require oxygen. According to macrobiotic teacher Michio Kushi, electrical cooking diminishes, rather than enhances, a food's energetic composition. The best way to test this is by a simple taste comparison.

- *Microwave Cooking*—Evolved for our "on-the-go," disposable society, microwave ovens are now used by one out of every two homes in the United States. Microwaving is a questionable method of cooking food for health on a regular basis. The advertised "convenience" factor reduces the attention we give to its potential harm. The microwave appeal of being able to boil water in "only seconds," as opposed to 45 seconds, seems to perpetuate our neurosis for getting the cooking process "over with." Microwave cooking diminishes a food's energy pattern by energetically disrupting its biomolecular structure. This form of nonionizing radiation, accelerated beyond electricity, makes a food's water molecules vibrate so rapidly that their motion is responsible for cooking the food.

CHOOSING A COOKING STYLE TO FIT YOUR NEEDS

Often, I've suggested that clients eat more vegetables. The common response is, "Great! I love salad—could eat it all the time."

"Salad" is not a vegetable category. It is a cooking style, and one of many. The following is a list and brief explanation of various cooking styles that offer a sense of variety and provide different qualities of nutrition and energy to your meals.

MICROWAVE WARNINGS

Available studies on microwaving have shown the following:

- According to the *Lancet,* Britain's premier medical journal, microwaved food, upon ingestion, can cause "structural, functional, and immunological changes in the body. It [microwave cooking] converts the amino acid L-proline into a proven toxin to the nervous system, liver and kidneys."

- Light and radiation researcher/author John Ott suggests that consumption of microwaved foods immediately reduces normal muscle strength.

- A study reported in the *Journal of the American Dietetic Association* concluded that microwave heating of human milk destroys vital immunoglobin A. Immunoglobin A is a protein necessary for a baby's essential physical development and for increasing natural immunity.

- Another study suggested that fats are denatured by microwave radiation, resulting in free radical formation—a highly carcinogenic occurrence.

- Andrew Weil, M.D., frequent media personality and author of numerous nutritional books, offers the following comments on microwaving:

    There may be real dangers associated with mircowaving food. We don't know enough about how microwaves affect our bodies to feel entirely safe with them. This longer-wave form of radiation can cook human tissues exposed to it directly, and even low doses may disrupt the delicate operations of biological control systems in our bodies. Weak electrical currents and electromagnetic fields are known to affect cellular growth and development, and to aid in the healing of tissue. Microwaves could have a negative effect on cell structures.

While there have been a number of studies that warrant concern, this is still an area of investigation that must be explored more thoroughly before conclusive claims can be made. However, discretion in choosing an established, healthy, and worry-free form of cooking might offer more mental comfort by not compromising long-term health.

- *Steaming*—Steamed food usually has a light taste, cooks quickly, and retains less water. The key to steaming vegetables is to bring the water to a boil before adding the vegetables. This can be done with a double-layered pot, with stainless steel steaming trays or Asian bamboo steaming baskets. An interesting variation is to use an approximate 2-foot square of white muslin that has been wrung out in pure cold water. The vegetables are placed in the cloth, which is then folded over the food and placed into the tray. After adding about 1 to 2 inches of water to the pot, bring to a boil; add the steaming tray(s) and cover. The steaming cloth absorbs excess moisture and keeps the vegetables fairly dry. Many items can be steamed or reheated with steam. Steaming works especially well for broccoli, cauliflower, cabbage, cut onions, and various root and ground vegetables.

- *Pressure Cooking*—Pressure cooking is an ancient form of cooking. This method may be used for different foods, but is most popular for cooking whole grain. The value of this type of cooking method, in regard to whole grains, is in the way high pressure penetrates the heat into the outer covering of the whole grain. This softens it, making it more digestible and easier to assimilate. Pressure-cooking often brings out a sweeter taste in most grains. It is one of many ways to cook grains and creates a healthy sense of variety.

- *Pot Cooking*—Used for stews, soups, and cooking grain. A covered pot, water, and ingredients are all that is necessary.

- *Soups*—Soups can be profoundly satisfying. Generally, they can be made by pot cooking or pressure-cooking methods and can include combinations of beans, vegetables, grains, or made with fish or chicken stock. A popular Asian technique for mineralizing soups is to add a small stick of a mild-tasting seaweed called kombu. I usually refer to kombu as oriental bay leaf since it is used in the same way as regular bay leaves are used in soups or sauces. A small (approximately 2 inch) piece of kombu makes a healthy addition to any soup and aids bean digestion by breaking down the starches responsible for gas.

- *Sauté (Water Stir Fry/Oil Stir Fry)*—Water fry means simply sautéing with water. Oil sauté uses oil. Instead of the common sauté style where the oil is heated in a skillet and the food fried, try the Chinese method of water-oil frying—add a little oil toward the end of the cooking. Very short-term, low-heat doesn't negatively change the chemical nature of the oil, as prolonged dry heat does, and preserves the natural flavor of the oil. Water frying is one of the best ways to prepare hard leafy greens to bring out their natural sweetness.

- *Raw*—Predominantly popular in the Western world, raw food is a refreshing addition to any vegetable plate. It is especially balancing to eat with animal protein (cooked animal meats with raw vegetable foods) and can be easier to digest if chopped into chewable sizes. For people with digestive disorders, poor assimilation, anemia, or high acidity, vegetables that are slightly cooked are often easier to digest.

- *Boiling*—In different culinary traditions there are many styles of boiling. There's quick boiling (usually known as *blanching*), where the vegetables are cooked in boiling water for 15 to 60 seconds. Although they still keep their "crunch" and maintain color, they can be easier to digest than raw vegetables. Another cooking style, used frequently during cold weather, is long simmering. In this cooking method the vegetables, usually starchy root varieties (squash, radish, turnip, carrot, onion, etc.), are cooked in a very small amount of water. A light sprinkle of sea salt helps the vegetables surrender additional water. The vegetables can be cooked until they are tender. This style of cooking, called *Nishime* by the Japanese, is used to restore vitality.

- *Pressing/Marinating*—While it might sound quite strange to eat a salad that has been "pressed," this style of food preparation has been a staple in many parts of Eastern Europe and Asia. Using a sea-salt, herbal, and/or spice marination, hearty vegetables such as cabbage, wild greens, onions, radish, cucumber, endive, etc., are finely shredded, torn, or grated, then crushed and kneaded with a slightly salty seasoning. Made in a ceramic crock and covered with a plate and heavy weight on top, these salads are pressed for 24 hours before serving. You can usually obtain a plastic "pickle press" from most Asian markets or a reliable cooking supply store. These small commercial presses have screw-down lids and, while smaller, are more convenient than conventional crocks. This style of cooking creates crispy, crunchy raw vegetable textures that are easier to digest. Pressed salad is usually served as a small side dish to larger portion main vegetable dishes.

- *Baking*—Commonly used for preparing hearty root vegetables, ground varieties (squashes and pumpkins, casseroles) and other dishes. Baking brings out the natural sugars in these vegetables, giving them a rich, syrupy sweet taste. Some vegetables can be baked in their whole state, such as squashes or onions, or cut and baked in a covered glass or ceramic dish. Cookbook author Aveline Kushi writes, "Baking requires longer cooking but gives strength and flavor. In most other cooking methods, such as boiling, energy goes from the bottom of the pot to the top. In baking, vegetables absorb energy evenly and radiate it from the center."

- *Broiling*—Broiling gives vegetables a distinctive bitter or slightly burnt flavor and allows soft vegetables to retain their natural shape. Vegetable shiskebabs with onions, carrots, summer squash, peppers, or tempeh (bean product) make wonderful side dishes. Broiling can also be used to prepare fish or chicken.

THE TWIN MENACES OF GRILLING: PAHS AND HCAS

Whenever fat drips on a flame, heating element, or hot coals, chemicals called PAHs (polycyclic aromatic hydrocarbons) form. The PAHs waft up in the smoke and land on the food. They can also form directly on food when it's cooked to a crisp.

"If you throw a steak or hamburger on the grill and let it get really brown—where the fat's dripping off it and flames and smoke are shooting up—that's the stuff you don't want to do," says National Cancer Institute epidemiologist Rashmi Sinha.

As early as 1775, PAH-containing soot was linked to cancer of the scrotum in chimney sweeps. Today, grilled meat is the major source of PAHs in our food.

Of more than 100 PAHs found in the environment, at least 19 have been identified in cooked food. As many as 12 of the 19 PAHs found in cooked food have been found to cause cancer in laboratory animals. Proof that they can cause cancer in humans is yet to be confirmed. Preventing PAHs is simply a matter of keeping the fat from dripping on the heat, which is why broiling (using a heat source above the food), or any type of cooking in a pan (e.g., stewing or baking), results in few if any PAHs. That's also why grilled fatty meats like pork contain more PAHs than leaner cuts.

Cooking meat, poultry, or fish at high temperatures can also present a problem. There are about six potentially cancer-causing chemicals called HCAs, or hetercyclic amines, which are created when animal meats are cooked at high temperatures.

"We know these compounds can probably cause cancer in humans," says Elizabeth Snyderwine, Chief of the Chemical Carcinogenesis Section at the National Cancer Institute (NCI) in Bethesda, Maryland. "What we don't know yet is how significant a problem they are in the American diet."

Until there's more evidence, you're better off being cautious. "It makes sense to avoid [HCAs] when we can," says Mark Knize of the Lawrence Livermore National Laboratory in Livermore, California.

"Meat and poultry produce the most HCAs because they contain the most amino acids and creatine, which are converted into HCAs," comments Lawrence Livermore's James Felton. "Seafood produces much less, and plant foods like veggieburgers, fruits and vegetables little or none."

Cooking with liquid—as in boiling, steaming, poaching, or stewing—generates no HCAs because the temperature never tops the boiling point of water.

THE FIVE SAVORY TASTES

The Five Savory Tastes are not a singing group. They are the recognized basic five tastes that are naturally contained in all foods. In traditional Asian medicine, each taste is correlated with a season, a type of warming or cooling energy, and a specific body organ or system. Theoretically, each taste nourishes a specific organ or organ system.

Practically speaking, the more you consciously include a variety of the five tastes in food preparation, the more satisfying and nutritionally enhanced your meals will be. Sometimes just a small amount of a "taste" can contribute significantly (e.g., a sprig of bitter-tasting parsley leaf).

The five tastes are bitter, salty, sweet, sour, and pungent. A food will never contain one exclusive taste; there will always be a predominance of tastes. Here are some examples of food sources and Asian medical organ connections for each taste. It is said that a little of a particular taste can strengthen an organ system, whereas excess can weaken it.

- *Bitter*—Associated with the early and mid-summer season, bitter foods are thought to stimulate the heart and small intestine. These foods include dandelion, parsley leaves, mustard greens, collard greens, burdock root, sesame seeds, cereal grain coffee substitute, and some types of corn.

- *Salty*—Associated with the winter season, salty food imparts strength and is thought to influence the kidneys and bladder. These foods include sea vegetables, miso, soy sauce, sea salt, umeboshi salt plum, and natural brine pickles.

- *Sweet*—Associated with the late-summer season, sweet food is thought to influence the pancreas, spleen, and stomach—organs of sugar absorption and distribution. Its nourishing effect is centering and relaxing. The sweet taste refers to natural whole foods and not the excessively refined sweet we know from white sugar. Sweet foods make up the largest percentage of our meals. These foods include whole grains, vegetables—especially, cabbages, carrots, onions, squashes, and parsnips—as well as sweet potato and chestnuts.

- *Sour*—Associated with the spring season, sour-tasting food has a constrictive effect, giving quickening energy. It is thought to influence the liver and gall bladder. These foods include sourdough bread, vinegar, wheat, sauerkraut, and lemon/lime.

- *Pungent*—Associated with the autumn season, the pungent taste gives off a hot, dispersing energy and is said to be beneficial to the lungs and colon. However, an excess of these foods can irritate the intestines. Pungent foods have been known to stimulate blood circulation and, according to Asian folk medicine, have a natural ability to help break down accumulation in the body. In most culinary cuisincs, they are commonly combined with animal protein and with foods high in fat. These foods include scallions, daikon radish, ginger, peppers, wasabe (dry mustard), and horseradish.

HOW FOODS FIT THE FIVE TASTES

For convenient referencing, the following chart lists some basic foods that fall into each category:

Bitter	Salty	Sweet	Sour	Pungent
Kale	Sea salt	Corn	Lemon	Ginger
Collards	Tamari	Cooked onions	Lime	Garlic
Mustard greens	Miso	Squash	Sauerkraut	Raw onions
Parsley	Sea vegetables	Yams	Umeboshi plum	White radish
Endive	Sesame salt	Cooked grain	Fermented dishes	Red radish
Celery	Umeboshi plum	Cooked cabbage	Pickles	Scallions
Arugula	Pickles	Carrots		Wasabi
Grain beverage		Parsnips		Spices
		Fruits		

While most of your meals will contain a minimum of 60 percent sweet foods (whole grains, vegetables, beans, and fruit), aim for a full range of other tastes with major meals. The other tastes can be represented in side dishes, sauces, and condiments, emphasizing a particular taste you may crave. There is a definite art to meal balancing.

The combination possibilities are plentiful with cancer-fighting qualities. The underlying principle dictates that these flavors, while seeming antagonistic (not compatible), are actually, by virtue of meal balancing, complementary.

Meals that include the five tastes will prove more satisfying, in terms of limiting cravings, and more fortifying. Many of the recipe suggestions in Chapter 12 take this into account. An example of this balance factor can be seen in recipes that call for oil; pungent or sour flavors taken in combination with oil help make oils easier to digest. Other examples of this might be mustard (pungent) and tamari (salty) with fish, or salt added to water-fried (or sautéed) onions. Eventually, this will become a natural practice as you develop your cooking efficiency and planning ability and comfortably ease into your new way of eating.

THE MEANING OF BREAKFAST

According to a recent statistic, one in four Americans never eats a morning meal, while 12 percent does so only "occasionally." The most frequent offenders against this traditional ritual are teens and young adults. Adults over 50 are the most likely to eat a morning meal. Over 72 percent of men and woman over 50 claim to eat a daily breakfast.

Modern researchers report that individuals eating ample morning meals have less tendency to gain weight, when compared with those who skip the morning meal and dine later. Their findings also indicate that those who eat a daily breakfast repeatedly outperform those who abstain from breakfast in both physical and mental activities.

The familiar morning ritual of "breaking the fast" has become less popular due to a number of reasons: long morning commutes to work, extended schedules arranged around the obligations of work, large dinner meals with no activity afterward and late-night eating. Late eating or snacking causes digestion to occur during times when our bodies should be resting and distributing the daily intake of nutrients—as opposed to digesting in a static horizontal position. Late-night eating frrequently results in fatigue the following day.

Our digestion is especially sensitive as our body awakens and the blood begins to speed its circulation. It is best to do light exercise before taking food and not to burden the body by overeating. Regular meal times beginning with consistent breakfasts will ensure minimum cravings for overeating and foods that are not health supportive.

Other conditions associated with late-night eating are unwanted weight gain, morning sluggishness, depression, and a lack of mental clarity. One important factor in cancer recovery is keeping the immune system is top shape. Weight gain, insulin swings, and high blood acidity contribute to nutritional depletion and can hinder immune function.

Avoiding breakfast frequently leads to a mild low blood sugar level that can bring on fatigue and irritability. It can also instigate strong cravings for sugar or refined foods that are capable of quickly elevating the blood sugar level. Breakfast skippers usually reverse the order of eating, having little or nothing for breakfast, average lunches, and large dinners instead of a healthy opposite pattern.

My Yugoslavian friend, Ruska, tells me that growing up in her country, familial wisdom suggested "to eat breakfast like a king, lunch like prince, and dinner like a pauper"—or Queen and Princess, as it may apply.

Good advice for any culture.

"I'd rather poke a stick in my eye then eat vegetables for breakfast."

A cancer client of mine half-jokingly uttered this colorful statement after I recommended limiting sweet-treat breakfasts and including a morning side dish of vegetables. That statement was logical coming from him—a fiercely loyal Harley Davidson motorcyclist who wore a T-shirt saying, "I'd rather eat a can of worms then ride a Honda."

By his facial reaction to my vegetable suggestion, you'd think I was asking him to sacrifice his first-born child.

"Vegetables? For breakfast? Are you kidding?" he asked, astounded.

"Absolutely!" I shot back. "Hey, man have you ever eaten an omelet with mushrooms, green peppers, tomatoes, and onions, or with spinach? And maybe had a small glass of tomato juice with it? We're talking vegetables, aren't we?"

He nodded grudgingly, looking as though I'd snatched his favorite toy.

Culturally and worldwide, our American breakfast habits are considered strange and unusual. Up to recently, traditional fare in the British Isles included an oat cereal, cooked all night with a side of local sea vegetables. Throughout Asia, you'll find cooked vegetables with grain porridges for breakfast and, in certain countries, pickles are offered as an alkaline morning side dish—presumably to counter accumulated acids from the previous evening's dinner.

In China, the popular breakfast is called "congee," a traditional morning dish of long-cooked grains with a porridge texture, often containing additions of pickled egg, small amounts of various kinds of meats, cooked vegetables, spices, raw scallions and sometimes, brine pickles. Eaten with relish, this nourishing stew fortifies one with energy throughout the morning—a stark contrast to the modern American machine-blown, enriched, colored, artificially flavored, and highly sugared puffed cereals, soaking in milk, to which we compound the sugar content by adding fruit. To some, it's initially a savory meal, but fatiguing in the long run.

Occasionally, I'll have a natural food equivalent of a popular commercial dry cereal with some soy milk and perhaps a piece of fruit, which I fully enjoy. It serves as a sentimental throwback to memorable childhood breakfasts, where additional entertainment was provided by reading the back of the cereal box. But unlike a wholesome hot cereal with a small side dish of vegetables, I am left unsatisfied and soon tired. By late morning, my biggest craving is to take a nap.

Rarely did older established cultures pour sweet syrups, refined sugar, or even milk into their morning porridges. Now, many people find a morning bowl of fresh fruit appealing as a breakfast. Although this may be initially satisfying, the simple sugar of fructose cannot sustain our needs for endurance energy. Such a breakfast, contrary to a number of fad diets which speak glowingly of fruits as "cleansing foods," can result in a late morning energy slump. Perhaps you'll want to use a little bit of raisin or cinnamon with rolled oats, but don't limit yourself to only what is familiar. Experiment with other, more nourishing and whole possibilities, such as dark leafy greens, orange or yellow-colored vegetables, or round vegetable varieties to meet your nutritional needs.

"THINKING ABOUT BREAKFAST GIVES ME A HEADACHE ..."

I once consulted with a woman in her mid-forties who continually nodded her head, positively acknowledging every sentence I uttered. I went over the dietary lists carefully and made sure she understood my suggestions. More nods. Before she left, I closed my notebook and addressed her directly.

"Now, before you leave, I want to make sure that I've answered all of your concerns, so if you have any lingering questions ..."

"No. Absolutely. You've made everything very clear. It's really not very complicated," she shrugged. "I think I can handle it," she assured.

"Well, I just like to be sure because it might seem complicated, but as you become more familiar with it, you'll realize it's actually quite simple."

"I'm sure," she said confidently.

She smiles and leaves. The following morning I get a frantic telephone call.

"I feel so overwhelmed! There's so much to do ... oh, my ... just thinking about breakfast gives me a headache—what do you do for breakfast? I'm so used to ..."

The trick to enjoying such a breakfast is learning to chew. Thorough chewing of whole grains brings out their subtle, whole, and natural sweetness—a sweetness that is not overwhelming and that energizes. Whole grains can also be soaked for several hours (or overnight) in a small amount of water to minimize the acid content held in their vitamin-charged, seven-layer covering. This makes the assimilation of fiber nutrients easier and more nourishing. A pinch of sea salt also increases the grain digestion by making it less acidic and bringing out more of the grains natural sweetness, in the same way that a dash of salt can make an apple slice sweeter.

Become a willing adventurer and experience vegetables as a small part of your breakfast. They make a delicious complement to combined grain porridges, garnished with seeds or nuts and other condiments.

GENTLY BREAKING YOUR BREAKFAST HABITS

Most of us eat specific foods for certain meals. We generally like something soft for breakfast, because few of us want to jump up from a deep sleep and begin the work of chewing. So our established custom is to have soggy cereal with fruit, gooey oatmeal, or soft and easy eggs accompanied by a popular breakfast addition that contrasts the soft texture of eggs with its own coarseness—the ubiquitous toast. For lunch, we typically eat a sandwich with maybe a cup of soup. Dinner is commonly reserved for a protein "main entré." I've found that most people can handle lunches and dinners creatively, but when it comes to breakfast, anything that deviates from the traditional norm, for some people, can be very stressing (see sidebar).

The three breakfast items just mentioned are pretty much the staple in America, unless you're like a cousin of mine, who, in defiance of the common rules, likes to jumpstart his morning with two colas and a pizza. It must be the rebel in him.

Because of typical breakfast traditions, you might find yourself missing what has been familiar to you. Therefore, if this morning meal becomes the struggle of the day, I'd suggest you fashion it as much as possible with what has been familiar to you—except for using better-quality ingredients.

Here are some examples:

TYPICAL BREAKFAST

NATURE'S CANCER-FIGHTING FOOD PLAN BREAKFAST

- Instant, flavored oatmeal with sugar,

Rolled oats, flavored with some fruit, and milk cinnamon, small amounts of raisins and soy milk. Another type of oat called steel-cut oats make a delicious and chewy breakfast. You can also cook any whole grain with extra water for a longer period (often the night before) of time and eat it the following morning after warming. Different toppings can be roasted nuts or seeds, sesame salt, or cinnamon. Sometimes I recommend diluting a level teaspoon of miso paste and mixing it into hot cereal, along with nut toppings. Cereals such as this are naturally sweet, warming, and nourishing. It might be more satisfying to have a piece of toast with a thin spread of nut/seed butter along with the soft grain if you miss that familiar texture combination.

- Eggs with toast and bacon

Egg-white omelet with vegetables, or tofu scramble (see recipe section), and/or fried/baked tempeh strips.

- Commercial dried breakfast

Select a natural version of dried cereal with milk, sugar, and cereal—use soy, rice, oat, or almond fruit milk in place of dairy milk along with fresh fruit.

COOKING TIMES FOR COMMON GRAINS

- **Quick-Cooking Grains** (up to 15 minutes): Rolled oats, buckwheat, basmati rice, couscous, corn grits, steel-cut oats, quinoa, teff, amaranth.
- **Medium-Cooking Grains** (20 to 35 minutes): Millet, sweet brown rice and white rice.
- **Long-Cooking Grains** (45 minutes +; these can be soaked for added nutritional benefits): Brown rice, wild rice, unhulled barley, pearl barley, oat groats, kamut, rye, spelt, and wheat.

"GRAINS ARE SOOOOOO BLAND-TASTING!"

Not exactly. Only seems that way. The real problem is our taste buds; they have become dulled by concentrated sweet foods. We've forgotten how to taste and chew and savor our food. That's principally because the food we're eating today has little real taste. It's an addictive overwhelm of sweetness, or flavor-trapped-in-fat quality; however, the more you chew poor-quality (non-health-supportive) food, the worse it tastes. Real food offers the opposite; its taste becomes increasingly sweet the more it is chewed and as the inherent sugars are gradually reduced to simpler forms. When mothers complain their children never eat vegetables, I point out that due to the sheer high volume of their child's sugar intake, the more subtle sweetness of vegetables cannot be appreciated. Maybe that's why you'll never find broccoli-flavored ice cream.

Gandhi's famous quote about chewing underlines the need to break everything down to practically a liquid in the mouth: "Drink your food, and chew your drink," he was fond of saying. The first stage of digestion is when the saliva can begin to break down nutritional component. It all begins in the mouth. Still, many of us of us bolt and inhale our food. In fact, "food inhalation," literally, has been ranked as the sixth major cause of accidental death in the United States—just ahead of airplane crashes—death, by choking on your food.

Don't swallow your food before you taste it.

SAVORY GRAIN AND VEGETABLE COMBINATIONS

If eating whole grains is new to you, or if you'd like the sensation of more complex tastes, consider combining whole grains with finely cut vegetables (as in pilaf recipes), either precooked in water-sauté style or cooked together with grains. Toasted nuts, or even chestnuts, make a flavorful or naturally sweet addition to grains. The greater variety of tastes you can experience, the more satisfying this transition can become.

There are an infinite number of ways to prepare grains for taste, variety, and increased nutritional protection. Here are some favorite basic combinations.

- Brown rice with brown sweet rice, onions, and shiitake
- Brown rice with wild rice, fresh corn, and roasted pumpkin seeds
- Brown rice with millet or polenta and roasted almonds
- Brown rice with minced radish, parsley, and sunflower seeds
- Brown rice with lentils and onions
- Brown rice with chestnuts
- Brown rice with chickpeas, minced carrots, and onions
- Brown rice with millet and chickpeas
- Brown rice with barley and leeks and carrots
- Brown rice with quinoa, watercress, and walnuts
- Brown rice with sweet brown rice, black beans, and scallions
- Brown rice with aramanth
- Brown sweet rice with black beans and onions
- Brown sweet rice, millet, and almonds
- Brown sweet rice, millet, leeks, and black beans
- Brown sweet rice and sesame seeds
- Millet with minced onions, cube-cut carrots and finely chopped cabbage

- Millet with squash or sweet potato
- Millet with cauliflower and tahini
- Millet with squash and azuki beans
- Rolled oats and quinoa with sesame salt
- Barley with mushrooms, carrots, celery, and onions
- Quinoa with black beans and onions
- Quinoa with Chinese greens and roasted cashews
- Quinoa with dried cranberries and walnuts
- Quinoa with squash and sautéed onion
- Quinoa with onion, kale and lime

Additionally, to any grain you can add the following:

- A second grain—Any two or even three whole grains
- A seed or nut—Roasted seeds or nuts as a garnish or cooked into the dish
- A bean or legume—Prior cooked beans, or bean products (tofu, tempeh)
- A vegetable—From "sweet" category, or otherwise, cut into small pieces
- Condiments—Sesame salt, sea vegetable flakes, spices, herbs

The possibilities are plentiful. With a little planning and variety in combining, grain, vegetable, and bean dishes can become delightful standard fare full of new sensory discovery, meal enjoyment, and positive health benefit adding to your culinary repetoire.

REGARDING RECIPE INGREDIENT AMOUNTS

In contrast to Western cookbooks, which give very specific amounts, many traditional Asian cookbooks just list approximations. They leave it up to you to figure your specific needs. This is considered a matter of personal intuition. Instead of a "pinch" of salt, you'll be advised to "add salt to taste." This can drive some people crazy if they're approaching cooking mechanically. So, while I try to provide specific amounts, please keep in mind that these are suggestions, as opposed to doctrine. Trust your intuition. If your recipe seems to flop, remember the words of Benjamin Franklin: "I haven't failed, I've just found 10,000 ways that it did not work."

REGARDING SUBSTITUTIONS

In some recipes vegetables are oil-sautéed. According to current research, short-time low heating of oil is not harmful. High heating of oils, especially to the point of "smoking," creates potentially harmful free radical elements that are considered carcinogenic. In the event you are restricting oil or are not comfortable with heating oils, or for whatever reason do not want to "cook" oil, by all means feel free to eliminate this step in your recipes. Water can be substituted in place of oil to create a "water-fry" style of cooking.

KELP IS ON THE WAY!—INTRODUCING SEA VEGETABLES

It's not a very glamorous picture. Hear the word *seaweed* and you immediately picture slimy green stuff, encrusted with sand and assorted ocean debris. Mmmm, good!

While such a picture might be the stuff of an average dirty beach wash-up, the real picture is one of numerous ocean varieties of sea vegetables with varied shapes and rich colors ranging from emerald green to electric black. Most of the worlds' coastal cultures ate vegetables from the ocean, while inland cultures stored and prepared them in dried form.

Sea vegetables are extremely low in calories, low in fat, high in protein, and contain anywhere from 10 to 20 times the mineral content of land vegetables. They also have an alkalinizing effect on blood, helping to neutralize acid conditions.

Sea vegetables are excellent sources of omega-3-fatty acids and contain a form of fiber that can bind steroids and carcinogens. Extensive research has documented their ability to cleanse and detoxify the body, extracting wastes and toxins from our tissues to be discharged by elimination.

You might not be aware of this but you've probably been consuming a small amount of these vegetables for years, as essential ingredients in common prepared foods often unmentioned on commercial labeling. Caragheenan, an extract from seaweed, is used to thicken many processed foods, including ice cream, puddings, soups, sauces, dressing mixes, and packaged desserts. In fact, if you've ever eaten in an Asian restaurant, you've definitely had a taste of seaweed. Sea vegetables are used in numerous foods from soup stocks to side dishes to stir-fried dishes and, most popularly, sushi rolls.

With a wide variety of flavor and texture, sea vegetables (the politically correct version of *seaweeds*) have a great number of uses. Sea vegetables such as hiziki, kombu, wakame, and nori have been part of the Japanese diet for centuries. Usually harvested in tested waters under strict supervision, sea vegetables have very little fat content, which makes them less likely to retain potential pollution, as opposed to food higher in fat content.

Six sea vegetables are widely available from health food stores and markets:

1. *Nori*—Nori is a greenish-color sheet seaweed that is commonly wrapped around rice to create sushi rolls. It can be bought already toasted and used as a crumble in soups and side dishes or as a condiment. I used to buy delicious-tasting Nori that had been harvested from British Columbia Native tribes when I lived in British Columbia. They used it abundantly in their cooking and the kids used to walk around munching on it as a snack. It was probably the best Nori I've ever tasted.

2. *Kombu*—I usually refer to this as oriental bay leaf, because it is used in much the same way—as an addition to soups and bean dishes or baked and ground up to be used as a condiment for mineral-deficient conditions.

SEA VEGETABLES AND CANCER PREVENTION

Numerous studies have linked sea vegetable consumption to reduced cancers and tumor inhibition:

- Several studies have shown that the consumption of brown sea-weed, Laminaria, is directly related to a lower incidence of breast cancer. Other sea vegetables have also demonstrated to be protective against other forms of cancer.

- A processed product frequently sold in health food stores made from the sea vegetable wakame has been demonstrated to result in regression of lung cancer in laboratory animals.

- In a study at McGill University in Montreal, the role of polysac-charides from brown seaweed (kombu) showed it to inhibit the intestinal absorption of radioactive strontium: "brown seaweed's are unique agents because they selectively bind strontium." Earlier studies at McGill showed that the alginic acid in sea veg-etables bound to toxins in the body, including heavy metals, through a process commonly known as chelation.

- Studies at the Harvard School of Public Health discovered that animals fed only 5 percent of their diet in kelp (kombu) showed resistance to laboratory-induced cancers. In animals that already had cancerous tumors, kelp-fed groups showed partial and, in some cases, complete tumor regression.

3. *Wakame*—A pretty deep-green-colored sea vegetable, wakame is a light-tasting sea vegetable similar to spinach, frequently used in soups. In some markets, you can purchase dried wakame, which is great for travel-ing—it makes a great instant soup mix.

4. *Hiziki*—A thick hairlike sea vegetable, richly black with 10 to 12 times the amount of calcium as contained in equal 100-gram portions of milk. Hiziki is usually com-bined in Asian cooking with sweet vegetables (onions, carrots, and cabbage) to reduce its "sea" flavor. As weird as it might sound, an oriental family I used to live with frequently made a baked dough roll containing cooked hiziki inside with onions and roasted almonds. I had to

practically beg for the recipe and to this day make it for friends and family. The reaction is usually similar:

"Wow, this is really great! What is it?"

"Seaweed."

"Seaweed? I'm eating seaweed?"

"That's right. How does it taste?"

"Wonderful!—I can't believe it. You have a recipe?"

"You'll have to beg …"

5. *Arame*—Arame is a kinder and gentler version of hiziki. It's lighter, less "seaweedy " tasting, and usually enjoyed without complaint, often being mixed with carrots and onions for added sweetness.

6. *Dulse*—A popular Northeastern Canadian and Irish sea vegetable. It has a very distinctive strong taste and is frequently used as a dry condiment. I've included it in various soup recipes and green or corn dishes with very enthusiastic responses.

Get adventurous! Try some sea vegetables in your cooking. Instead of beginning with a solo seaweed dish, make some a small portion of arame, as a start, with sweet vegetables. You can also try some wakame or a small piece of kombu in your next soup.

RETHINKING SALT

Blood, sweat, and tears share a common ingredient: salt. We cannot function without it. The functions of heart, liver, kidneys, digestion, and adrenal glands are dependent on some percentage of salt. Yet we have been told repeatedly that salt will elevate blood pressure. In most minds, this has become an established connection; salt = high blood pressure.

From the variety of opinions regarding salt in the diet, it would seem fitting that beside the word *controversy* in the dictionary would be a picture of a salt shaker. Opinions on salt run the gamut from black to white: It's bad. It's good. It's unnecessary. It's vital.

For years, physicians have pointed their fingers at salt and attributed numerous degenerative conditions to our excessive intake. *Excessive* is the key word here; some Japanese researcher claimed that salt excess in Japan varies from 6 to 8 teaspoons daily, while in America, conservative estimates put our excesses at 4 to 5 teaspoons—on a daily basis! Considering that the American Heart Association recommends healthy Americans adults maintain an average of 1 to 1¼ teaspoons daily (2400 milligrams), this consumption of salt redefines the meaning of excess.

Today, most low-salt diets are prescribed to relieve kidney problems and hypertension. In hypertension, the blood vessels are constricted by overconsumption of salt. This forces the heart, in a Herculean effort, to pump blood through strangled capillaries (with an incredibly small diameter of approximately 4 microns). The sodium also draws water from blood cells and blood vessels, shrinking surrounding tissues and causing dehydration in the process. Lower back ache (kidney pain), thirst cravings, and eye-facial edema (puffiness) are also characteristic of excess salt.

Such reactions are, obviously, due to excessive salt consumption and warrant restriction. But the need for salt cannot be overlooked or devalued; a lack of salt can lead to poor intestinal muscle tone and symptoms of loose bowel (diarrhea). Salt helps to keep blood vessels and cells slightly contracted and keep the body warm. This is one of the reasons more salt is consumed in the winter by most cultures in temperate climates. However, an excess of salt can restrict circulation and create more vulnerability to cold.

A more comprehensive look at the mechanism of what makes blood pressure rise is given attention in *Lot's Wife—Salt & the Human Condition,* by Sallie Tisdale:

> *It is an astonishingly widespread belief that salt causes high blood pressure and a low-salt diet relieves it; that once a person's blood pressure begins to climb they are doomed to salt-free soup for life. Clearly, sodium is involved, and the renin-angiotensin-aldosterone system is intricately related to sodium metabolism. The kidneys are involved. Blood volume is*

involved. But what happens, really, when a person with high blood pressure cuts back on sodium? With some people, their blood pressure rises. The research is new, for no one had considered this possibility until a few years ago. There is a cautious consensus beginning to appear that only about 40 percent of the hypertensive population will have lower blood pressure on a low-salt diet. Thirty out of a hundred people will stay the same—a vain sacrifice—and the other 30 will have higher blood pressure.

The need for salt is well known. What is not well known is the poor and harsh quality of ordinary "table" salt. All salt is actually sea salt, or, at least, at one time was sea salt. Inland, rock salt deposits were once dissolved in the great ocean that covered our earth over 300 million years ago, before shifts in the earth's crust buried parts of the original sea. Rainfall over eons has leached some of the nonsodium chloride minerals out of rock salt deposits and washed them into the sea. As a result, sea salt is somewhat higher in "trace minerals" (silicon, copper,

---

WHAT'S WRONG WITH COMMON TABLE SALT?

Mass-produced and refined table salt is 99.99 percent sodium chloride, regardless of its origin. This refined salt is made of uniformly fine crystals—made fine by a 1200° F oven heating process and then flash-cooled. To add insult to injury, refined salt is then combined with a number of additives; potassium iodine is added to salt to "iodize" it, providing "antigoiter" comfort. Iodine is essential to the formation of thyroid hormones. However, iodine is very volatile and oxidizes immediately when exposed to light. Because of this, dextrose, a simple sugar, must be added to stabilize the iodine in iodized table salt. This gives birth to another problem: Adding only the two ingredients of potassium iodide and dextrose would turn the salt purple. This is not considered marketable; therefore, a little sodium bicarbonate is mixed in to bleach the color. Finally, the crystals are coated with a compound such as sodium silico aluminate (note all the extra sodium compounds in "table" salt) to make sure that the salt will be "free flowing" in humid conditions.

calcium, nickel, etc.) than common rock salt. In fact, there are approximately 84 buffering elements in natural, solar-dried sea salt to protect our bodies from the harshness of pure sodium chloride.

Natural salts, those dried by a solar evaporation process, are made of larger crystals and still contain their matrix of valuable trace minerals. However, natural salts do not "free flow." Since they are not coated with a water-repelling chemical, salt naturally attracts moisture from the air. Sun-dried, solar sea salt cannot be shook evenly from a salt shaker. You can't pour it on your food as you converse over the dinner table. This is one of the characteristics of good-quality salt; it appears "damp."

Suddenly, the slogan "When it rains, it pours" has renewed meaning.

Sea Salt Versus Table Salt—The Taste Test

Naturally solar-evaporated sea salt has a uniquely different taste, but don't believe me. Be your own judge by taking a simple taste test: Put a couple of table salt grains directly on your tongue. Notice that the initial taste is sharp, salty, and acrid with a lingering flavor that can be harsh, metallic, and distinctly unpleasant.

Now, rinse your mouth and try several grains of sea salt. Notice a difference? Its taste is slightly sweet, smooth, pleasant, and satisfying. It's amazing to realize how sensitive taste buds can be. They have an ability to distinguish subtle differences of artificial ingredients versus natural ingredients from two separate salts in an identical sodium chloride base. Good-quality sea salt has the natural advantage of being able to enhance the flavor of other ingredients.

The Vegetarian Dilemma

For people who have been on a high-fat, average meat-and-potato diet and decide suddenly to change their habits, the need for salt is minimal, if not unnecessary, in the beginning. Their bodies are usually clogged with salt and they would do well to avoid the substance for a period of time. Therefore, there is no one-size-fits-all paradigm for salt use.

For vegetarians, it's another story. Biochemist and author of two books on sea salt, Jacques De Langre offered the following observation regarding vegetarians:

> [Vegetarians] … have so much ingested potassium from the green leafy vegetables, this cannot be neutralized by sodium— if potassium is excessive in relation to sodium. This can also make the body lose its ability to produce hydrochloric acid, which can produce digestive problems, quite common in vegetarians.

The blood relationship of sodium to potassium is essential. Potassium always predominates; however, if we take an excessive amount of sodium, potassium can restore the balance. Heavy meat eaters (obtaining salts via the animal muscle) who become vegetarian on a no-meat, no-salt diet tend to feel almost euphoric at first. They feel lighter, more energetic, and experience greater mental clarity. However, while there are exceptions, excessive potassium can result in these initially positive conditions changing to their opposite; people become lethargic, mineral deficient, emotionally negative and depressed. They begin craving meats (for the salts contained within the meat tissue), or salt, itself. Since they've usually been indoctrinated to this point about the negative effects of meats and salt, they invariably end up replacing these cravings with fats and stimulants—stimulants, such as honey, sugar, or juices, to maintain declining energy, and fats, such as oils, nut butters, or avocados, to keep satisfied with meals. For the type of vegetarian wishing to remain vegan, a little salt cooked into the food or fermented salt products, along with sugar restriction, works wonders.

Sea salt added to the diet, either in its direct form or in fermented preparation as miso or tamari (natural soy sauce), can be highly alkalizing. It can also help to alleviate fatigue.

There is a sister fruit to the apricot called the *Ume* plum in Japan. The Japanese pickle this plum in salt for a number of

HOW MUCH SALT IS TOO MUCH?

How can you determine when you've taken too much salt? Here are six symptoms that might indicate you're taking beyond your needs:

1. *Thirst*—Excessive salt will inspire thirst. Your thirst becomes insatiable. If you drink fruit juice in an attempt to satisfy this craving, you'll notice that the sugar will also create increased thirst. Drink water. Sometimes a little lemon juice squeezed into water is a quick way to "de-salt."

2. *Overeating*—Often, salt will increase your desire for greater amounts of food. This is especially true for individuals who avoid sugar. Their craving becomes transferred to one that demands volume.

3. *Sweet Cravings/Alcohol Cravings*—Salt and sugar—a perfect union in its own way. Either extreme will create cravings for the other. A salty meal's compliment is a sweet dessert; burger, fries, *and* a shake.

   Alcohol is a distillation of sugar—it's concentrated sugar. Remember this the next time you might be in a tavern or bar and notice the owner making certain the nuts, chips, popcorn, or other salty snacks are well supplied to patrons. It's rarely because he's considerate. It's about increasing the desire for alcohol.

4. *Irritability*—Excessive salt may produce irritability. This may be due to the physically constricting effects of salt (a person we call "uptight"), its lowering of blood sugar, or its effect on the nervous system.

5. *Swelling*—In some people, swelling of ankles and hands or puffiness around the eyes may be due to excess salt.

6. *Coloring*—While there are many reasons for darkness beneath the eyes, I suspect one of them might be excessive salt. This is a personal observation. In Chinese medicine, this area relates to the kidneys. Excessive salt can be troublesome to these organs.

The Power to Fight Cancer Program suggests small amounts of salt that range from 500 milligrams ($1/4$ teaspoon) to 1500 milligrams ($3/4$ teaspoon), give or take. The salt recommended is natural, solar-dried sea salt that should be cooked into the food, as opposed to adding it to an already cooked dish.

months and package them as *Umeboshi* salt plums. Highly salty with strong citric acid properties, they are excellent for neutralizing digestive acidity. In Mexico, a similar salty plum is called salitos.

Umeboshi are handy to have when traveling for cases of indigestion, or from fatigue whose probable cause is acidity.

Avoiding "Windy" Days

I've kept in touch with a former British neighbor for years. When I was a teenager, he was somewhat of a mentor to me, being over 25 years my senior. He once attended a lecture of mine and sat in the back of the hall, taking it all in. Afterward, we had dinner and throughout the meal he kept saying, "I couldn't believe all those people had came to hear you. I am, indeed, very proud. Good show, it was." He'd seen me on television, heard me on the radio, and when I visited him in the hospital, when he was recovering from an acute condition, gave him an earful on changing his diet and lifestyle. He always listened but never made a move to change.

One day, after returning from a business trip, he telephoned me and announced, "Well, lad, I'm ready to go to one of 'your' restaurants." Naturally, he was ready—he'd just begun dating a woman 15 years younger who was a yoga teacher and very health oriented. Love had made him into a convert.

I suggested an upscale natural foods restaurant. Later that evening, he left me a telephone message on my answering machine: "Verne, absolutely smashing dinner. Ate like a soldier—although I must have looked more like a pig! I could dine like that all the time. Yes! I can do this. Thanks a lot . . ."

Nice message. However, the following morning, while on a bike ride, I came home to a second, and very contrasting message:

"Hey, Boyo, you can have the lot of that food! Man, I am suffering! Been up most of the night full of wind—dog gassy to you Americans. I must have passed enough wind to fill the Hindenberg. Should have warned me, lad—I'm afraid to leave the house. I can just see me on the tennis court this afternoon! Call me, would you?

My friend had learned his first lesson in food combinations, overeating, drinking with his meals, rushing, and poor chewing. The Gas Gods were in top punishing form.

I've never bought the standard reasoning for gas: the "swallowing" of air. Thirty years of personal and professional experience have taught me otherwise. Here are eight practical strategies for avoiding gas. You can thank me later.

1. *Volume*—If you overeat you're likely to run the risk of acidity and subsequent gas. Portion your volume beforehand and take your time. You can always eat more later.

2. *Simple Sugar and Complex Sugar Combinations*— Everyone has different tolerances; however, simple sugars digest (e.g., fruit) quickly, and often, if they're eaten with complex sugars (e.g., grain), they can end up fermenting the slower-digesting grain that's still digesting in the stomach. Gas is the result. In the story about my British friend, one of the things he did was rush through a large meal and then stuff down a dessert immediately afterward. Not a good idea. Especially on an important date—unless you want to make it an early evening. In the beginning, until you become accustomed to these foods and have the opportunity to experiment and learn about your own tolerances, I'd suggest that you eat dessert separately, not with the meal, or as long as you can wait after completing the meal, providing you've saved some room.

3. *Bean Volume*—I found that when clients began eating beans, they would have an amount just short of a fiesta plate; mounds and mounds of beans! Beans have two difficult starches that do not easily break apart in the human intestine. Generally, in bean cooking, there are a number of things a cook can do to minimize gas potential. However, the four most important are (1) keeping volume down, (2) thorough chewing, (3) making sure the beans have been cooked with sea salt, or adding some yourself, and (4) not eating anything sweet at the same meal.

YOUR KITCHEN, COOKING, AND COOKWARE

The more you practice healthy cooking, the more you'll come to respect your cooking environment. Here are some basic tips for getting the best from your cooking efforts:

- Keep your working area clean and orderly.

- Minimize aluminum or chemically treated, "nonstick" cookware. Some finishes can eventually dissolve into food. Enamel, glass, cast iron and stainless steel offer safer quality.

- Store whole grain inside of an airtight jar or container and in a cool area. Placing 1–2 fresh bay leaves in each grain jar can usually ward off bugs. Be sure to rinse all grains several times before cooking.

- Remember that your feelings and attitudes have a subtle influence in cooking. Cultivate a peaceful attitude when preparing food as well as when eating.

- Live plants offer a kitchen (as well as other parts of your home) beauty, a sense of freshness, and oxygen.

- Grains, beans, soups, and desserts can often be prepared in advance. Vegetables are usually better if prepared fresh.

- Try to clean as you cook, in order to avoid a sink full of dishes after meal time.

- Commit to making one new recipe each week from a cookbook.

- Consider taking a natural foods cooking class or ethnic cooking class and learn to substitute natural ingredients for common ones that are not health-supportive.

- Remember that cooking for yourself and others can be an expression of your love and friendship

4. *Thorough Chewing*—The predominant macronutrient in Nature's Cancer-Fighting Food Plan is carbohydrate. Carbohydrates digest in the mouth. When they hit the stomach, they cease digesting, until eventually passing into the duodenum, and then resume breaking down, which could take hours. Therefore, you must chew these foods thoroughly. Becoming a good chewer does not mean you have to do this slow cow dance with your jaw and take forever at the table. Chewing can be very active work; the human jaw not only moves up and down but

laterally as well. Gandhi once said, "Chew your drink and drink your food." He meant to allow your drink to pass slowly through your mouth without gulping, but mixing the drink with your enzyme-digesting saliva before swallowing, and to chew your food well enough so that it can almost become a liquid so that it feels like you're "drinking" it. If you diligently chew just one meal per week, your chewing will improve with every meal thereafter.

5. *Tension*—Our digestive secretions become inhibited when we're upset. At this point it would be better to excuse yourself, take a brief walk, sort out your thinking, and do some deep breathing before returning to the table and attempting to eat. Tension is not conducive to digestion and could account for poor digestion.

6. *Drinking with Meals*—This might be a minor gas factor but could account for poor assimilation, inadequate nutrition, and residual acidity. Ideally, it is best to drink moderately, after meals.

7. *No-Salt Meals*—Many foods are easier to digest with the alkalinity of sea salt, such as protein (fish, chicken, bean and bean products), cruciferous vegetables (cabbage, broccoli, and greens), and most other grains.

8. *Combining Proteins and Carbohydrates*—For years I rolled my eyes when I heard people claiming they could not digest protein and carbohydrates together. However, eventually I realized that certain people, particularly those who are allergy prone or big sweet-eaters, do tend to have difficulty combining proteins with complex carbohydrates. In this case, if all else has failed in the pre-venting-gas department, I suggest eating protein and complex carbohydrate (specifically whole grain) separately, at different meals. So, when you have the bean soup, you avoid the grain for that meal and perhaps have a salad or side vegetable dish with it, instead. Eventually, you can build up a tolerance and enjoy these combinations again, as cultures have for thousands of years.

12
SALUD!
NUTRITIOUS, DELICIOUS, AND EASY-TO-MAKE RECIPES

salud (sah-lood') Sp. {orig f. }—A salutation of blessing for good health. *Pour tu' Salud* ("for your health!")

BREAKFAST MENUS

1

Roasted Almond-Raisin Quick-Time Oatmeal
Whole Wheat Toast with Almond Cream
Grain "Coffee" with Dash of Vanilla and Soy Milk

2

Oatmeal-Quinoa Porridge & Roasted
Sunflower Seeds
Sweet-Onion Kale
Rye Toast Brushed with Flax-Seed Oil
Dandelion-Chicory Root Lemon Tea

3

7-Minute Morning Miso-Vegetable Soup

Toasted Corn Tortillas with Tempeh, Corn,
& Onions in Parsley-Kuzu Sauce

Light Green Tea

4

Choice of Natural Boxed Cold Cereal with Seasonal Fruit

Sourdough Toast with Peanut Cream

Roasted Barley Tea

5

Scrambled Tofu & Vegetables over Sourdough Toast

Tempeh "Bacon"

Grain "Coffee"

BREAKFAST RECIPES

1

~ Breakfast ~

Roasted Almond-Raisin Quick-Time Oatmeal
Whole-Wheat Toast with Almond Cream
Grain "Coffee" with Dash of Vanilla and Milk

This is an easy and familiar breakfast. The raisins are an optional ingredient and best if added two-thirds of the way into the cooking, allowing them to puff up slightly. Add raisins to the oatmeal, as opposed to adding a little oatmeal to a bowl of raisins. The idea is to add a hint of sweet. I like to cook this recipe longer by continuously adding small amounts of water. Then it becomes a creamy consistency. Additions of condiments like roasted seeds or nuts, or a pinch of salt help to keep this standard breakfast from tasting like watery cardboard. The toast provides a satisfying texture to complement the oatmeal; the "coffee" is made from grains, contains no caffeine, and helps your appetite be satisfied at the end of the meal.

Serves—Approximately 3
Time—10 to 20 minutes

Ingredients

Oatmeal

4 cups (+) of filtered water
$1^1\!/_2$ to $1^3\!/_4$ cups of rolled oats
$^1\!/_8$ to $^1\!/_4$ tsp. of sea salt
Handful of chopped roasted almond bits
2 tbs. tablespoons organic raisins
Cinnamon

Toast with Almond Cream

1–2 slices whole wheat bread
1 tbs. almond butter
2 tbs. water
Dash of tamari

Note: For a one-person serving, use a total of $^3\!/_4$ cup of grain.

Method

Oatmeal

- Add 4 cups of water to a small pot with a pinch of sea salt, cover, and bring, as the British say, to a "fierce" boil.

- Gently stir in 1½ cups of oats as you lower the flame to a simmer. Cover the pot about ⅘ so steam can escape for a period of 10 to 15 minutes cooking.
- Check occasionally to make sure the water has not evaporated. If the oats are looking dry, gently stir in about ⅓ to ½ cup of water. You might have to repeat this step if your flame is too high or if you desire a creamier texture.
- After 10–15 minutes of simmering, add chopped roasted almonds (usually available already toasted in bins at natural food stores, or chop into bits and dry roast in a skillet for approximately 15 minutes) and raisins.
- Cook for another 10 minutes or so.
- Add cinnamon toward the end and serve.

Note: If you'd like a nuttier tasting oatmeal, try a 5-minute dry roasting (low–medium flame) to slightly brown the oats before adding the boiling water.

Whole Wheat Toast with Almond Cream

Try toasting some of the nonyeast breads, which are a bit more chewy but more substantial. To make a spread from any nut or seed butter, dilute with a small amount of water to make a "cream consistency." The purpose is to make the nut oil easier to digest and easier to spread.

- Take a heaping teaspoon of organic almond butter and add it to an empty cup with several tablespoons of water. Mix well to combine and create a creamy consistency. Spread on toast.
- Add approximately ½ teaspoon of natural soy sauce (tamari) or a pinch of salt, if your prefer. (Rarely have I met a person who did not roll their eyes with an expression of sensory delight at this simple mixture.) Spread evenly on the bread.

Condiment Options
Sesame salt, a dash of vanilla, 1 to 3 tablespoons of soy, oat, or almond milk.

Grain Coffee Beverage with Dash of Vanilla and Milk

One brand of cereal grain coffee I recommend is called Roma. Other brands, such as Cafix, Pero, Barley Brew, or Instant Yannoh, also work wonderfully. I prefer Barley Brew or Yannoh, but these are not always available.

- Add one teaspoon to ⅓ of a cup of soymilk and ⅔ cup of boiling water.
- Mix in a dash of vanilla with a sprinkle of nutmeg for an added treat.

2

~ Breakfast ~

Oatmeal-Quinoa Porridge & Roasted Sunflower Seeds
Sweet-Onion Kale
Rye Toast Brushed with Flax-Seed Oil
Dandelion-Chicory Root Lemon Tea

This hearty porridge is similar to the preceding oatmeal recipe with the addition of a quick-cooking South American grain called quinoa ("keen-wa"). Quinoa is a uniquely delicious small grain with a high protein content.

Serves—Approximately 3
Time—15 to 25 minutes

Ingredients

Oatmeal with Quinoa

¾ to 1 cup of rolled oats
¾ to 1 cup of quinoa
4 cups (+) of filtered water
Roasted sunflower seeds
Sesame-salt condiment ("gomashio")

Sweet-Onion Kale

One bunch kale
One large onion
¾ to 1 cup filtered water
Pinch of sea salt

Method

Oatmeal-Quinoa Porridge with Roasted Sunflower Seeds

- Assemble all ingredients. Then wash the quinoa to take away a slightly bitter outer coating. To wash, simply place the quinoa in an empty pot, fill with water, stir the quinoa with your hand to cleanse it, and then pour the water out, using your hand to keep the quinoa from spilling, or using a fine mesh strainer.

- Add water to a small pot with a pinch of sea salt, cover, and bring to a "fierce" boil. Gently stir in the oats and quinoa as you lower the flame to a simmer. Cover the pot about ⁴⁄₅ so some steam can escape and allow to cook for 15 to 20 minutes.

- Check occasionally to make sure that the water has not evaporated. If the grains are looking dry, add about ⅓ to ½ cup of water each time and stir.

- After 15 minutes of simmering, add roasted sunflower seeds (usually available already roasted in bins at natural food stores, or dry roast in a skillet for approximately 15 minutes, shaking the nuts to distribute the heat evenly.

- Cook for another approximately 10 minutes or until consistency is pleasing.

Note: For one person, use a total of ³/₄ cup of grain with 2¹/₄ cups of filtered water.

Sweet-Onion Kale

Sometimes a sweet vegetable like onions can be a perfect complement to greens.

- Slice the onions into crescents after removing skin.
- Bring approximately 1 cup of water to a boil in a large skillet. Add the onions and a pinch of sea salt and cover for 5 minutes.
- Rinse kale leaves and chop. Put aside.
- Remove skillet cover and add more water, allowing the onion cooking steam to evaporate completely. The onions will taste sweet as they become clear. The longer you cook them (which means adding a bit more water each time) the sweeter they'll become.
- Finally, add another ¹/₂ to ³/₄ cup of water, raise the flame until it boils, add the chopped kale, and adjust heat to low–medium. The kale will cook within 5 minutes. Remember that the remainder heat will continue cooking the kale, so be careful not to overcook.

Rye Toast Brushed with Flax Oil

Toast a slice or two of rye bread. Add a sprinkle of sea salt, or ¹/₂ teaspoon of tamari, to two teaspoons of flax oil and mix together. Brush on toast.

Condiment Options for Oatmeal-Quinoa Porridge

Sesame salt, or ³/₄ teaspoon of water-diluted miso paste, or, as strange as this might sound, I enjoy this dish with a sheet of toasted nori seaweed (the green sheet that's usually wrapped around sushi rolls). Rip the nori into small pieces and stir it in while the food is still steaming.

Dandelion Chicory Root Lemon Tea

A favorite tea among older Italians. You can purchase roasted dandelion root tea bags (not dandelion leaf) from a number of companies, such as See-Lect, Alvita, and Frontier. This hearty tea, considered a tonic for the liver in American herbal medicine, is a nice finish to any meal, often naturally reducing the desire to continue eating afterward.

- Steep tea in boiled water.
- Add a pinch of roasted chicory.
- Add a squeeze of lemon juice (optional).

3

~ Breakfast ~

7-Minute Morning Miso-Vegetable Soup
Corn Tortillas with Tempeh, Corn, & Onions in Parsley-Kuzu Sauce
Light Green Tea

This quick miso soup recipe is a great way to begin your day! Tempeh, first fried under low heat and then combined with corn and onions in a kuzu sauce, makes for a delicious high-protein meal. Since it is fermented, the protein is easily broken down for absorbing maximum nutrition.

Serves—Approximately 4

Time 5 minutes for miso soup, 15 minutes for tempeh, corn, and onions

Ingredients

7-Minute Morning Miso-Vegetable Soup

5 cups of filtered water
One 3/4-inch piece of dried wakame sea vegetable
One large onion
Two carrots
1 3/4–2 tbs. barley miso paste diluted into 3–4 tbs. water to thin

Corn Tortilla with Tempeh, Corn, & Onions in Parsley-Kuzu Sauce

1 tbs. sesame oil
8 ounces of tempeh cut into 1-inch cubes
2 onions sliced wedge style
2 cups fresh or frozen corn kernals
3 cups filtered spring water
3/4 tsp. powdered ginger
1 tsp. umeboshi vinegar
1 1/2 tbs. kuzu (natural thickener—dilute in 1/8 cup cold water)
Minced parsley
Corn tortilla (packaged), lightly toasted to make warm and bendable, not crisp

Method

7-Minute Morning Miso-Vegetable Soup

- Soak the dried wakame until soft (7 to 10 minutes).
- Cut onion into thin crescent slivers to cook quicker.
- Cut carrots into thin half moon sections.
- Bring water to a boil in a medium saucepan over a medium range flame.
- Add the diced wakame and simmer for 1 minute.
- Add the onion and simmer for 4–5 minutes.
- Add carrots after onions.
- Stir diluted miso into broth and turn off the heat. Allow to remain for 1 minute.

Corn Tortilla with Tempeh, Corn, & Onions in Parsley-Kuzu Sauce

- Heat 1 tablespoon sesame oil in a heavy skillet with a low–medium heat until hot (do not burn or smoke!).
- Add tempeh cubes and sauté until crispy.
- Remove and place tempeh on a paper towel to drain excess oil. Set aside.
- In a medium-sized soup pot, layer onions, corn, and the tempeh. Add water and bring to a boil.
- Lower heat and cook until onions are fairly soft—approximately 5 to 7 minutes.
- Lightly season with tamari and ginger. Simmer for another 5 minutes.
- Add a small amount of fine chopped fresh parsley and 1 teaspoon of umeboshi vinegar.
- Stir in dissolved kuzu while continuously stirring, until the sauce begins to thicken. Empty ingredients into a serving bowl.
- Briefly toast the corn tortillas and serve on the side.

Light Green Tea

Enjoy a cup of lightly steeped green tea.

4

~ Breakfast ~

Choice of Natural Boxed Cold Cereal with Seasonal Fruit
Sourdough Toast with Peanut Cream
Roasted Barley Tea

This breakfast is a familiar one to millions across the country, only substituting healthier ingredients. Common boxed breakfast cereals contain anywhere from 22 percent to 58 percent refined sugar and a host of other unnecessary artificial ingredients. Choose healthier ones from your natural foods stores that are fruit sweetened. Milk can be substituted for with better-quality and healthier soy, oat, almond, or rice milks. This makes a good start for creating a transition breakfast.

Serving—One bowl per individual
Time—3–5 minutes; as long it takes to mix ingredients and chop fruit!

Ingredients

Dry Cereal

Choice of natural dry cereal (Oatio's,™ Brown Rice Krispies™, etc.)
Small amount of soy, almond, oat, or rice milk
Fresh fruit

Sourdough Toast with Peanut Cream

Variety of grain bread, toasted if desired
Organic peanut butter (diluted with water, as detailed in the recipe for whole wheat toast with almond cream)

Method

Dry Cereal with Soy/Grain Milk

- Mix dry cereal with nut or grain milks.
- Add chopped fruit.
- Spread peanut cream on toast.

Roasted Barley Tea

This is a rich, full-bodied, and soothing after-meal tea.

- Add one teaspoon roasted barley tea (available at choice natural food stores or Japanese markets—this tea is called "mugi-cha") per cup to boiling hot water.
- Simmer for 3 to 5 minutes.

5

~ Breakfast ~

Scrambled Tofu & Vegetables over Sourdough Toast
Tempeh "Bacon"
Grain "Coffee"

This breakfast is a mock American-style breakfast. The scrambled tofu recipe is adapted from New Zealand cookbook author Cheryl Beere, who, in preparing this dish for friends, is always asked if this recipe, (which has the color and taste of eggs), actually contains eggs. It's a great egg substitution dish with varied tastes. The delicious tempeh "bacon" recipe was adapted from cookbook authors Mary Estella and Lenore Baum.2

Serves—Approximately 4
Time—Approximately 15–20 minutes

Ingredients

Scrambled Tofu with Vegetables

2 blocks of firm or medium-firm tofu
2 tbs. dark sesame oil
Diced carrot
Diced celery
Diced onion
2 tsp. tamari soy sauce
1/4 cup finely chopped coriander
1/4 tsp. tumeric
1/4 tsp. ground black pepper
Toasted sesame seeds
Sourdough toast

Tempeh "Bacon"*

2 tbs. sweet, white miso
1/2 cup boiling water
1 tsp. prepared natural mustard
2 bay leaves
2 garlic cloves, thinly sliced
1/4 tsp. white pepper
1/2 lb. tempeh cut into small strips

*A similar commercial product is sold in natural food markets under the brand name of "Fakin' Bacon."

Method

Scrambled Tofu

- Heat a large cast-iron skillet or frying pan and add toasted sesame oil. When hot (*not* burning) add diced carrot, celery, and onion and oil-sauté until soft—approximately 5 minutes.
- Add grated ginger and then crumble in tofu with your fingers.
- Stir slightly and add the coriander, tumeric, pepper, and tamari. Cover and cook for 3 minutes.
- Remove from heat and serve over sourdough toast.
- Sprinkle lightly with toasted sesame seeds and serve immediately.

Tempeh "Bacon"

- In a saucepan, puree miso in water with a spoon. Add remaining ingredients (natural mustard, bay leaves, minced garlic, and white pepper) except for the tempeh. Stir gently.
- Add cut tempeh strips. Simmer covered for 20 minutes.
- Drain tempeh strips. Place on an oiled baking dish. Discard marinade.
- Broil until crisp and browned for 6 to 8 minutes. Turn over and broil for an additional 5 minutes.

Note: Tempeh "bacon" can also be added to stews, sandwiches, stir fry, and salads.

Variation: For a juicier "bacon," add 1 teaspoon of toasted sesame oil when first adding all remaining ingredients before adding tempeh.

Grain "Coffee"

Grain beverage of choice

LUNCH MENUS

1

Arisha's Lemon Red Lentil Soup
Brussel Sprouts with Ginger-Plum Glaze
Leafy Green Salad with Lemon-Parsley Dressing
Chilled Mandarin Orange Wedges
Twig Tea

2

Tofu & Vegetable Sesame Stir Fry
Walnut Rice
Assorted Greens in Citrus-Sparkle Dressing
Dandelion Root Tea

3

Rebecca's Grilled Millet & Butternut Squash Cakes
Miso Glazed Carrots
Pronto-Blanched Watercress
Chamomile Tea

4

Cream of Celery-Leek Soup
Tempeh "Reuben"
Plain & Easy Steamed Broccoli
Chef St. Jacques Spice Cookies
Twig Tea

5

Sweet Rice & Chestnuts
Refried Beans
Avocado Vinaigrette & Chopped Mixed Greens
Light Green Tea

LUNCH RECIPES

1

~ Lunch ~

Arisha's Lemon Red Lentil Soup
Brussel Sprouts and Ginger-Plum Glaze
Leafy Green Salad with Parsley-Lemon Dressing
Chilled Mandarin Orange Wedges
Twig Tea

This delicious soup recipe comes from the inspiring kitchen of Arisha Wemhoff in Omaha, Nebraska. Television cooking show host and cookbook author Christina Pirello's elegant side dish stew of brussel sprouts with ginger-plum sauce offers a nice complement and a rosemary-mustard dressing adds a unique flavor to a wild green salad.

Servings—4
Time—Approximately 30–35 minutes

Ingredients

Arisha's Lemon Red Lentil Soup

1 cup dried red lentils

2 onions, sliced thin into moons

2 garlic cloves, minced

1 tsp. ground cumin

4 cups filtered water

1 bay leaf

1 tbs. lemon juice

2 strips lemon rind

1 tbs. sesame oil

1/2 tsp. sea salt

Brussel Sprouts and Ginger-Plum Glaze

4–5 cups of trimmed, whole brussel sprouts

1–2 sweet onions, cut into wedges

Dash of tamari

1 cup of filtered water

2–3 tsp. fresh ginger juice

2 heaping tsp. kuzu diluted in cold water

2 tsp. umeboshi vinegar

Leafy Green Salad with Parsley-Lemon Dressing	**Chilled Mandarin Orange Wedges**
Mix wild greens	Sliced and chilled wedges

Dressing: concentrated vegetable stock (boiled down from one cup to 5–6 tbs.)
1 tbs. lemon juice
1/3 cup of finely chopped fresh parsley
1 tbs. balsamic vinegar

Method

Arisha's Lemon Red Lentil Soup

- Into a 4-quart pot, heat 1 tablespoon of sesame oil.
- Add chopped onions and sauté until translucent.
- Mash 2 garlic cloves into 1/2 teaspoon sea salt and add to onions with 1 teaspoon of ground cumin.
- Cook ingredients for 7 minutes.
- Add red lentils and water to onion mixture and boil. Skim off any foam.
- Reduce heat, add bay leaf and lemon rind, and simmer covered for 25–30 minutes.
- Add lemon, stir, and serve hot.

Brussel Sprouts and Ginger-Plum Glaze

- Into the base of each brussel sprout (use 4–5 cups of brussel sprouts), cut a shallow cross (this is not religiously significant—it's for even cooking).
- Into a heavy pot, layer cut onion wedges (from 1–2 medium-size onions) and then add the brussel sprouts.
- Sprinkle tamari (approximately 1 to 1 1/2 teaspoon) into mixture.
- Add 1 cup filtered water, cover, and bring to a slow boil over medium heat. Simmer for 25–40 minutes.
- Season to taste with tamari, add fresh ginger juice, and simmer for an additional 5 minutes.
- Gently stir in kuzu that has been thoroughly diluted in cold water and cook, stirring vegetables gently to avoid breaking them, as a thin glaze forms over the vegetables. This should take about 2 to 3 minutes.
- Remove from heat and sprinkle lightly with umeboshi vinegar or brown rice vinegar.
- Place into a serving bowl and serve warm.

Leafy Green Salad with Parsley-Lemon Dressing

Dressing:

- In a 1-quart saucepan, boil down vegetable stock to reduce it to 5–6 tablespoons.
- Add ingredients of vegetable stock (5 tablespoons), 1 tablespoon fresh lemon juice, 1 tablespoon of Balsamic vinegar, 1/3 cup fine-chopped parsley, and 1/4 teaspoon sea salt to screw-top jar. Shake to mix. Pour into blender and blend thoroughly.
- Mix into wild greens.

Chilled Mandarin Orange Wedges

- Remove orange wedges from refrigerator and serve.

Twig Tea

Brew Kukicha twig tea in loose form or tea bag version.

2

~ Lunch ~

Tofu & Vegetable Sesame Stir Fry
Walnut Rice
Assorted Greens in Citrus-Sparkle Dressing
Dandelion Root Tea

A delicious and energy-packed lunch menu for any season. The tofu dish can also go equally well with long-grain brown rice as a dinner. A friend described the citrus dressing as something that "sparkles" on your tongue! A similar version of this dressing appears in Christina Pirello's *Cooking the Whole Foods Way.*

Servings—4

Time—Actual kitchen work: 15 minutes; however, the rice will take approximately 45 minutes to cook thoroughly. This can be put up 1/2 hour prior to beginning to cook other ingredients. During the last 15 minutes of rice cooking, you can begin to assemble other dishes and ingredients.

Ingredients

Tofu & Vegetable Sesame Stir Fry	Walnut Rice
2 carrots	3/4 cup shelled walnuts
1 onion	2 cups long-grain brown rice

1 cup corn kernels (fresh or frozen)
5 bok choy leaves
1½ cups snow peas
1 tbs. safflower oil,
2 blocks (2 lbs.) fresh tofu
1 tbs. tamari (or can substitute Braggs Amino)
1 clove minced garlic
½ inch fresh minced ginger

4 cups filtered water
⅓ cup minced parsley
½ tsp. sea salt

Assorted Greens in Citrus-Sparkle Dressing:

Dressing:
⅛ cup olive oil
Juice of one lemon
Juice of one orange with grated orange peel
Grated scallion
¼ roasted bell pepper, finely minced
1 tsp. soy sauce
3 tbs. balsamic vinegar
Pinch of sea salt
½ tsp. powdered ginger

Method

Tofu & Vegetable Sesame Stir Fry

- Heal oil in a large skillet.
- Add wedged cut onions and cook for 2 minutes on medium–high heat.
- Add diagonally cut carrot and corn kernels to this mixture and cook for another 2 minutes.
- Add cube cut tofu, cover, and continue to cook on medium–high heat, stirring frequently.
- After 4 minutes, add thinly sliced bok choy, snow peas, ginger, and chopped garlic. Stir for several minutes to bring to a finish. Add soy sauce to mixture and serve hot.

Walnut Rice

- Dry pan roast or oven roast walnuts, 15–20 minutes until fragrant and golden.
- Add rinsed rice and all ingredients, except for parsley, in a medium-sized pot.
- Cover and bring to a boil. Lower heat and simmer for 45 minutes—or until the rice is tender.

- Remove from heat and fluff gently while mixing in the parsley.

Note: If the top of the rice appears dry, gently mix it beneath and continue cooking over a low heat for another 5 to 10 minutes.

Assorted Greens in Citrus-Sparkle Dressing (makes approximately 1 cup)

- Squeeze juices of 1 lemon and 1 orange.
- Grate a small amount of orange.
- Roast ¼ of one bell pepper, finely minced.
- In a small saucepan, warm oil and soy sauce for 2 minutes.
- Whisk together all ingredients until blended.

Dandelion Root Tea

Steep tea bags and add a bit of lemon.

3

~ Lunch ~

Rebecca's Grilled Millet & Butternut Squash Cakes
Miso Glazed Carrots
Pronto-Blanched Watercress
Chamomile Tea

This delicious grilled millet recipe comes from old friend and award-winning author Rebecca Wood, and the miso glazed carrot dish is a simple favorite of mine from Arisha Wemhoff's kitchen. Blanching greens is a speedy way to heat a vegetable for better assimilation without cooking it limp and still retain its rich green color. Blanched greens can be added to salads, tossed in sandwiches, or simmered in the last 3 minutes of soup making. Alternate greens for blanching are kale, collards, mustard greens, bok choy, dandelion, broccoli raab, turnip tops, and daikon greens.

Servings—4

Time—Actual cooking time is approximately 10 minutes; however, making fresh millet requires approximately 25 minutes to cook. Leftover millet that has been warmed by steaming will also work for this recipe to reduce cooking time.

Ingredients

Rebecca's Grilled Millet & Butternut Squash Cakes

1 cup millet
1 tsp. mustard seeds
2½ cups filtered water
2 cups peeled and diced butternut squash
1 tsp. dried (or minced) ginger
½ tsp. sea salt
½ cup fresh chopped cilantro

Miso Glazed Carrots

3 cups carrots cut to ½-inch slices
½ cup finely chopped onion
3 cups vegetable broth or water
1 tbs. sesame oil
1 tbs. light miso paste
2 tsp. grated orange zest
1 tsp. grated ginger
⅓ tsp. toasted sesame oil

Pronto-Blanched Watercress

1 stalk watercress
Pinch of sea salt
Lemon juice
Umeboshi vinegar

Method

Rebecca's Grilled Millet & Butternut Squash Cakes

- Dry pan roast the millet for approximately 4 minutes on medium–high heat, constantly stirring. When the first seed pops, roasting time is over.
- Wash the millet with a water rinse, drain, and set aside.
- Toast the mustard seeds and curry powder for 1 minute or until their aroma is released.
- Mix the millet and spices, water, squash, ginger, and sea salt in a medium saucepan. Over a high heat, bring to a boil. Lower the heat and simmer, covered, for 25 minutes, or until the millet has absorbed all the water.
- Remove from heat and allow to cool.
- Preheat the grill.
- Add the cilantro to the millet mixture. Wet your hands and blend the millet mixture to a good uniform consistency. Form into 12 cakes.
- Place the cakes on the grill and grill for approximately 3 minutes on each side, or until golden. Serve hot.

Miso Glazed Carrots

- Heat sesame oil, add onions and carrots, and sauté until onions are softened and translucent.

- Cream miso with ¼ cup of broth.
- Add vegetable broth, zest, and ginger to vegetables.
- Reduce heat and simmer uncovered until liquid is reduced to a glaze and carrots are tender-crisp.
- Stir in toasted sesame oil, season with salt, and turn off heat.

Pronto-Blanched Watercress

- Mix 2 teaspoons of fresh lemon juice with 2 teaspoon of umeboshi vinegar, 1½ teaspoon flax oil, and ¼ cup water.
- Wash 2 bunches of watercress well and soak for 15 seconds to scan for bugs (watercress is notorious for being a bug haven). Drain and chop into small sections.
- Bring 1 quart of water to a hearty boil. Add a pinch of salt.
- Drop watercress into the boiling water and remove after 20 to 30 seconds.
- Transfer to small storage bowl and mix in lemon-umeboshi dressing.

Chamomile Tea

Steep chamomile tea (loose or tea-bag form) in boiled water. A squeeze of lemon adds a nice tart taste.

4

~ Lunch ~

Cream of Celery-Leek Soup
Tempeh "Reuben"
Plain & Easy Steamed Broccoli
Chef St. Jacques Spice Cookies
Twig Tea

A noncream soup that gets its creamy consistency from using rolled oats! Of the many tempeh reuben recipes I've tried, this one from Lenore Baum seems to be the most popular in my kitchen. Sometimes it's important simply to enjoy the natural taste of vegetables without feeling like you have to improve on nature and add some culinary pizzazz by making a sauce, glaze, or dip. I've also included Asheville, North Carolina Chef Benoit St. Jacques's Spice Cookies recipe from cook and friend Merle Davis. (Mrs. Davis informs me, at present, that there is no known cure for Chef Benoit's Spice Cookie addiction—yum!)

Servings—4

Time—Prep time amounts to 20 minutes; however, the Rueben recipe will take a total of 40–45 minutes to cook.

Ingredients

Cream of Celery-Leek Soup

2 small leeks, sliced lengthwise, rinsed, diced
¾ cup sliced celery
4–5 cups filtered or spring water
⅔ cup rolled oats
2 tbs. white miso
Garnish with fine chopped parsley and thin scallion slices
Optional garnish: Dulse (sea vegetable) flakes

Plain & Easy Steamed Broccoli

Cut stems and flowers of broccoli

Tempeh "Rueben"

½ tsp. toasted sesame oil
½ lb. tempeh, cut into 1-inch strips
1 tsp. prepared natural mustard
1 tsp. barley miso
½ cup water
2 garlic cloves, minced
1 tbs. mirin
4 cups green cabbage, finely shredded
1 cup low-salt sauerkraut and juice
4–5 tbs. uncooked plain mochi, grated

Chef St. Jacques Spice Cookies

Dry Ingredients:
1 cup oatmeal
1 cup walnuts
1½ cups pastry flour
½ tsp. each of cardamom nutmeg, allspice, and cinnamon
1 tsp. baking soda
Pinch of sea salt
½ cup currants

Twig Tea
Kukicha twigs, or kukicha tea bags

Wet Ingredients:
2 tbs. lemon Juice
⅓–½ cup safflower oil
½ cup maple syrup

Method

Cream of Celery-Leek Soup

- Over medium heat, add enough water to cover leeks and bring to a boil. Add celery and reduce heat to a simmer. Cook for 3 to 4 minutes.
- Add remaining amount of water and bring to a boil.
- Add oats to boiling broth and cook over low heat for 15 minutes.
- Remove ¼ cup of liquid broth to dilute miso and stir until dissolved.

- Add miso to soup pot and simmer 1–2 minutes. Turn off heat.
- Add parsley, scallion, and dulse powder (optional) garnish to soup bowls after pouring soup.

Tempeh "Rueben"

- In a cast-iron skillet or nonstick pan, heat oil. Add tempeh strips and sauté until golden brown—about 5 minutes on each side.
- In a small bowl combine mustard, miso, and water. Pour this mixture over the miso.
- Add garlic, mirin, cabbage, and sauerkraut and its juice. Mix together gently.
- Simmer with full cover for 20 minutes. Add additional water as needed.
- In the meanwhile, preheat broiler or oven to 350°.
- Transfer mixture to a 2-quart casserole dish. Sprinkle grated mochi over top.
- Melt under broiler, or bake covered until golden brown for approximately 25 minutes.

Plain & Easy Steamed Broccoli

- Rinse and soak broccoli for one minute in a large bowl of cold water. Look for little critters—broccoli often contains bugs. Rinse again.
- Chop broccoli stems and flowerets.
- Bring water to boil in a covered medium pot with a steaming tray.
- Add broccoli and cover.
- Steam for 4 to 6 minutes. Do not overcook.

Chef St. Jacques Spice Cookies

- Combine oatmeal and nuts in food processor or blender until coarsely chopped. Add all other dry ingredients. Combine all wet ingredients and add dry to wet. Shape into cookies. Bake at 350° for 15–20 minutes. And don't be a cookie pig. Share them.

Twig Tea

Brew kukicha twig tea in loose form or tea-bag version.

5

~ Lunch ~

Sweet Rice & Chestnuts
Refried Beans
Avocado Vinaigrette & Chopped Mixed Greens
Light Green Tea

Author Aveline Kushi of Boston made this simple rice dish in a home cooking class I attended in 1971. It is generally a holiday dish reserved for New Year's day. Unlike other "nuts," chestnuts have a low fat content that other nuts would kill for—about 3 to 5 percent. The best part is the unique sweetness they add to rice. Brown sweet rice is a unique variety of brown rice containing a little higher protein and water percentage than ordinary brown rice. Once cooked, it comes out slightly "sticky." I've never grown tired of this dish. The classic Mexican dish of refried beans—*refrito*—doesn't mean "fried twice," but "fried well." Using a very small volume of oil, this dish is a traditional staple. You can cook these from scratch or, more conveniently (until ambition or time presents itself), purchase organic cooked beans in enamel-lined, lead-free cans from a number of natural food companies. Generally, I've used Eden® brand. The avocado vinaigrette comes courtesy of cookbook author and writer Cheryl Beere.

Servings—4

Time—Prep time amounts to 15–20 minutes. Total cooking time is approximately 60 minutes.

Ingredients

Sweet Rice & Chestnuts

2 cups brown sweet rice
1/2 cup dried chestnuts or 1 cup fresh
2 cups water
1/3 tsp. sea salt

Refried Beans

2 cups cooked pinto beans
1 diced carrot
1 bay leaf
1/3 tsp. sea salt per cup beans
1 to 1 1/2 cups diced onions

Avocado Vinaigrette & Chopped Mixed Greens

1 1/2 tbs. olive oil
1 level tsp. dried oregano

Choice of chopped mixed greens
1 onion, minced
¼ cup rice vinegar
1 clove garlic, peeled
1 tbs. mirin
½ tsp. salt
1 tbs. lemon juice
1 level tsp. black pepper
1 ripe avocado, peeled
⅓ cup of olive oil

1 level tsp. dried basil
2 tsp. ground cumin

Light Green Tea

Loose, or tea bag form

Method

Sweet Rice & Chestnuts

- Soak dried chestnuts the night before in about three times the amount of water to chestnuts. The chestnuts will swell, so be sure to use ample water. This will soften the chestnuts and make them more digestible for tomorrow's cooking.
- In cool water, wash rice.
- Add the rice and chestnuts in a medium-sized pot with heavy lid.
- Add sea salt.
- Cover completely with lid and bring to boil. Then lower heat and simmer for 50 to 60 minutes.
- Transfer to serving bowl and mix rice and chestnuts together.

Refried Beans

- With a medium–high heat, bring ½ to ¾ cup water to boil in a small pot. Add ⅓ teaspoon sea salt per cup of beans.
- Open prepared, canned beans, or leftover beans, and add to pot. Stir water and beans thoroughly.
- Add diced carrot and bay leaf.
- In a separate skillet, heat oil, add onions, and sauté over a medium heat for 6 to 8 minutes or until soft.
- Add oregano, basil, and cumin.
- Continue to sauté for 5 additional minutes, adding some of the bean liquid to prevent onions from burning.

- When the onions are sweet and soft, add the beans and mash to a thick paste. Cook over low heat, uncovered, for about 5 to 8 minutes, adding bean liquid continuously to prevent burning. Serve hot.

Avocado Vinaigrette & Chopped Mixed Greens

- In a blender, combine the garlic and onion.
- Puree together until smooth.
- Add vinegar, mirin, sea salt, lemon juice, black pepper, and avocado and puree again until thick.
- Add the olive oil to combine.
- Mix in thoroughly with chopped greens and serve.

Light Green Tea

Steep loose, or tea-bag form of tea.

DINNER MENUS

1

Creamy Cauliflower Soup
Linguini with Orange Roughy, Portobello Mushroom, & Sun-Dried
Tomatoes
Mixed Baby Green Salad with Tahini-Tart Dressing
Fruit Kanten
Mint Tea

2

Seven Minute Savory Broccoli-Cauliflower Miso Soup
Wild Rice, Corn, and Pecans with Shiitake-Onion-Corn Topping
Roasted Root Vegetables
Peach Mousse
Barley Tea

3

Dilled Corn Chowder
Millet-Mashed Potatoes with Caraway
Mesclun Salad & Creamy Lemon Dressing
Almond Drop Cookies
Twig Tea

4

Aztec Butternut-Squash Soup
Native American Holiday Rice
Ginger Salmon Bake
Water-Sautéd Bok Choy, Swiss Chard, & Napa Cabbage
Apple Glaze
Grain Coffee

5

Broiled Halibut with Lemon & Capers
Simply Baked Onions
Mixed Green Salad with Roma Tomatoes in Basil-Garlic Vinaigrette
Apricot Slices with Mint Leaf Garnish
Herb Tea

DINNER RECIPES

1

~ Dinner ~

Creamy Cauliflower Soup
Linguini with Orange Roughy, Portobello Mushroom,
& Sun-Dried Tomatoes
Mixed Baby Green Salad with Tahini-Tart Dressing
Fruit Kanten
Mint Tea

This delicious "pasta meets sea" dish was made by a friend at an event dinner I attended in the eastern United States.

Servings—4
Time—Approximately 25 minutes. Kanten needs approximately 30 minutes setting time.

Ingredients

Creamy Cauliflower Soup

1 large cauliflower
¼ cup white miso
¼ cup umeboshi vinegar
3–4 large sprigs parsley
½ tsp. nutmeg
1 tsp. toasted sesame oil
Filtered spring water to cover

Mixed Baby Green Salad with Tahini-Tart Dressing

Choice of mixed salad greens and assorted raw vegetables (carrot, white radish, tomato, cucumber, etc.).

Dressing (to vary, use equal parts)
2 tbs. umeboshi paste
2 tbs. toasted tahini butter
2 tbs. grated onion with juice
3 sprigs diced parsley
Water—to desired consistency

Linguini with Orange Roughy, Portobello Mushroom, & Sun-Dried Tomatoes

4 (5-ounce) cut orange roughy filets
1 cup sun-dried tomatoes

Fruit Kanten

2½ cups apple, or desired fruit juice

2 cloves garlic, minced

10 thinly sliced, fresh basil leaves

2 green onions, finely chopped

1 cup thinly sliced Portobello mushroom

3/4 cup rice or soy milk

1 lb. linguini or spaghetti

1/4 cup filtered or spring water

1 tbs. tamari

Basil stems for garnish

Sea salt

3 level tbs. agar-agar flakes

1 1/2–2 cups of bite-size fresh fruit

Note: Tempeh or fried tofu can be used in place of fish.

Mint Tea

Loose or tea-bag form

Method

Creamy Cauliflower Soup

- Wash cauliflower and divide into flowerets.
- Pressure cook with 3/4 covered in water (add a pinch of sea salt) for 10 minutes, or longer (until tender) in pot with heavy lid.
- Add white miso, umeboshi vinegar, and sesame oil and cook for additional 5 minutes.
- Place contents of pot into blender and puree.
- Allow to cool.
- Sprinkle with fresh nutmeg and garnish with a sprig of parsley for each bowl.

Mixed Baby Green Salad with Tahini-Tart Dressing

- Mix equal parts umeboshi paste, tahini, and grated onion with juice into small bowl.
- Add water to thin for desired consistency.
- Add dice parsley garnish.
- Mix into salad greens.

Linguini with Orange Roughy, Portobello Mushroom, & Sun-Dried Tomatoes

- Heat oil in a skillet over medium heat.
- Add the portobello mushroom and a pinch of salt and sauté for approximately 5 to 6 minutes.

- Add tamari.
- Add sun-dried tomatoes and garlic. Stir cook for 2 to 3 minutes.
- Add basil leaves, water, rice milk, and onions.
- Add a pinch of sea salt.
- Top with fish sections and continue cooking over a low heat for 4–6 minutes.
- As your fish is cooking, cook the linguini in a large pot for boiling water until it's al dente'—nearly tender (usually 5 to 7 minutes at a fierce boil), but slightly firm.
- Drain linguini, but avoid rinsing.
- Place linguini into the cooking pot; add roughy and sauce.
- Mix contents thoroughly but gently.
- Garnish with basil sprigs, and serve hot.

Fruit Kanten

Light and refreshing, this is the nearest thing to a natural version of chilled fruit gel—also known as Jell-O®

- Combine juice, salt, and agar-agar in a saucepan. Bring to a slow boil over a low heat. The most common mistake people make is boiling the agar too quickly, making it sink to the bottom of the pot still intact.
- Simmer 10–15 minutes, stirring frequently until the agar-agar is dissolved.
- Place fruit pieces into a glass serving dish and delicately pour the mixture over the fruit.
- Allow to stand 30 minutes, garnish with a mint leaf, and refrigerate.

Note: Softer fruits such as cherries, berries, peaches, or melons do not require being cooked in the kanten mixture. However, more firm textures, such as apples or pears, need to be cooked within the agar-agar and juice mixture in order to soften.

Mint Tea

Serve hot mint tea, from tea bags or in loose form for a zesty finish.

2

~ Dinner ~

Seven-Minute Savory Broccoli-Cauliflower Miso Soup
Wild Rice, Corn, and Pecans
with Shiitake-Onion-Corn Topping
Roasted Root Vegetables
Peach Mousse
Barley Tea

This simple and 7-minute quick (all right, maybe ... 12 minutes) soup is a nice complement to the entrée grain dish, made deliciously fragrant by the blending of mushroom and roasted pecans. The baked root vegetable dish brings out a unique and natural sweetness that satisfies.

Servings—4
Time—Approximately 20 minutes prep (45 minutes total cooking time)

Ingredients

Seven-Minute Savory Broccoli-Cauliflower Miso Soup

1 large cauliflower, chopped
1 bunch broccoli, chopped
4 cups filtered or spring water
2 cups vegetable stock
1 stick dry kombu sea vegetable
1 scallion stalk garnish
1½–2 tbs. barley miso paste
3 tbs. grated mochi
2 tbs. kuzu

Roasted Root Vegetables

2 beets
2 parsnips
2 rutabagas
Safflower oil
Sea salt
2 tsp. tamari

Wild Rice, Corn, and Pecans with Shiitake-Onion Corn Topping

1 cup wild rice
2–2½ cups filtered or spring water
½ cup fresh (or frozen) corn
1 tbs. sesame oil
¼–⅓ tsp. sea salt
½ cup roasted pecans
Topping:
1 cup minced onion
1 cup fresh shiitake, diced
1½ cups water (approximately)

Peach Mousse

2 bars agar-agar, rinsed
4 cups peach juice
2 peaches finely chopped
2 cups water
Pinch sea salt
2 tbs. almond butter
1 tsp. vanilla

Method

Seven-Minute Savory Broccoli-Cauliflower Miso Soup

- Bring 4 cups of water to a rapid boil with one stick of kombu at the pot bottom.
- Add chopped cauliflower and broccoli. Bring to a boil, cover, and simmer for approximately 6–8 minutes.
- Add vegetable stock to this mixture and transfer to blender. Put aside several broccoli and cauliflower flowerets. Blend mixture to a puree.
- Transfer back to pot. Bring to near boil. Add several pieces of cooked but uncut broccoli and cauliflower flowerets for decorative purpose.
- Add 2 tablespoons kuzu to 1/4 cup cold water and dissolve by stirring into the heated soup for 1–2 minutes. This amount of kuzu will add a slightly thicker quality to your soup.
- Remove 1/4 cup of soup into a mug and dissolve 1 1/2–2 tablespoons barley miso paste. Add to soup and turn off heat.
- Add finely grated mochi as a floating topping for a cheeselike quality.
- Garnish with fine chopped scallion.

Wild Rice with Pecans & Shiitake-Onion Corn Topping

Shiitake-Onion-Corn Topping:

- Dice an onion and water fry in approximately 1 1/2 cups water until onion becomes clear.
- Add diced shiitake and stir. Make sure there is at least 1 cup of water remaining to cook the mushrooms. Cook for 3 to 5 minutes.
- Add frozen corn or fresh corn chopped from the ear.
- Add in 2 teaspoons tamari and remove from heat. Put aside.

Wild Rice with Pecans:

- Oven roast or dry pan roast chopped pecans until browned and fragrant. Put aside.
- Rinse wild rice in a colander under cold running water. Allow to drain.
- Place water and salt in a heavy saucepan over high heat and bring to a boil.
- Add rice when the water boils and lower to a simmer.
- Simmer rice for approximately 40 minutes. The kernels will usually split open.
- Add the roasted pecans and allow to steam with the cover on for another 10 minutes.
- Add shiitake-onion corn topping and mix.
- Optional: Add fine chopped parsley as a garnish.

Note: While I recommend hand-harvested varieties of wild rice (as opposed to darker-color commercial varieties), they are harder to come by and usually more expensive. Hand-harvested wild rice has a distinct nutty and woodsy taste and require less water. See resources section for U.S. distributors.

Roasted Root Vegetables

- Preheat oven to 375°.
- Cut beets in circles, parsnips on an angle, and rutabaga in cubes.
- Rub each piece with oil and dust with sea salt.
- For golden vegetable edges, have each piece touch the pan surface.
- Bake 30–45 minutes, turning once or twice.

Peach Mousse

- Place the juice, water, and salt in a pot.
- Add the agar-agar—shred into small pieces.
- Cook on a medium flame until the agar-agar dissolves.
- Pour into a serving dish and allow to set in the refrigerator.
- After the kanten has set, place in a blender.
- Add the almond butter and vanilla.
- Blend to a smooth cream.
- Fold in the chopped peaches.
- Serve in individual glasses and garnished with chopped, roasted almonds

Barley Tea

A mellow finishing touch. Steep loose dark roasted barley ("mugi-cha") in boiling water for 5 minutes to desired strength.

3

~ Dinner ~

Dilled Corn Chowder
Millet-Mashed Potatoes with Caraway
Mesclun Salad & Creamy Lemon Dressing
Almond Drop Cookies
Twig Tea

This delicious millet recipe can be made to have the taste and texture of mashed potatoes. Originally, this dish was created for people who wanted to avoid potatoes but missed that familiar taste and texture. As a part of the nightshade family of vegetables, some research has indicated that potatoes might be problematic for arthritis and similar conditions. Whether or not this may apply to you, try this unique way to enjoy millet. The flourless, oil-free almond cookies are full of delicate flavor with the subtle sweetness of barley malt.

Servings—4
Time—Approximately 20 minutes prep, 35 minutes of total cooking.

Ingredients

Dilled Corn Chowder

Corn kernels from 4–5 ears
2 stalks of minced celery
2 small carrots, minced
3 tbs. cornmeal
Pinch of sea salt
1 tbs. fresh dill
1½ tbs. "mellow miso"
Optional: 1 tbs. barley malt

Mesclun Salad & Creamy Lemon Dressing

2 tbs. avocado
1 tbs. umeboshi paste
1 tbs. fresh lemon juice
¼ cup soft tofu
6 tbs. water

Millet-Mashed Potatoes with Caraway

1 cup millet
3 cups filtered or spring water
1 small onion, diced
½ head cauliflower, cut in chunks
⅛ tsp. sea salt
1 tbs. fresh parsley, fine cut
1 tbs. caraway seeds
1 tbs. tamari

Almond Drop Cookie

(This recipe makes 18 cookies)
3 cups almonds
⅓ cup apple juice (approx.)
Juice of 1 orange
1 tsp. vanilla extract
½ tsp. cinnamon
1 cup rice syrup or barley malt
⅓ tsp. sea salt

Twig Tea

Kukicha twigs, or Kukicha tea bags

Method

Dilled Corn Chowder

- Heat water, add chopped corn cobs you've sliced corn kernels from, sea salt, and cornmeal, stirring constantly to prevent lumps.
- Place a "flame diffuser" beneath pot to prevent burning the cornmeal.

- Simmer for 10 minutes.
- Remove corn cobs; add vegetables and barley malt (optional).
- Simmer 15 minutes.
- Remove a bit of the broth and dilute the miso. Add the diluted miso broth to the pot.
- Simmer 1–2 minutes—do not boil!
- Add dill and remove from heat. Serve hot.

Millet-Mashed Potatoes with Caraway

- Bring water to boil in a pressure cooker (or pot with heavy lid*).
- Rinse millet through a strainer. Drain.
- Add diced onion, millet, cauliflower, caraway, and salt to pressure cooker and lock lid in place securely. Over a high heat, allow pressure to rise.
- Place a flame diffuser beneath the pot to spread heat evenly. Maintain high pressure, but reduce heat. Allow to cook for 20 minutes. Remove from stove.
- Reduce internal pressure by running cold water over pot.
- Release stem latch to allow remaining pressure to escape.
- Remove lid after all pressure has been released.
- Mash millet in the pot by using a potato masher.
- Add 1 tablespoon tamari and mix in.
- Serve warm.

Pot Cooking: Use 1/2 cup extra water and cook for 30 minutes using a heavy or weighted lid.

Mesclun Salad & Creamy Lemon Dressing

- Combine avocado oil, umeboshi paste, fresh lemon juice, soft tofu, and water.
- Mix thoroughly and add to mixed green salad medley.

Almond Drop Cookie

- Preheat oven to 325°.
- Grind the almonds in a blender to make almond meal.
- Add enough apple juice to make a smooth paste.
- Combine the almond paste with remaining ingredients.
- Drop this mixture by tablespoons onto a well-oiled baking sheet and press each cookie lightly with a fork.
- Bake on a high rack for 10 minutes or until the cookies look golden. They are easy to burn and require careful attention.

Twig Tea

Brew kukicha twig tea in loose form, or tea bag version.

4

~ Dinner ~

Aztec Butternut-Squash Soup
Native American Holiday Rice
Ginger Salmon Bake
Water-Sautéd Bok Choy, Swiss Chard, & Napa Cabbage
Apple Glaze
Grain Coffee

This variation of Aztec soup, inspired by Jody Main, is best served in a carved-out pumpkin for that gourmet touch. The native rice dish is my holiday staple (any holiday will do, especially Thanksgiving). The ginger salmon bake is a simple, no-frills recipe anyone can master in minutes. The green vegetable combination is a nutritious and subtly sweet mixture.

Servings—4

Time—Approximately 25 to 30 minutes of prep time, with a little over an hour of actual cooking.

Ingredients

Aztec Butternut-Squash Soup

$2/3$ cup raw pumpkin seeds
1 medium butternut squash
2 onions, chopped
1 chile, seeded and chopped
3 cloves crushed garlic
1 tsp. sunflower oil
5–6 cups water
$1/3$–$1/2$ tsp. sea salt

Native American Holiday Rice

1 cup brown rice
$1/2$ cup wild rice
2–3 cups corn kernels
$1/3$ cup minced watercress
Optional: 2 tbs. tahini, water thinned
with 2 tsp. tamari

Ginger Salmon Bake

4 (5 ounce) salmon filets
2 tbs. fresh ginger juice
2 tbs. tamari
4 tbs. water
2 scallion stalks

Apple Glaze

4 ripe apples
1 cup apple juice
1 tbs. kuzu, dissolved in cold water
1/2 tsp. fresh ginger juice
Pinch of sea salt

Grain Coffee

Choice of grain coffee

Water-Fried Bok Choy, Swiss Chard, & Napa Cabbage

1 bunch bok choy
1 bunch swiss chard
1/2 napa cabbage
Water
Toasted sesame seeds

Method

Aztec Butternut-Squash Soup

- Preheat oven to 350°.
- Toast pumpkin seeds in a heavy skillet over medium heat for a few minutes, stirring constantly until they are puffed, popping, and deliciously fragrant.
- Set aside half the seeds for garnish, and blend remaining half in blender until finely ground.
- Poke several holes in the squash with a fork and set on a baking sheet. Bake for 30 to 40 minutes until tender.
- Remove squash from oven, scoop out seeds and fibers, and cut into cubes.
- In a skillet on medium–low heat, sauté onions, chile, and garlic in sunflower oil for 8–10 minutes.
- Bring water to a boil; add the squash and sauteed vegetables. Cover, reduce heat, and simmer gently for 15 minutes or until vegetables are tender.
- Add the gound pumpkin seeds and sea salt. Simmer for another 15 minutes. The soup will thicken.
- Serve in a tureen (or hollowed-out pumpkin) and sprinkle with remaining seeds.

Native American Holiday Rice

- Pressure cook ($1\frac{1}{2}$ cups grain to 2–$2\frac{1}{4}$ cups water) or boil with heavy lid ($1\frac{1}{2}$ cups grain to 3 cups water) brown rice and wild rice together with sea salt.
- Bring up to pressure (or full boil) and allow to simmer for 45–55 minutes (boiled grain, at least 60 minutes). Remove from heat and transfer to mixing bowl.
- Quick boil fresh corn kernels (or frozen) for 2 minutes. Add minced watercress for the last minute of cooking.
- Combine corn and watercress with brown and wild rice.
- Optional: Thin 2 tablespoons of roasted tahini butter in 5 tablespoons of water. Add 2 teaspoons of tamari to make a grain sauce and mix into grain and corn dish.

Ginger Salmon Bake

- Fine grate approximately a half-thumb size amount of fresh ginger root to extract 2 teaspoons fresh ginger juice. Add 2 teaspoons tamari and 4 tablespoons water. Into this, add finely chopped scallion, using two stalks. Mix cooking marination together. Set aside.
- Rinse 4 (5 ounce) salmon filets in cold water.
- Place in glass baking dish. Add ginger-tamari mixture with scallion.
- Bake at 400° for 15–20 minutes. Sample a small piece of salmon after 15 minutes to test.

Water-Fried Bok Choy, Swiss Chard, & Napa Cabbage

- Toast sesame seeds for approximately 10 minutes in a dry skillet using a medium flame on your back burner. Stir frequently to avoid burning. Make extra to have handy as garnish for other dishes.
- Wash all greens thoroughly in a colander.
- Chop greens in uniform small pieces.
- Bring 1 to $1\frac{1}{2}$ cups water to a boil and add greens. Cover with some exposed area ($\frac{1}{3}$ covered) and cook with medium flame for 4 to 6 minutes.
- Garnish with toasted sesame seeds.

Apple Glaze

- Preheat oven to 350°.
- Cut the apples in half and remove cores.
- Lay apples in shallow baking dish, cut side up, and dust with sea salt.
- Cover and bake for 15 minutes.
- As the apples are baking, heat apple juice over low heat until fairly hot.

- Stir in dissolved kuzu, stirring until mixture thickens and clears. This should take about 4 minutes. Add ginger juice and pour over the cooked apples.
- Increase oven heat to 400° and return apples to oven, uncovered, for 15 minutes to set glaze.
- Serve warm.

Grain Coffee

Choice of brewed grain coffee with rice or soy milk.

5

~ Dinner ~

Broiled Halibut with Lemon & Capers
Simply Baked Onions
Mixed Green Salad with Roma Tomatoes in Basil-Garlic Vinaigrette
Apricot Slices with Mint Leaf Garnish
Herb Tea

A "meaty" fish recipe enhanced with a tart lemon taste, "effortless" baked onions, and tangy vinaigrette of basil and garlic over mixed greens.

Servings—4

Time—Approximately 20–25 minutes (not including the 2 hours for baked onions)

Ingredients

Broiled Halibut with Lemon & Capers

4 (4–5 ounce) halibut filets
2 leek stalks, thin-cut lengthwise
1–2 tsp. tamari
2 tbs. capers, thoroughly drained
1 carrot, strand or matchcut style
Spring or filtered water
Juice of two lemons

Simply Baked Onions

4 medium-size yellow onions

Mixed Green & Tomato Salad with Roma Tomatoes in Basil-Garlic Vinaigrette

Mixed greens

Roma tomatoes

Dressing:

2 tbs. brown rice vinegar

5 tbs. olive oil

½ cup fresh basil leaves

½ tsp. sea salt

1 garlic clove, coarsely chopped

Method

Apricot Slices with Mint Leaf Garnish

Sliced apricots

Mint leaf garnish

Herb Tea

Choice of herb tea

Broiled Halibut with Lemon & Capers

- Heat olive oil over a medium heat.
- Add leeks and tamari and sauté for 2 to 3 minutes.
- Add capers and sauté for 1 minute.
- Add strand cut carrots and continue sautéing for another minute.
- Evenly layer the vegetables across the bottom of the skillet and lay halibut on the vegetables. Add a small amount of water to cover the skillet bottom.
- Cover and cook for 10 to 12 minutes, until halibut is tender.
- Transfer to serving dish and pour lemon juice over the entire fish.
- Serve warm.

Simply Baked Onions

This is a very simple recipe that requires advance planning since it has to bake for 2 hours. It has an appealing texture and very satisfying sweetness. When my daughter was very young, I used to have her make this for me. It gave her an incredible feeling of kitchen competence. (Maybe too much; almost every time she entered the kitchen, she'd ask: "Daddy, should I bake some onions for you?")

- Preheat oven to 350°. Wait 5 minutes.
- Lay onions, still in their brown wrapper skins, on a cookie sheet and place in oven.
- Allow to cook for 2 hours. Of course, you don't have to stand there waiting, but 2 hours later, you'll have incredibly sweet onions.
- Simply, peel skins off, slice in quarters, and serve.

Mixed Green Salad with Roma Tomatoes in Basil-Garlic Vinaigrette

To a mixed green vegetable add chopped Roma tomatoes and the dressing.

Dressing:
- Combine dressing ingredients in a blender and smooth.
- Toss into salad and mix.

Apricot Slices with Mint Leaf Garnish

- Slice fresh apricot slices.
- Garnish with fresh mint leaves.

Herb Tea

Choice of fresh or dried tea bag of herb tea

RECIPE PRODUCT GLOSSARY

Agar, Agar-Agar (Ah-gahr)—Also known as kanten. Kanten's complex carbohydrate quality acts as a gelling agent. Agar has been use for years by the confections industry. It is the vegetarian alternative to gelatin, which is made up from animal parts, including ground horse hooves.

Barley Malt Syrup—Similar in appearance and taste to molasses. Barley malt is composed chiefly of maltose sugar and is made by the cooking of sprouted barley until it's concentrated into a sweet syrup. It has a minimal mineral content.

Brown Rice Syrup—A thick syrup that is amber colored and used in numerous natural food dessert recipes.

Brown Rice Vinegar—This unique vinegar has a smooth and mild flavor and is traditionally brewed. Most superior brands will ferment their vinegar for one year.

Chestnuts—Despite being extremely low in fat (4 to 8 percent), chestnuts offer a unique texture of unusual sweetness. Their season is the fall. (Being brought up in New York City, a fond autumn memory was purchasing warmed chestnuts from street vendors on cool winter days.) Dried chestnuts can be found in many natural foods markets as well as Asian groceries. They are best soaked overnight, drained, and cooked with grain dishes.

Daikon (Dye-kon)—A long white radish popular in Asian markets. According to the dietary traditions of Asian medicine, daikon has strong healing properties. It aids in the breakdown and digestion of fat and protein and, for this reason, often is served with many fish dishes. It has a subtle diuretic effect.

Fresh Ginger Root—A pungent tropical vegetable typically used in stir fries, with animal protein dishes, and in many Asian medicinal preparations. Ginger juice can be easily extracted by grating the root on a porcelain or stainless steel grater, gathering the small ginger fragments, and squeezing them to liberate the juice.

Gomashio (Goh-mah-shee-o)—Also known as "sesame salt," this condiment is a delicious blend of toasted sesame seeds and sea salt, usually made in a large proportion of 20:1, or 24:1—that is, 20 teaspoons of toasted sesame seeds to 1 teaspoon of sea salt. The seeds are roasted, mixed in a surbachi (Asian mortar and pestle with serrated edges), and ground until the sesame seeds are crushed and their oil covers the salt. If made properly, it should not inspire thirst. You can buy this product commercially prepared, but it pales next to the freshly homemade version.

Grain "Coffee"—There are many grain coffees on the market. What they have in common is that they are made with whole grain and do not contain any caffeine. To some, they taste like coffee, to others, vastly different. Their hearty taste makes a nice finish to most meals. They can be purchased in individual packets for traveling or jars. I often pack some into a baggie for trips, which allows me to customize how strong I want it.

Kombu (Kom-boo)—This dried sea vegetable, also know as sea kelp, has always sounded to me like it should have been the name of a circus clown. I like to refer to kombu as "Asian bay leaf" since it is used much like a bay leaf—in soup stocks, medicinal preparations, and bean dishes. Known as the original and natural form of MSG, kombu is a natural flavor enhancer. Its mineral content is helpful to reducing the gas-producing starches in beans.

Kukicha Twig Tea (Ku-key-cha)—It might sound very strange to drink from a brew of twigs, but this tea is a very popular Asia tea and, since its introduction to the natural foods markets during the mid-1960s, has become quite popular. It is a mild, very-low-caffeine tea, high in minerals and made from the stems and twigs of tea bushes. It is generally roasted, and this reduces its caffeine content further. Most of the caffeine from the tea bush is concentrated in the leaves. Make sure the label on your tea says "Twigs Only."

Kuzu (Coo-zoo)—Also known in the U.S. south as "kudzu," this valuable chalky white root starch is usually used as a thickening agent in sauces and icings. It only dissolves in cold water and must be gradually stirred into a warm liquid in order to thicken. According to Asian folk medicine, kuzu makes the blood alkaline, is beneficial to the intestines and stomach, and helps to relieve muscle pain. It has far more medicinal properties than arrowroot starch powder. One tablespoon of kuzu will thicken one cup of liquid.

Mirin (mihr-ihn)—A unique cooking wine from Japan that is made from sweet brown rice, koji rice, and water. It has a light and sweet taste. Often used to complement stronger flavors such as miso, tamari, or vinegar, mirin is a nice addition to many dishes. Purchase only naturally brewed versions that can be found in natural food stores.

Miso (Mee-so)—Miso (see Chapter 8) is an aged, fermented soybean paste that is typically made from grain, soybean, and sea salt. There are an amazing array of miso products, but generally two types: dark and light. In most cases, the darker the natural miso the longer it has been fermented, which is considered more strength building and medicinal. Light miso tends to be sweeter, contains less salt, and is fermented for a shorter period of time.

Mochi (moh-chee)—Mochi is a product that is made from cooked sweet brown rice that has been pounded, formed into square cakes, and dried. It has an energy-producing effect and naturally sweet taste. In Asian folk medicine, mochi was added to miso soup to produce more milk for nursing mothers. Mochi is very versatile; it can be grated and added to dishes to produce a cheeselike effect, it can be used in waffle-irons to produce a flourless and sweet waffle, and it can be used in soups, or as a side dish with other foods.

Rice Milk—A mildly sweetened (usually with barley malt) grain beverage that can be substituted for milk.

Sea Salt—The difference between mine (land) salt and sea salt is a matter of mineral content and bioavailabity. The best sea salt is slightly "damp," indicating that it has been solar, and not oven, dried. Sea salt is best added during the cooking process, which helps to "digest" the salt.

Shiitake Mushrooms (Shee-tah-kay)—Prized for their medicinal qualities (see Chapter 8), shiitake mushrooms are delicious and help to neutralize animal protein by reducing cholesterol. Dried mushrooms can be purchased and soaked for 10 minutes to an hour, before cooking. Generally, buy loose mushrooms and not those that have been packaged in plastic-wrap cartons.

Sea Vegetable Flakes—Many of the more common sea vegetables used worldwide can be purchased in dry, flake form to be used as a mineral supplement or to neutralize excessive acids in the diet. Some of them are nori, dulse, wakame, and kombu. While the idea of eating "slimy seaweed" may be repulsive, there are so many delicious ways to prepare these as an accent to a meal instead of a main taste.

Sesame Oil—Sesame oil is a light and nutty-flavored oil that can be used in many dishes. The "toasted" version is generally used as a flavoring accent and not cooked for any real period of time.

Shoyu—Shoyu is the Japanese term for soy sauce that is naturally fermented and made from soybeans, roasted wheat, and salt. It is fermented in wooden kegs for a period of 18 months to 3 years. See *Tamari* to understand the differences between these soy sauces.

Soy Milk—Soy milk is a good milk transitional food. I suspect that many people think it's the saving grace of all dairy reformers, however, based on new research, moderate use of soy milk might be the best bet. It has lower fat and chemical residue than regular milk, small molecular structure (to prevent allergy reactions), fewer calories, and virtually no cholesterol. It can be diluted to add to dry cereals.

Soy Sauce—This is the standard term for that dark and very salty liquid on every Asian restaurant table. Unfortunately, commercial soy sauces are not brewed with traditional methods, or fermented for a period of many months, or even years. Chemicals and/or yeast are frequently used to speed this process, and the commercial soy sauces often contain sugar, corn syrup, and artificial flavors and colors.

Tahini (Tah-heee-nee)—Made from the ground hulls of sesame seeds, tahini has a nutty flavor and is high in oil content. Canned tahini is often bitter and grainy and rarely organic. Arrowhead Mills®, Westbrea®, Maranatha®, and Tohum® all make and distribute organic, quality tahini butters. Roasted tahini has a fuller flavor and is used more frequently for recipes.

Tempeh (temp-pay)—This is a fermented soybean product originally from Indonesia. Containing more than 50 percent the protein volume of hamburger, tempeh is cholesterol free. It has a very appealing texture and is frequently mixed with strong seasonings such as ginger, vinegar, soy sauce, mustard, and garlic. It can be grilled, steamed, sautéed, or baked. Tempeh can be found in the refrigerated section of your natural foods market.

Tofu (Toe-fu)—Tofu is made from soybeans and is a healthy source of calcium and vegan protein. Traditionally, tofu was eaten in small quantites, in soups and side dishes. Its blandness makes it a good candidate for mixing with other foods due to its ability to absorb flavors (this is especially true of dried tofu). It comes in soft styles and firm white blocks. Soft tofu is more frequently used in soups and for creamy sauces. Firm tofu is best for frying, baking, and grilling. You can enhance the degree to which tofu will absorb flavors by creating a two-board tofu press: Place tofu between two small wooden cutting boards for 20 to 25 minutes to drain excess water. Tofu is found in the refrigerated section of your natural foods market.

Umeboshi Paste (Uhmm-ee-bou-she)—Umeboshi plums are a fruit similar to the apricot. They are bright pink, have a combination salty and sour taste, and are high in iron. The plums are picked when they are still unripe and fermented in a wooden keg for nearly one year. They have exceptional natural antibiotic qualities and are used in many Asian folk remedies. The paste is the meat from the plums that has been pureed. Umeboshi paste is most frequently used in salad dressings, sushi, and sauces. A level teaspoon of umeboshi paste in one cup of "twig-only" tea can usually remedy an upset or acid stomach fairly quickly.

Umeboshi Vinegar—This vinegar is a byproduct of the umeboshi process and is actually more of a salt brine liquid than a vinegar. It is delicious and most frequently used on salads, pastas, and cooked greens.

Zest—This is another word for "peel," the colored, outer layer of citrus fruit skin. The white part (the "underskin") usually contains a bitter aftertaste. Avoid it. When a recipe calls for "lemon zest," it is suggesting that the skin be carefully grated for it's "zest essence."

RESTAURANT AND TRAVELING TIPS

It doesn't require Herculean will to stay on your healthy program. It may require a bit of compromise, but there are a number of options whether you're at a company event, a wedding, a cruise, on an airplane, or on the road. Here are some things that have worked for me and numerous clients:

Breakfast

- Usually, oatmeal is available from most restaurants. What can transform this "bland breakfast" into something more interesting is bringing along a couple of condiments—some roasted nuts/seeds, perhaps a bit of cinnamon, or the grain condiment called sesame salt (a.k.a. "gomáshio"). In some restaurants, corn grits are available.

- It is also helpful to travel with your own tea bags. They take up little room and help digestion. You can also obtain instant grain coffee (with no caffeine) packets or just put one or two teaspoons into a small zip lock baggie before you leave the house. I use a couple of drops of lemon in mine for a bit of a taste kick.

- Whole wheat or buckwheat pancakes are now more widely available. Use syrup moderately. If only artificial syrup is available, I opt for a small amount of honey on the side of my plate, where I dip my forkful before eating.

- When I used to travel across Canada by rail, I'd take a wide mouth soup thermos and, before retiring, place ¾ of a cup of toasted rolled oats (lightly dry pan fry the rolled oats before packing them into 1-cup portions in baggies with a pinch of salt) with 2 cups of water that has been boiled. Tighten the cap, shake once or twice, and allow to remain overnight. In the morning, instant oatmeal. I'd bring this to the dining car and, regardless of what ever else I would order, I'd feel a sense of mental comfort by having my morning grain, ensuring me of endurance energy, regular eliminations, and more satisfaction with my meals.

Restaurant Lunches

- Use your tea bag, or order herbal tea with an orange, lemon, or lime wedge.

- Ethnic restaurants usually offer healthy choices as long as you specify to go easy on the oil. Avoid MSG and sweetened dishes.

- Usually, some kind of "veggie burgers" are available, as are salad dishes, vegetarian soups, a steam vegetable plate, bean dish, or a pasta and vegetable dish.

Ethnic Choices

Please remember this—for *any* restaurant you dine in: You are the patron. You keep these places in business by frequenting their establishment or referring friends, family, and coworkers. Get over feeling timid about customizing your order. Do it politely, with diplomacy and a smile. Sound firm, but not expectant. Ask. This usually works. Generally, better-quality restaurants will go out of their way to please you—within reason. A generous tip ensures repeat service. They may forget what you order, but rarely will they forget that your gratitude was reflected in your tip.

- **Chinese:** I have found that most of the servers in Chinese restaurants will humor my requests—rarely will I get what I order, so I usually preface my ordering by telling them that I will send back what I have not ordered. I also ask them to repeat my order after I've finished. I know this must sound condescending, but my experience has not been all that positive over the years, so I've become slightly militant as a patron. I usually specify no MSG, chicken stock, sugar, or eggs and low, low oil. What does that leave? Steamed moo shu vegetables, rice, lo mein noodles with vegetables, and, sometimes, baked vegetarian spring rolls. Read your fortune, but don't eat the fortune cookie.

- **Japanese:** Order vegetarian sushi and choose your own vegetables from what may be available. Eda mame (steamed soybeans in the pod) makes for a nice, filling appetizer. Sometimes, if raw fish is not appealing, many sushi chefs (for counter patrons) will bake a small piece of salmon in their toaster ovens and make a baked sushi salmon roll with cucumber, sesame seeds, and nori. In more traditional restaurants, you can order soba noodles with vegetables (nabe mono) and ask for some wakame (a light sea vegetable that tastes like spinach) and scallions mixed in. This is very satisfying. Another option is to ask for miso broth instead of their standard soup broth. I do this to avoid their stock soup, which is usually sweetened with mirin, a rice wine. Most commercial miso soups that you order in Japanese restaurants contain MSG and other chemicals. If you order tempura, ask for some raw daikon (white radish), as this helps to digest oil. The salty dip they provide can help with the digestion of oil.

- **Mexican:** Make certain that they use vegetable oil for the frying of beans, chips, or rice. (More economical restaurants often use beef lard to fry foods.) Request corn tortillas instead of white flour. Use guacamole in place of sour cream. Order a bowl of beans with onions, cilantro, and tomato. In many places you can order a custom burrito and fill it with rice, beans, lettuce, and a bit of guacamole. Fresh fish tacos are usually baked with vegetables and make a nice entrée.

- **East Indian:** My favorite dish in Indian restaurants is vegetable biryani (stir-fried vegetables with rice, nuts, and small pieces of fruit), without eggs. I'll also ask that they use minimum oil when making this dish. Along with this, I'll often order a cauliflower-potato dish (aloo gobi), some chickpea stew (channa masala), or a side of cooked lentils (dahl). This is a very satisfying meal, composed mostly of complex carbohydrate. Although the rice is usually white, the added oils do not cause it to elevate blood sugar. Once in a while I'll treat myself to their onion wheat chappati (flat bread) and finish with some tea—my bag or theirs.

- **Mid-Eastern:** As appetizers, tabouli (cut wheat grits, olive oil, and parsley), lentil soups, and hummus (chickpeas and tahini) make for satisfying appetizers. Usually a Greek platter or some sort of vegetarian appetizer is also available and can be easily shared. I'm not a fan of feta cheese; however, a little bit might add a flavorful addition to your meal. Popular entrées like couscous vegetable stew or lentils and bulgur (mjadra) can be ordered as well as a baked (instead of fried) falafel platter.

- **Thai:** I'll often order a thin rice noodle dish (pad thai) and ask to have it prepared with vegetables and tofu instead of meat. They look at me as if I'm from another planet when I ask them to make it without sugar. "Why? No taste!" warned my waiter. "Oh yes, wonderful taste. It's OK. No sugar, please," I have to repeat. If the broth is vegetable based, I'll order an entrée-sized bowl of tom yum vegetable soup with or without noodles. I'll also order some vegetable curry and ask them to either hold the coconut milk or add "just a little bit."

- **Ethiopian:** If there's an Ethiopian restaurant in your town, you're in for a treat. A healthy meal of grain, vegetable, and greens is tastefully available, attractively prepared, and economical. The injera bread is a spongy bread made from their traditional grain, teff. You can order a chickpea salad (buticha), rice dishes, fish plates, or a vegetarian combination platter with yellow split peas (kik alitcha) and different greens (usually collard greens).

- **American Deli:** In most delis you can still get a traditional vegetarian mushroom-barley soup. You might be able to order kasha (cooked buckwheat—sometimes cooked with chicken broth), a plate of steamed vegetables, and some boiled fish or a salad with dressings on the side. Herbal teas are usually available.

Traveling

One of the best resources for traveling is to have one of the national natural food restaurant guides to help make healthy selections. I usually check with local natural food stores or look at their bulletin board. In most restaurants, you can get some type of vegetable soup, a salad, a steamed vegetable plate, some broiled fish, a bean dish, or something from their specials or entrée list. It's also handy when traveling to take along a baggie of tea bags and some toasted seeds or condiments that can be added to foods to enhance nutrition and satisfaction. In restaurants, ask for what you want—substitute, suggest, be creative. Your meals merely enhance the journey.

AFTERWORD

*"It is not death or pain that is to be dreaded,
but the fear of pain or death."*

—Epictetus, Discources (2nd c.)

In the Preface to this book, I described what it was like for me, as a young boy, to see my mother die of cancer—and how it led me to the search for answers in the years that followed. But the story would seem unfinished if I didn't describe, briefly, where that search led me. And, at the same time, I feel that this book would be incomplete if I did not describe some of the other clues that I have uncovered along the way—in pursuit of the foe that took my mother's life.

I left home just after my sixteenth birthday.

We used to call it "running away."

I continued schooling while living with relatives, working temporary jobs, dabbling in the theater and finding myself, naturally drawn to health issues. Not surprisingly, I was dreadfully fearful of becoming sick. My pervasive fear throughout adolescence was that I might suddenly develop this mysterious fatal disease my emotions bolstered my motivation to change. In the recesses of my young mind, anything relating to health, except for the conventional medicine that failed my mother, had appeal. And, in 1970, you couldn't get further away from convention than the exotic construct called "macrobiotics," a philosophy, lifestyle and diet based on the teachings of traditional cultures.

311

I began to encounter people who regarded macrobiotics almost like a religion—a unifying solution to all the ills of the world. After meeting a friend who had cleared a long-standing case of acne with the diet, I began to read everything available on the subject. The more I read, the more I felt assured of my new direction.

I moved from California to the "macrobiotic Mecca" of Boston and into a communal house with students of all ages who came from a wide variety of backgrounds. We followed the eclectic teachings of George Ohsawa, the founder of the macrobiotic movement, and his most popular students: Michio and Aveline Kushi, who taught in Boston, and Herman and Cornelia Aihara, who led the macrobiotic movement in the San Francisco area.

For a four year period, I took courses at Kushi's East West Foundation in Oriental Medicine and participated in seminars. The curriculum included acupuncture theory, nutrition, physiology, massage, folk remedies, martial arts and world philosophy. After leaving Boston, I applied for a part-time apprenticeship with a well-respected New York City Chinese doctor who was in his late seventies. I had a year of private tutoring, during which I assisted with his patients.

Macrobiotic philosophy—and the standard diet that was an essential part of the macrobiotic lifestyle—had definite benefits for me at that time. I was finally able to break an obsessive sugar habit. My body strengthened, my skin cleared, my sleep became shorter and deeper, and my stamina improved. Best of all, my fear of sickness gradually diminished, as I grew confident that a healthy and long life was something we could realize thorough choice.

LESSONS FROM TEACHING

I began to teach and, with an entrepreneurial eagerness, organized seminars that I promoted around the country. The seminars allowed me to refine many of the concepts explored in this book while offering several introductory approaches for beginning dietary change. Frequently, after seminars, participants scheduled private sessions to have this information personalized for their individual needs. Before fax and email arrived. I would do follow-up telephone sessions to receive feedback and offer additional recommendations. The follow-up results helped me shape an effective and practical program that people could consistently follow without complaints of deprival.

For the next ten years, I traveled non-stop. I spoke at symposiums, expositions, chiropractic colleges, prisons, medical facilities, Universities and health organizations. I was interviewed for television and radio, and wrote numerous articles for national publications.

But a teacher is always learning. From listening to my students concerns, I learned to address things that were never emphasized in my macrobiotic studies. Through counseling experience, I learned about the emotional connections that most Americans have with their eating habits. I had the opportunity to witness, first-hand, how stress influences dietary choices. I observed how certain individuals would be more motivated when they knew the "why" of things—that is, why a particular food or nutrient produced a predictable reaction from the immune system or an improvement in over-all health.

As my clients asked more questions, I became increasingly motivated to understand the specific role certain nutrients had in degenerative disease. I wanted to be able to support my recommendations not only from a philosophical viewpoint, but with the certainty that I was offering practical advice with tangible outcomes.

I also realized the need to make this information more flexible in scope, more westernized in reference, and more inclusive of mind and spirit teachings. I wanted to achieve a balanced approach, but without compromising the integrity of my recommendations.

So, my views expanded. At the start, inspired with idealistic fervor, I held to the belief that "diet was everything." But when I was able to identify obsessive adherents of one type of limited diet, it became very clear to me that dietary measures did not necessarily result in the best health. There had to be more to it than that.

And so, my focus shifted somewhat. Above all, I wanted to motivate people with a new love and respect for their bodies while offering a fresh perspective about the need to create more meaning to life, instead of attempting to motivate them by instilling a fear of sickness. I began to see problems not only from the standpoint of nutritional deficiency, but a "passion-for-life deficiency," a "love deficiency," a "sense-of-meaning deficiency."

Today, I advocate a broader program. The nutritional information that you find in this book is a starting point, but I can't end this book without acknowledging the mental and spiritual realms of health, which also play a role.

THE BIGGER PICTURE

Beginning in the late eighties, I had a four-year association with two medical groups. The physicians in this group became extremely supportive of my work as they saw their patients (whom I call my clientele) making the transformation to healthier lives. I offered general suggestions focusing on reducing cravings for sugar and fat while gradually adding whole foods on a weekly basis.

Structuring our work as a "one-month experiment," we initially concentrated on reducing stimulants (sugar, caffeine, salt), while adding whole grain, beans and bean products, plentiful amounts of vegetables, reducing animal protein and late-night eating. Exercise recommendations and stress management suggestions were also included. The physicians gradually reduced certain medications as the health of our people noticeably improved.

The transformations were often dramatic. In the span of weeks, we saw elevated blood pressure numbers drop, cholesterol counts plummet, skin conditions clear, desirable weight-loss, and improved endurance among a large percentage of clients, as well as a decline in insulin use and reduced depression. Interestingly, the physicians I worked with began to pay more attention to their own diets as well as that of their patients, taking more time with them and following their progress. Eventually, the physicians began to focus their practices on illness prevention, relying primarily on diet and lifestyle changes.

At the same time, I continued to explore a number of holistically oriented healing approaches that include the ancient and sage medical traditions of China, Tibet and Native America. In my associations I was able to witness the power of these traditions in preventing, treating disease and alleviating suffering. I was also inspired by some truly amazing spiritual teachers whose influence is strong and stabilizing.

MANY ROADS OF THE HEALING JOURNEY

"There is no journey to healing. Healing is the journey."

—Greg Anderson, *Healing Wisdom*

The healing path is composed of many roads all leading to the same destination: the place where body, mind and spirit are resurrected. The road, or roads we choose to adventure on should be based on fulfilling the incomplete areas of our lives, areas we've neglected, calling for greater nurturence and expression.

Those roads may be named: Faith, Purpose, Nutrition, Love, Honesty, Compassion, Immunity, Passion, Spirit, Forgiveness, or Gratitude. In the relatively young field of allopathic medicine—the kind that's practiced by most conventional medical doctors today—we've only recently recognized that healing efforts must not only be personalized for the patients special needs, but must offer some semblance of control, encouraging him or her to make informed choices instead of being hi-pressured by "experts" who claim to do it all for them.

There is no one-size-fits-all solution, or "universal cure," be cause illness is more than a simple viral assault; illness can be fed and bred by any number of factors, including those psychological and stress-related.

There are many "selves" we must consider in our quest for healing from physical, spiritual and psychological selves, to the subdivisions of each of these categories. This collective embodiment of selves reminds me of those historically-famous Russian

Matryoshka nesting dolls. These symbols of Russian creative artistry are hand-painted, traditionally made from thin wood and snugly fit inside each other. They begin at one size and each doll, in order to fit within the other, must be proportionately smaller down to the very last doll, which can sometimes be the size of a pea. Similarly, our own "selves" are layered within us and dependent on each other. True healing honors each one.

Clinical research, as well as anecdotal testimony, has repeatedly shown that the people who survive cancer often have many of the following ten traits:

1. Life Purpose
2. Positive Attitude
3. Good Nourishment
4. Healthy Lifestyle
5. Manageable Stress
6. Sense of Humor
7. Love and Social Support
8. Emotional Expression
9. Physical Exercise
10. Strong Faith

These ten traits can have vital healing influence. In seminars where I speak on these self-healing characteristics. I usually ask participants to consider which areas they need to emphasize for more comprehensive healing. I suggest initiating a personal dialogue that questions everything about the way we live, love, and care for ourselves.

Here are many questions to ask: What dietary factors are making us more susceptible to sickness? What psychological issues have we ignored that have now graduated into hidden sources of habitual stress? Can we strengthen our faith to deal with the escalating fears that are typically less significant for people with strong spiritual direction? What gives us joy?

Our hope for healing begins when we commit ourselves to examining and integrating those missing ingredients, which are essential for more passionate, healthy, and vital lives.

Verne Varona

ACKNOWLEDGMENTS

*"The only end of writing is to enable the readers
better to enjoy life or better to endure it."*

—Dr. Samuel Johnson (1709–1784)

At the end of the play, the audience applauds the actors. The actor's bow and point to other cast members, including them as recipients of the applause. However, behind the scenes, so many others have a hidden and equally important part of realizing this production.

In writing this book I have been advantaged by the loving and supportive influence of family members, teachers, friends, colleagues, and clients. The reader will kindly indulge me while I offer a public thanks to those who have made a difference in my life and have helped me to realize this book. I am rich in friendships and fortunate to have this way of expressing my gratitude:

To my beautiful and loving daughters, Sara, Desire, and Haley. I pray for you all to have long, healthy, happy, loving, and creative lives. And thank you Sara, for your culinary efforts and for late night awakening shoulder massages that kept me from banging my head against the keyboard.

To Robert Davis, CEO of YellowOnline.com, whose incredible faith, brotherly counsel, and constant support allowed me to devote full-time efforts to researching and writing this book. You are a gift, Robert. Thank you for helping me to realize a dream. Please know that you have made a difference. I pray in some way that this book can serve you as your support has served me.

To my teachers, Michio and Aveline Kushi, Herman and Cornelia Aihara, Jacques and Yvette de Langre, Duncan Sim, Nomboro Muramoto, and Anthony Channing. My deep gratitude for your hard-earned wisdom and generosity in sharing it.

I have had the benefit of thousands of clients that over the years motivated (and in some cases, *forced*) me to broaden my perspective in the face of ideology. They are truly teachers of the most noble and enduring kind. I have learned much from your suffering, your pain, your revelations, and your joy. Thank you for sharing such precious insight and most of all, for your continued feedback. This book is the result of your collective efforts.

To Margaret Hollander, a beautiful and altruistic soul whose encouragement, support, and positive feedback inspired and sustained me at just the right time. Big hug, Margaret.

To George Mulek for his generous Vancouver assistance and support of my work.

To Peter and Brenda Gignac for their unwavering support and dear friendship.

To my high school buddy, Jack Bone, who initially encouraged me, over 30 years ago in a Culver City health foods store, to investigate alternative medicine. See what you started, Jack!

To my brother-in-spirit, Eduardo Longoria for his continued friendship and for optimistically holding a vision of possibility when it was needed most.

To Martin Fallick for your committed caring of my mother and for being present when I reached out.

To Mildred Nieves, for your loving dedication to my father Carl during the last five years of his life. You demonstrated a quality of love I have always drawn on for inspiration. Thank you.

To Barbara DeAngelis for help with my "Tribute" and the lessons we shared.

To Glenda Wolchuk for your dear friendship and indefatigable promotion of my work throughout Texas. May you find true inspiration in a chocolate-free life. Thanks so much, Glenda.

To Jack and Dora Ledbetter for thoughtful support and encouragement.

To Olivia Cerco for assisting in research, overwhelming me with newsletters and for those four annoying words that I secretly found inspiring: "Is it finished, yet?"

To Amanda Cori for being the loving and exceptional mother that you are to Haley and for your constant love and support. I promise to always use the spell-check.

To my Omaha sister-in-spirit, Sandy Acquila, of Omaha Healing Arts, for your treasured friendship, media-efforts, title brainstorming over the telephone, feedback (whether I wanted it or not), wonderful workshop promotions, and for having the comic insanity to put a picture of Elvis on 5,000 copies of my flyers instead of my own.

To Alex McIntryre for her supportive assistance in helping me to refine my audio materials which laid the initial groundwork for developing the Exceptional Health Program.

To Tom De Silva of Erewhon, Inc., for his unyielding efforts to popularize whole foods and for his faithful and gracious support.

To Susan Marque for early chapter feedback, constant support and recipe-testing and proofing. Your enthusiasm has been a gift, Susan. Big thanks.

To Diane Bradshaw of Utah School of Hypnosis for a wonderful 15 year friendship, seminar promotion, and introducing me to hypnosis.

To Ruska Porter for her absolute optimism, constant encouragement, and the opportunity to speak at the Monday night Hollywood sessions. You continue to be the energizing influence behind many by your radiant example and faith in healing.

To my good friend, Phil ("Bass-Man") Chen for being a one-man support team, endless video taping of my seminars, audio sessions, the French Meadows camp, and your special brand of Chinese-Jamaican wisdom that uniquely distills everything into prose that sings.

To Monique Guild for your loving encouragement, intuitive insight, Intro suggestions, and for knowing when to make fun of me at those times most necessary.

I am honored to have been touched and inspired by the presence of the following individuals who have passed from this life: Octavia Serina, Herman & Becky Hertzovitz, Sydney Bruder, David Hertzovitz, Max Cohen, Gertrude Meyer, Duncan Sim, Herman Aihara, Amos Consilvio, Midge Henry, Megan Beyhan, Strother Martin, Jennifer Greene, Andy Sherbine, Cecile Tovah Levin, Stanley Ralph Ross, Dr. Charles E. Shields, Pat Rico, Joe Sonner, Lilly Kushi, Murray Schneider, Benjamin Spock, M.D., and Cesar Chavez.

The following friends have acted as seminar organizers in numerous cities throughout the country. Your social conscience and eagerness in assisting me has been a source of continued growth and passion toward reaching more people. Thank you: Susan Avinar, New Jersey; Patricia Becker, Menlo Park, CA; Krista & Reed Berman, Winter Park, Florida; Diane Bradshaw, Salt Lake City, Utah; Greg Burns of Super Slow, Woodland Hills, CA; Terry Rex Cady, Seattle; Davaid & Anita Catron, Salt Lake City, Utah; Jan Ste. Germaine, KCK; Suzy Gillespie, Omaha; Carol & Jim Gordon, British Columbia; Judy Grill, Alexandria,

Virgina; Will Hoglund, Fargo, ND; Joel Huckins, Oakland, CA; Majorie Keyser, Saskatchewan; Sunny Matthews, Miami, Florida; Patrick McDermott, Omaha; Carolyn McGarraugh, Oklahoma City; The Monday Night Palo Alto Alto Group faithfully directed by Gerard Lum, Ilona Pollack and Gary Alinder; Trudy Novack, Montreal; Ocean & Intaba of Ahimsa Sanctuary, Courvalis, Oregon; John & Barb Purdie, Saskatchewan; Mary Schmidt, D.C., Evertt, WA; Mary Tataryn, Winnipeg, Manitoba; United Farm Workers, La Paz, CA

A very warm thank you to Professor Jeffery Rockwell, D.C., of Parker Chiropractic in Dallas, Texas for the opportunity to guest teach classes and for the special assembly student body presentation.

I want to thank the following organizations for their seminar sponsorship: Larry Cooper and his wonderful *Annual Health Classic* (Santa Barbara), organizer extraordinaire, Carl Ferrer, who directs the *French Meadow's Annual Summer Camp*, in Lake Tahoe and Phyia Kushi with David Kirshner from the annual *KI Summer Conference* in Westfield, MA. Thank you all so much for such consistent support.

For their culinary contributions, I am grateful to: Aveline Kushi, Cheryl Beere, Rachel Albert-Matesz, Arisha Wemhoff, Susan Marque, Adela Pedroza, Ann Sherman, Merle Davis, Christina Pierello, Lenore Baum, Meredith McCarty, Julia Ferrer, Debra Singletary, Sara Varona, and Robert Pezdirtz.

I am grateful to my friends, Timothy Kitz and Daniel Zimbaldi, of ZONA Film Productions for our writing projects, their cinematic support and for an inspirational association I am proud to be a part of.

I would like to thank some friends who have contributed suggestions along the way or have just been there when needed: David Briscoe, Chih Chien Lin, Bob Ligon, Hugh & Diana Tingling, Tom "Big Sam" Sweeney, Bob Mattson, Sheri Demaris, Jimmy Israel, Julian Israel, and Ranier and Alex of AR Motorsport, L.A for keeping me cruising happily and safely.

Thank you Lino Stanchich, comrade, brother (and occasional parent), all rolled into one for a twenty-five year friendship and especially for those unsolicted pep talks—your enthusiasm is always appreciated.

I also want to thank Alfred Ramsey for being a man of true integrity and returning my lost laptop from the commuter jungle of Mid-Way Airport—you are outstanding, Alfred!

I am indebted to a number of medical practitioners for their support and encouragement:

—Thank you Michael Brown, M.D., for taking the bold initial step and including me in your practice at Calabasas Medical Group. That was a working demonstration of faith.

—Thank you Joshua Leichtberg, M.D., for the opportunity of working together, your faith, and the Summa Medical Group experience. That was an inspiring experience for me.

—Thank you Theresa Dale, N.D. of The International College of Naturopathy, for featuring me in your programs and supporting my work with an entire student body.

—I wish to thank Dennis Kessler, OMD for sharing our offices together in Beverly Hills and for his endless patience and flexibility with my scheduling.

—I am also grateful to Jim Bleckman, M.D., for your support of my work and counseling.

—For his dedication and outstanding research, I also wish to deeply thank Keith Block, M.D. of Block Medical in Evanston, Illinois for chapter suggestions, the quality and dedication you bring to your work, and for personifying "cutting-edge" in both conventional and alternative fields.

—I am also indebted to the kindness and critical eye of Doris Kanter, who graciously cheered me through each chapter with savvy commentary and interminable optimism about the need for this material to reach many hands. Thank you, Doris for your charitable heart and all the cheerleading. I'll miss those penciled micro-print margin notes and the accompanying

Underwood typewriter explanations on the back of Hal's television scripts. Now, get *your* book done!

—My warm experience with being accepted into the Prentice Hall family has soothed and healed my cynicism and concerns about working with a major publishing house. In Executive Editor Ed Claflin, I have found a gifted professional whose gentle, but firm critique and editorial wisdom kept me on track and continually focused. Thanks for immediate and constructive feedback, thorough notes and most of all, patience and flexibility beyond the call of duty.

—My thanks to editor Barry Richardson for his painstaking review of the manuscript and superb editorial work.

—A special thank you goes to editor Doug Corcoran, who initially green-lighted this book for Prentice Hall and recognized its potential. I wish you well, Doug.

—Finally, I wish to say a heartfelt thanks to my super literary agent, Bob Silverstein of QuickSilver Books whose persistent efforts found a wonderful home for this book with the folks at Prentice Hall. Your sage counsel and rallying faith has supported me for almost ten years. I am grateful for your management, your patience and our good friendship. Live long and prosper, Bob!

—... and finally, I wish to thank you, dear reader, for getting this far. It is my prayer that this work be instrumental in helping you positively transform your health, so that you may reach out to others and do the same.

RESOURCE GUIDE

Alternative Physician Organizations

- Physicians Committee for Responsible Medicine

  5100 Wisconsin Avenue, NW—Suite 404, Washington, DC 20016; 202-686-2210. Promotes preventive medicine, whole foods nutrition, ethical research practices, and compassionate medical policy. *Publishes Good Medicine*, a quarterly journal.

Alternative Approaches to Cancer: Patient Services

- Ralph Moss's *Healing Choices*: 206-437-2291
- Patrick McGrady's *CanHelp*; 3111 paradise Bay Road, Port Ludlow, WA 98365, 206-437-2291

Cancer Organizations

- *Cancer Control Society*, 2043 North Berendo Street, Los Angeles, CA 90027, 800-227-2345
- *CaPCURE*, 1250 Fourth St., Suite 360, Santa Monica, CA 90401, 310-458-2873 / 800-757-2873
- *Commonweal,* Cancer Help Program, P.O. Box 316, Bolinas, CA 94924, 415-868-0970

- *Wellness Community National Headquarters,* 2716 Ocean Park Boulevard, Suite 1040, Santa Monica, CA 90405—310-314-2555

Alternative Approaches to Cancer: Journals

- *The Cancer Chronicles*, Equinox Press, 144 St. John's Place, Brooklyn NY, 11217

Alternative Medicine Publications

- The Townsend Newsletter for Doctors & Patients (www.tldp.com)
- Alternative Medicine Magazine
- Natural Health Magazine

Alternative Approaches to Cancer: Recommended Books

- *Save Yourself from Breast Cancer: Life Choices That Can Help You Reduce the Odds,* Robert Kradjian, M.D. (New York: Berkeley Books, 1994)
- *The Cancer Prevention Diet*: Michio Kushi's Blueprint for the Relief and Prevention of Disease, Michio Kushi (New York: St. Martin's Press, 1993)
- *Definitive Guide to Cancer*, by Burton Goldberg, John W Diamond, M.D., Lee W. Cowden (Tiburon, CA: Future Medicine Publishing, 1997)
- *The Truth About Breast Cancer*—A 7 Step Prevention Plan by Joseph Keon, Ph.D. (Mill Valley, CA: Parissound Publishing, 1999)
- *Alternatives in Cancer Therapy*—*The Complete Guide to Non-Traditional Treatments* by Ross Pelton, Ph.D. and Lee Overholser, Ph.D. (New York, Fireside Books, 1994)
- *The Healing Path*—*A Soup Approach to Illness* by Marc Ian Barasch (New York: Arkana, 1995)

- *Remarkable Recovery—What Extraordinary Healings Tell Us About Getting Well and Staying Well* by Caryle Hirshberg and Marc Ian Barasch (New York: Riverhead Books, 1995)

- *Antioxidants Against Cancer*, by Ralph Moss, Ph.D. (New York: Equinox, 2000)

- *The Cancer Industry: the Classic Exposé of the Cancer Establishment*, Ralph Moss, Ph.D. (New York: Paragon House, 1989)

- *Choices in Healing: Integrating the Best of Conventional and Complementary Approaches to Cancer*, by Michael Lerner, Ph.D. (Cambridge, MA: The MIT Press, 1994)

- *Beating Cancer with Nutrition* by Partick Quillin, Ph.D. with Noreen Quillin (Tulsa: Nutrition Time Press, Inc., Revised Edition: 1998)

- *Eat to Beat Cancer* by J. Robert Hatherhill, Ph.D. (Los Angeles: Renaissance Books, 1998)

- *Cancer as a Turning Point*, by Lawrence LeShan, Ph.D. (New York: Plume, 1994)

- *Whole Healing,* by Elliot S. Dacher, M.D. (New York: Dutton, 1996)

- *Reclaiming Our Health-Exploding the Medical Myth and Emracing the Source of True Healing*, by John Robbins (Tiburon: HJ Kramer, 1996)

- *Return to Wholeness: Embracing Body, Mind and Spirit in the Face of Cancer,* by David Simon, M.D. (New York: John Wiley & Sons, Inc., 1999)

- *Chicken Soup for the Surviving Soul: 101 Stories of Courage and Inspiration from Those Who Have Survived Cancer,* by Jack Canfield, Mark Victor Hansen, Patty Aubery and Nancy Mitchell, RN (Deerfield Beach, FL: Health Communications, Inc., 1996)

- *Healing Wisdom: Wit, Insight and Inspiration for Anyone Facing Illness,* by Gred Anderson (New York: Penguin Books, 1994)

General Nutrition: Related Books

- *Healing with Whole Foods—Oriental Traditions & Modern Nutrition*, by Paul Pitchford (Berkeley: North Atlantic Books, 1993)
- *Food & Healing* by Annemarie Colbin (New York: Ballantine Books, 1986)
- *Hawaii Diet* by Terry Shintani, M.D. (New York: Pocket Books, 1999)
- *Basic Macrobiotics* by Herman Aihara (Oroville, CA: GOMF Press, Revised Edition, 1998)
- *Diet for New America*, by John Robbins (Walpole, NH: Stillpoint Publishing, 1987)
- *The McDougall Plan*, by John A. McDougall, M.D. and Mary A. McDougall (New Jersey: New Century Publishing, 1983)
- *Sugar Blues*, by William Dufty (New York: Warner Books, 1975)
- *Lick the Sugar Habit*, by Nancy Appleton, Ph.D. (New York: Warner Books, 1986)
- *The Book of Miso*, by William Shurtleff & Akiko Aoyagi (New York: Ballantine, 1981)
- *Diet for a Poisoned Planet*, by David Steinman (New York: Ballantine Books, 1990)
- *Total Wellness*, by Joseph Pizzorno, N.D. (Rocklin, CA: Prima Health, 1998)
- *Woman's Bodies, Woman's Wisdom,* by Christiane Northrup, M.D. (New York: Bantam Books, 1994)

Herbal Nutrition Books / Schools

- *Herbal Medicine, Healing & Cancer* by Donald R. Yance, Jr. with Arlene Valentine (Chicago: Keats Publishing, 1999)
- *Herbs Against Cancer; History and Controversy* by Ralph Moss, Ph.D (New York: Equinox Books, 1998)

- *The Way of Herbs,* by Michael Tierra, C.A., N.D. (New York: Pocket Books; 1990)
- *Back to Eden,* by Jethro Kloss (Coalmont, Tennessee; Longview Publishing House; 1965)
- Herbs for Health (magazine)—Available at newsstands (www.discoverherbs.com)

Herbal Schools
- The School of Natural Healing—800-372-8255 (www.schoolofnaturalhealing.com)
- The Australasian College of Herbal Studies—800-487-8839 (www.HerbEd.com)

Specific Nutrition: Related Books

Hazards of Dairy Food
- *Don't Drink Your Milk*, by Frank Oski, M.D. (New York: Health Services, 1983)
- *Milk: The Deadly Poison*, by Robert Cohen (Englewood Cliffs: Argus Publishing, 1998)
- *Moooove Over Milk,* by Vicki B. Griffin, Ph.D., Diane J. Griffin and Virgil Hulse, M.D. (Hot Springs, NC, "Let's Eat!," 1997)—1-800-453-8732

Hazards of Meat
- *Mad Cowboy: Plain Truth from the Cattle Rancher Who Won't Eat Meat*, by Howard F. Lyman (New York: Scribner, 1998)

Cookbooks

- *Cooking the Whole Foods Way*, by Christina Pirello (New York: HP Books, 1997)
- *Fresh from a Vegetarian Kitchen*, by Meredith McCarty (New York: St. Martin's Press, 1995
- *The Self-Healing Cookbook*, by Kristina Turner (Grass Valley, CA: Earthtones Press, 1989)

- *Lenore's Natural Cuisine*, by Lenore Baum (Farmingham Hills, MI: Culinary Publications, 2000)

- *Aveline Kushi's Complete Guide to Marcobiotic Cooking*, by Aveline Kushi with Alex Jack (New York: Warner Books, 1985)

- *The Splendid Grain*, by Rebecca Wood (New York: William Morrow & Co., 1997)

- *The Book of Whole Meals*, by Annemarie Colbin (New York: Ballantine, 1986)

- *Sweet & Natural*, by Meredith McCartey (New York: St. Martin's Press, 1999)

Related Healing Books: Stress Management, Psychology, Spirituality

- *Man's Search for Meaning*, by Viktor Frankl (New York: Touchstone Books, Revised Edition: 1984)

- *Close to the Bone,* by Jean Shinoda Bolen, M.D. (New York: Scribner, 1996)

- *Making Loss Matter*, by Rabbi David Wolpe (New York: Riverhead Books, 1999)

- *Love Medicine & Miracles*, by Bernie Siegel, M.D.(New York: Harper & Row, 1986)

- *How to Live Between Office Visits*, by Bernie Siegel, M.D. (New York: Harper Collins, 1993)

- *Happiness is a Serious Problem,* by Dennis Prager (New York: Regan Books, 1998)

- *Taking Responsibility,* by Nathaniel Branden, Ph.D. (New York: Simon & Schuster, 1996)

- *Healing Words—The Power of Prayer & the Practice of Medicine,* by Larry Dossey, M.D. (New York: HarperCollins, 1994)

- *The Little Prince,* by Antoine de Saint-Exupery (New York: Harcourt Brace & Company, 1943, 1971)

- *Homecoming: Reclaiming and Championing Your Inner Child*, by John Bradshaw (New York: Bantam Doubleday Dell Pub., 1992)

- *The Self-Healing Personality,* by Dr. Howard S. Friedman (New York: Plume Books, 1992)

- *The Healing Mind—The Vital Links Between Brain and Behavior, Immunity and Disease,* by Dr. Paul Martin (New York: St. Martin's Press, 1997)

- *Peace Is Every Step: The Path of Mindfulness in Everyday Life,* by Thich Nhat Hanh (New York: Bantam Books, 1991)

- *Even in Summer the Ice Doesn't Melt,* by David K. Reynolds (New York: William Morrow, 1986)

- *Living Beyond Limits: New Hope and Help for Facing Life-Threatening Illness,* by David Spiegel, M.D. (New York: Random House, 1993)

- *Love & Survival: The Scientific Basis for the Healing Power of Intimacy*, by Dean Ornish, M.D. (New York: HarperCollins, 1998)

- *Light's Out—Sleep, Sugar and Survival*, by T. S. Wiley (New York: Pocket Books, 2000)

Books on the Hazards of Medical Radiation

- *Questioning Chemotherapy* by Ralph Moss, Ph.D. (New York: Equinox Books, 1995)

- *Radiation-Induced Cancer*, by John Gofman, M.D. (San Franciso: CNR Books, 1990)

- *Health Exposure to Low Levels of Ionizing Radiation*, by Beir, Committee on the Biological Effects of Ionizing Radiation (National Academy Press, 1990)

Environmental Health Books

- *The Ecology of Commerce,* by Paul Hawken (New York: Harper, 1993)

- *Nontoxic & Natural,* by Debra Lynn Dadd (Los Angeles: Tarcher, 1984)

Visualization and Guided Imagery Books

- *Getting Well Again*, by O. Carl Simonton, Stephanie Mattnhews and James Creighton (New York: Bantam, Revised Edition: 1992)

- *Staying Well with Guided Imagery: How to Harness the Power of Your Imagination for Health and Healing*, by Belleruth Naparstek (New York: Warner Books, 1994)

- *Healing*, by Belleruth Naparstek (New York: Warner Books, 1994)

- *Creative Visualization*, by Shakti Gawain (New York: Bantam Books, 1983)

- *Visualization for Change: A Step-by-Step Guide to Using the Powers of Your Imagination for Self-Improvement, Therapy, Healing, and Pain Control*, by Patrick Fanning (Oakland, CA: New Harbinger, 1988)

- *Rituals of Healing: Using Imagery for Health and Wellness*, by Jeanne Achterberg, Ph.D., Barbara Dossey, RN, MS and Leslie Kolkmeier RN (New York: Bantam New Age Books, 1994)

- *Thirty Scripts for Relaxation Imagery & Inner Healing, Volume 2*, by Julie T. Lusk (Duluth, MN: Whole Person Associates, Inc., 1993)

Audio Tapes

1. *Health Journeys: For People with Cancer*. Belleruth Naparstek. Time Warner AudioBooks. Los Angeles, CA, 1993

2. *Health Journeys: For People Undergoing Chemotherapy*. Belleruth Naparstek. Time Warner AudioBooks. Los Angeles, CA, 1993

3. *Self-Healing: Creating Your Health, Loving Yourself*. Louise L. Hay. Hay House Audio. Carlsbad, CA, 1983

4. *The Miracle of Mindfulness: A Manual on Meditation*. Thich Nhat Hanh. Abridged Audio Casettes: Harper Audio. 1995

5. *Meditation for Beginners*. Jack Kornfield, Sounds True. Louisville, CO, 1998

6. *How to Meditate*. Lawrence LeShan. Audio Forum. Gilfrod, CT, 1987
7. *Effective Meditations for Health and Healing*. Meditations Contemporary. Effective Learning Systems, Bonita Springs, FL, 1995

Visualization and Meditation Workshops

- Simonton Cancer Center, P.O. Box 890, Pacific Palisades, CA 90272; 213-454-4434

Kusa Seed and Research Foundation

- Founder, Lorenz K. Schaller. Kusha is dedicated to safeguarding and distributing seed and educational information for endangered grains. KUSA—P.O.Box 761, Ojai, CA 93024 -Tel: 805-646-0772

Mail Order Natural Food Company's

- *Diamond Organics*—Organically Grown Fruits & Vegetables Direct to Your Door: 1-888-ORGANIC (888-674-2642)—Call for Catalogue
- *Gold Mine Natural Foods*—1-800-475-FOOD (3663)—Call for Catalogue

Handforaged Natural Wild Rice—100% Organic

Two sources are available:
- Leech Lake Wild Rice, Route 3—Box 100, Cass Lake, MN, 56633
- Manitok Wild Rice—Box 97, Callaway, MN, 56521. 1-800-726-1863

Grain Coffee (caffeine-free)

- Lima Co. Organic Instant "Yannoh"—Original— Available at most natural food outlets
- Sundance "Barley Brew"—Sundance Roasting Company, PO Box 1886, Sandpoint, Idaho, 83864—Available at most natural food outlets or via mail order.

Sea Salt

- Philippe & Selina deLangre continue to promote Jacque
  deLangre's work on sea-salt. They produce a unique publication called "A Grain of Salt," and run *The Grain &
  Salt Society*—273 Fairway Drive, Asheville, NC, 28805.
  Telephone: 800-867-7258. High quality mineralized
  celtic sea-salt can be ordered directly or from their website: www.celtic-seasalt.com. It can also be found in
  major natural food markets.

Alkalinizing Products

- Proprietor, Jim Karnstedt has a unique company that
  distributes numerous personal and commercial products
  related to increasing alkalinity, including drinking water
  ionizers. Contact: The Ion & Light Company, 2263 1/2
  Sacramento St., San Francisco, CA, 94115. Telephone:
  415-346-6205—800-426-1110. Their web site is: www.ion
  light.com

Specific Alternative Cancer Approaches Mentioned in Nature's Cancer-Fighting Foods

- **Hoxsey:** BioMedical Center, P.O. Box 727, 3170 General
  Ferreira, Colonia Juarez, Tijuana, Mexico 220000; 011-
  52-66-84-9011
- **Essiac:** Resperin Corporation; 613-820-9311—"Original
  formula" Available at most natural food outlets
- **Macrobiotics:** Kushi Institute, P.O. Box 7, Becket, MA
  01223; 413-623-5742
- **Mistletoe** (aka *Iscador*): Widely used in Europe as an
  immune enhancer. For more info: www.cancernet.nci.nih.
  gov/index. Additional info: Physicians Association for
  Anthroposophical Medicine, P.O. Box 269, Kimberton, PA
  19442. There are a few US physicians who obtain and
  administer Iscador in this country. Suggest contacting
  Dr. Immaculada Marti, M.D. at Davies Medical Center in
  San Francisco. Telephone: 415-565-6000.

Additional Alternative Cancer Therapies

- **Stanislaw Burzynski, M.D.:** 12000 Richmond, Suite 260, Houston, Texas 77082; 713-531-6464

- **Gerson:** Gerson Research Organization, 7807 Artesian Rd., San Diego, CA 92127-2117; 800-759-2926

- **Keith Block, M.D.:** Individualized cancer programs utliizing a comprehensive blend of conventional and alternative approaches. Block Medical Center, 1800 Sherman Avenue., Suite 515, Evanston, IL 60201; 708-492-3040

- **The Immune Institute:** Offering a variety of alternative cancer programs under the direction of Darryl See, M.D. 18800 Delaware St., Suite 900, Huntington Beach, CA 92648. Telephone: 714-596-8822. Website: www.immuneinstitute.com

Specific Nutrients Mentioned in Nature's Cancer-Fighting Foods

- **Maitake D-Fraction** Mushroom extract and capsules. Available at natural food markets.

- **Maitake Dried Whole Mushroom:** Gold Mine Natural Foods—800—475-3663

- **MGN-3**—Lane Labs. Available at natural food markets.

- **IP-6**—Enzymatic Therapy/Phyto-Pharmica. Available at natural food markets.

- **MilkThistle**—Brands: Jarrow Formulas/Source Naturals/Mariposa Botanicals

- **NAC**—Brands: Jarrow Formulas/Shiff/Source Naturals

- **Sun Chlorella**—Available at natural food markets.

Specific Miso Brands

- *Miso:* South River, Miso Master, Ohsawa, Mitoku (preferably 2–3 year old batches)

- *Soy Sauce*—with wheat (Shoyu): Nama Shoyu from Ohsawa, Westbrea, Mitoku, Eden—without wheat (Tamari): Ohsawa, Eden, Westbrea, Mitoku

Information Sources on the Internet

- *National Center for Complementary and Alternative Medicine*
  http://nccam.nih.gov
- *Center for Alternative Medicine Research in Cancer*
  http://www.sph.uth.tmc.edu/utcam
- *Alternative Health News Online*
  http://www.www.altmedicine.com
- *Wellness Web Alternative / Complementary Medicine*
  http://www.wellweb.com/alternativecomplementary
  _medicine
- *Commonweal*
  http://www.commonweal.org
- *Ralph Moss, Ph.D*
  http://www.ralph.moss.com
- *CancerGuide: Steve Dunn's Cancer Information Page*
  http://www.cancerguide.org
- *Investigative Journalist, Peter Barry Chowka's articles on Alternative Medicine*
  http://www.chowka.com
- *David & Cindy Briscoe's comprehensive website on macrobiotics for Americans*
  http://macroamerica.com
- *The Kushi Institute's official website*
  http://www.macrobiotics.org/KI
- *George Ohsawa Macrobiotic Foundation*
  http://www.gomf.macrobiotic.net
- TV cooking show personality Christina Pierello's website
  http://www.christinacooks.com
- *Cookbook author Meredith McCarty's website of cooking resources*
  http://www.healingcuisine.com
- *Health Classic Symposium—Santa Barbara, CA Seminar Retreat*
  http://healthclassics.com

ENDNOTES

INTRODUCTION

"... single required course in nutrition." Robbins, John—*Reclaiming Our Health*—HJ Kramer, Tiburon, California (1996), p. 3–4

"... of, *Foods That Fight Pain*, ..." Bernard, Neal, M.D.—*Foods That Fight Pain*—Three Rivers Press, New York(1998), p. xvi-xvii

"... of these deaths was avoidable." Epstein, S.—"Winning the War Against Cancer? ... Are they even fighting it?"—*The Ecologist*—Vol. 28:2, pp 69–80 (1998)

"... ingestion, and other environmental factors." Simone, Charles,—*Cancer and Nutrition*—McGraw-Hill, 1983: 1–237

"... The National Academy of Sciences, ..." National Academy of Sciences, National Research Council, Food and Nutrition Board (1989)—*Diet and Health; Implications for reducing chronic disease risk*—Washington, DC: National Academy Press.

"... of Health and Human Services, ..." The Surgeon General's Report on Nutrition and Health (1988).

"... The Cancer Institute, ..." Butrum, et al.—NCI dietary guidelines: Rationale—*Am J Clin Nutr*—(1988); 48:888–95

"... and The American Cancer Society." Simone, Charles, M.D.—*Cancer & Nutrition—A Ten-Point Plan to Reduce Your Risk of Getting Cancer*—Avery Publishing Froup, New York (1994), p. 1

"... does the incidence of cancer." Waller, R.—"The Diseases of Civilization"—*The Ecologist*—vol 1:2 (1970).

CHAPTER 1

"... heard physician Joe D. Nicols..." Nicols, Joe D., M.D., Presley, James. *Please, Doctor, Do Something!,* 1972.

"Here are seven ..." Author expanded list from Mhcio Kushi's Arlington Street Church Lecture Series; Boston, Massachusetts. A condensed version appeared in *Macrobiotic Diet* (Tokyo: Japan Publications, 1974).

". . . before it is medically detectable." Hatherill, Robert J. "Introduction," in *Eat to Beat Cancer* (Los Angeles: Renaissance Books 1998).

". . . the growth of cancer cells." Bernard, Neal. "Cancer Pain," in *Foods That Fight Pain* (New York: Three Rivers Press, 1998).

"According to Professor Campbell, . . ." Campbell, T. Colin. *Why China Holds the Key to Your Health,* March 2000, www.newcenturynutrition.com.

". . . population in general in California." Block, Keith I., Gyllenhaal, Charlotte. "Nutrition: An Essential Tool in Cancer Therapy," a report prepared for the Office of Technology Assessment, U.S. Congress, Washington, D.C., 1990.

". . . dairy products, eggs, and meats." Pusateri, D. J., Roth, W. T., J. K., Shultz, T. D. "Dietary and Hormonal Evaluation of Men at Different Risks for Prostate Cancer," *American Journal of Clinical Nutrition,* 1990;51:371–327.

". . . no milk at all." Block, Keith I., Gyllenhaal, Charlotte. "Nutrition."

". . . 50 percent, compared with nondrinkers." Willet, W. C., Stampfer, M. J., Colditz, F. A., et al. "Breast Cancer before Age 45 and Oral Contraceptive Use; New Findings," *American Journal of Epidemiology,* 1989;129:269.

". . . cancer risk of other women." Toniolo, P., Riboli, E., Protta, F., Charrel, M., Cappa, A. P. "Calorie-Providing Nutrients and Risk of Breast Cancer," *Journal of the National Cancer Institute,* 1989;81:278, referenced from Bernard, Neal, *Foods That Fight Pain* (New York: Three Rivers Press, 1998).

". . . times higher than for beef." Sinha, R., Rothman, N., Brown, E. D., et al. "High Concentrations of the Carcinogen 2-Amino-1-Methyl-6-Phenylimidazo-[4,5] Pyridine (PhIP) Occur in Chicken But Are Dependent on Cooking Method," *Cancer Research,* 1995; 55:4516–4519.

". . . smaller and fewer in number." Decosse, J. J., Miller, H. H., Lesser M. L. Effect of Wheat Fiber and Vitamins C and E on Rectal Polyps in Patients with Familial Adenomatous Polyposis," *Journal of the National Cancer Institute,* 1989; 81:1290–1297, referenced in Bernare, Neal, *Foods That Fight Pain* (New York: Three Rivers Press, 1998).

CHAPTER 2

"Different mutagens are formed . . ." Spingarn, N. E., Solcum, L. A., Weisburger, H. G. "Formation of Mutagens in Cooked Foods. II. Foods with High Starch Content," *Cancer Letters,* 1980; 9(1):7–12.

". . . World Health Organization (WHO) report . . ." World Health Organization Report 797, referenced in Melina, V., Davis, B., Harrison, V., in *Becoming Vegetarian* (Summertown, Tenn.: Book Pub. Co., 1995).

"A 1977 study . . ." Boyd, N. F., et al. "Effects at Two Years of a Low-Fat, High-Carbohydrate Diet on Radiologic Features of the Breast: Results from a Randomized Trial," *Journal National Cancer Institute,* 1977; 89(7):488–498.

"A study from Uruguay . . ." Yuan, J.M., et al. "Diet and Breast Cancer in Shanghai and Tianjain, China," *British Journal of Cancer,* 1995; 71(6):1353–1358, referenced in Patrick Holford, *Say No to Cancer* (London: Piatkus, 1999).

"A study by the National Cancer Institute . . ." Smith-Barbaro, P., et al."Carcinogen Binding to Various Types of Dietary Fiber," *Journal National Cancer Institute,* 1981; 67(2):495–497.

". . . study by Tomas M. S. Wolever, M.D., . . ." Wolever, Thomas M.S. "Glycemic Index: Flogging a Dead Horse?" *Diabetes Care,* 1997; 20(3):452–456.

". . . this exists in medical literature, . . ." Yu, D.T., Burch, H. B., Phillips, M. J. "Pathogenesis of Fructose Hepatotoxicity," *Laboratory Investigations,* 1974; 30(1):85–92.

". . . less than that in America." *Hippocrates,* May/June (1990), referenced in Gittleman, Ann Louise, *Get the Sugar Out* (New York: Crown, 1996).

". . . insulin levels and cancer potential." Yam, D. *Medical Hypotheses,* 1992; 38: 111, referenced in Quillin, Patrick, *Beating Cancer with Nutrition* (Tulsa, Okla.: Nutrition Time Press, 1998).

". . . in seven healthy human volunteers." Berstein, J., et al. *American Journal Clinical Nutrition,* 1973; 26:180, referenced in Quillin, Patrick, *Beating Cancer with Nutrition* (Tulsa, Okla.: Nutrition Time Press, 1998).

"Healthy human volunteers . . ." Sanchez, A., et al. *American Journal Clinical Nutrition,* 1973; 26:180, referenced in Quillin, Patrick, *Beating Cancer with Nutrition* (Tulsa, Okla.: Nutrition Time Press, 1998).

"An epidemiological (population) study . . ." Horrobin, D. F. *Medical Hypotheses,* 1983; 11(3):319, referenced in Quillin, Patrick, *Beating Cancer with Nutrition* (Tulsa, Okla.: Nutrition Time Press, 1998).

"In a study . . ." Hoehn, S. K., et al. *Nutrition and Cancer,* 1979; 1(3):27, referenced in Quillin, Patrick, *Beating Cancer with Nutrition* (Tulsa, Okla.: Nutrition Time Press, 1998).

". . . breast cancer than nondrinkers did." *Journal American Medical Association,* 1998; 279:535.

". . . Institute in Hungington Beach, CA, . . ." Alternative Medicine Magazine, "Cellular Mechanisms of 12 Anti-Cancer Strategies," (November, 2000).

". . . french fries (80 times . . ." This figure from Interview Magazine (1983) profile of Nathan Pritikin.

". . . higher part of the range." Bernard, Neal D. *Cancer and Your Immune System,* newcenturynutrition.com.

". . . supplements can increase LDL cholesterol." Harris, W. S., et al. "Effects of a Low-Saturated-Fat, Low-Cholesterol Fish Oil Supplement in Hypertriglyceride Patients," *Annals of Internal Medicine,* 1998; 109:465–470. See also Demke, D. M., et al. "Effects of a Fish Oil Concentrate on Patients with Hypercholesterolemia," *Atherosclerosis,* 1988; 70:73–80.

". . . was reduced by 20 percent." Regan, Timothy. "Myocardial Blood Flow and Oxygen Consumption during Postprandial Lipemia and Heparin-Induced Lipolyse," *Circulation,* 1961; 23:55–63, referenced in Whitaker, Julian M., *Reversing Heart Disease* (New York: Warner Books, 1985).

"In dozens of animal studies, . . ." Arnot, Bob. *The Breast Cancer Prevention Diet* (Boston: Little, Brown & Co., 1998), p. 36.

". . . the *British Journal of Cancer* . . ." Talamini, R. "Special Medical Conditions and Risk of Breast Cancer," *British Journal of Cancer,* 1997; 75(11):1699–1703.

"... same province in northwestern Italy." Bernard, Neal D. *Cancer & Your Immune System,* Ibid.

"Some studies . . ." Bernard, Neal D. *Cancer & Your Immune System,* New Century Nutrition Archives, www.newcenturynutrition.com/NCN/articles/cancerandimmune.shtml.

" . . . clients I will recommend fish," Contamination in freshwater fish is rampant. I generally eat only ocean varieties. Farm-raised fish (particularly for salmon, trout, sturgeon, catfish, and tilapia) are routinely given antibiotics, are also given poor quality feed, are confined to swimming in unnaturally crowded pens, and as a result are more susceptible to disease.

"... University of Illinois at Urbana-Champaign ..." Visek, William J. "Intestinal Cancer May Be Increased by Meat Ammonia," *Medical Tribune,* September 20, 1972, referenced in Thrash, A., Thrash, C., *Nutrition for Vegetarians* (Seale, Ala.: New Lifestyle Books, 1996).

". . . increased risk for colon cancer." Pellet, P.L. "Protein Requirements in Humans," *American Journal Clinical Nutrition,* 1990; 51:723–737, referenced in Bernard, Neal D., *Protein Myths,* PCRM Publication.

". . . link between cancer and protein." Committee on Diet, Nutrition, and Cancer of the National Research Council. *Diet, Nutrition, and Cancer* (Washington, D.C.: 1982).

"Case-control studies . . ." Anderson, J.W., Hypocholesterolemic Effects of Oat-Bran or Bean Intake for Hypercholesterolemic Men," *American Journal of Clinical Nutrition,* 40:1146-55, 1984.

". . . breast cancer under experimental conditions." Carlson, et al, "Prolactin stimulation by meal is related to protein content, *Journal of Clinical Endocrinology and Metabolism,* 1983; 57:334-338.

". . . breast cancer under experimental conditions." Carlson, Stimulation of prolactin secretion by protein is due to amino acids—*Clinical Res,* 1985;33:305A.

CHAPTER 3

". . . to stop cancer from developing." Cameron, E., Pauling, L. "Supplemental Ascorbate in the Supportive Treatment of Cancer: Reevaluation of Prolongation of Survival Times in Terminal Human Cancer," *Proceedings of the National Academy of Science,* 1976; 7:4538–4542.

". . . during an 11-week study." Study, *Circulation: Journal of the American Heart Association,* December 1999.

". . . cancer, and other medical conditions." Bloch, A., Thomson, C. A. "Position of The American Dietetic Association: Phytochemicals and Functional Foods," *Journal of the American Diet Association,* 1995; 95:493–496, referenced in Craig, Winston J., "Phytochemicals: Guardians of Our Health," Continuing Education Article, Nutrition Department, Andrews University, Michigan.

". . . inhibits the liver's detox mechanisms, . . ." Ohsake, Y., Ishida, S., Fujikane, et al. "Combination Effects of Caffeine and Cisplatin on a Cisplatin Resistant Human Lung Cancer Cell Line," *Gan to Kagaku Ryoho,* July 1990; 17(7):1339–1343.

". . . structural changes in animal DNA." Ibid, and Aeschbacher, H. U., Meier, H., Jaccaud, E. "The Effect of Caffeine in the in vivo SCE and Micronucleus Mutagenicity Tests," *Mutation Research,* 1986 May; 174(1):53–58.

"In a study on prostate cancer, . . ." Seattle Post-Intelligencer Reporter, "Vegetables Can Protect Against Prostate Cancer, Study Finds," by Tom Paulson, January 5, 2000.

". . . 1990s twenty-million-dollar study . . ." Caragay, A. B. "Cancer-Preventative Foods and Ingredients," *Food Tech,* 1992; 46(4):65–68, referenced in Craig, Winston, J., Phytochemicals: Guardians of Our Health.

". . . basil, cucumber, cantaloupe, and berries." Ibid.

"New phytochemical research . . ." Steinmetz, K. A., Potter, J. D. "Vegetables, Fruit and Cancer, II. Mechanisms," *Cancer Causes Control,* 1991; 2:427–442, referenced in Craig, Winston, J., Ibid.

"However, research has shown . . ." Schardt, D. "Phytochemicals: Plants against Cancer, *Nutrition Action Health Letter,* 1994; 21(3):1,9–11, referenced in Craig, Winston, J., Ibid.

"These phenolics . . ." Decker, E. A. "The Rrole of Phenolics, Conjugated Linoleic Acid, Carnosine, and Pyrroloquinoline Quinone as Nonessential Dietary Antioxidants," *Nutrition Review,* 1995; 53:49–58, referenced in Craig, Winston, J., Ibid.

". . . curcumins in ginger and tumeric." Zheng, G.-Q., Zhang, J., Kenney, P. M., Lam, L. K. T. "Stimulation of Glutathione *S*-Transferase and Inhibition of Carcinogenesis in Mice by Celery Seed Oil Constituents." In *Food Phytochemicals for Cancer Prevention, I. Fruits and Vegetables,* Hang, M. J., Osawa, T., Ho, C.-T., Rosen, R. T. (eds.). (Washington, D.C.: American Chemical Society, 1994), pp. 144–153, referenced in Craig, Winston, J., Ibid.

". . . of estrogen-stimulated breast cancer." Serrtaino, M., Thompson, L. U., Oka, K. "The Effect of Flaxseed Supplementation on the Initiation and Promotional Stages of Mammary Tumorigenesis," *Nutrition Cancer,* 1992; 17:153–59, referenced in Craig, Winston, J., Ibid; Hirano, T., Fukuoka, K., Oka, K, et al. "Antiproliferative Activity of Mammalian Lignan Derivatives against the Human Breast Carcinoma Cell Line, ZR-75-1, *Cancer Invest,* 1990; 8595–601, referenced in Craig, Winston, J., Ibid.; Serraino, M., Thompson, L. U. "The Effect of Flaxseed Supplementation on Early Risk Markers for Mammary Carcinogenesis," *Cancer Letter,* 1991; 60:135–142, referenced in Craig, Winston, J., Ibid.

". . . with established anti-cancer activity." Kennedy, A. R. "The Evidence for Soybean Products as Cancer Preventive Agents," *Journal of Nutrition,* 1995; 125:733S–743S, referenced in Craig, Winston, J., Ibid.

". . . consume soy or soy products." Messina, M. J., Persky, V., Setchell, K. D., et al. "Soy Intake and Cancer Risk: A Review of the In Vitro and In Vivo Data," *Nutrition Cancer,* 1994; 21(2):113–131, referenced in Craig, Winston, J., Ibid.

". . . lignans, ellagic acid, and saponins." Thompson, L. U. "Antioxidants and Hormone-Mediated Health Benefits of Whole Grains," *Crit Rev Food Sci Nutr,* 1994; 34:473–497, referenced in Craig, Winston, J., Ibid.

". . . in its phytochemical make-up." Thompson, L. U. "Potential Health Benefits of Whole Grains and Their Components," *Contemp Nutr,* 1992; 17(6):1–2; referenced in Craig, Winston, J., Ibid.

"... in particular, anti-HIV—properties." Herbbrief: Burdock Root, by Laurel Vukovic, *Natural Health* Magazine, April, 2000.

"... two servings of fruit daily." Patterson, B., Block, G., Rosenberger, W. F., et al. "Fruits and Vegetables in the American Diet: Data from the NHANES II Survey," *American Journal of Public Health,* 1990;80:1443–1449.

"According to Andrew Weil, M.D., ..." Weil, Andrew, M.D., *Eating Well for Optimum Health,* Knopf, New York, 2000, p. 157–158.

"... from large-scale intervention trials." Decker, E. A. "The Role of Phenolics, Conjugated Linoleic Acid, Carnosine, and Pyrroloquinoline Quinone as Nonessential Dietary Antioxidants," *Nutr Rev,* 1995; 53:49–58, referenced in Craig, Winston, J., "Phytochemicals: Guardians of Our Health"; Sies, H., Krinsky, N. I. "The Present Status of Antioxidant Vitamins and Beta-Carotene," *American Journal of Clinical Nutrition,* 1995; 62(suppl.):1299S–1300S, referenced in Craig, Winston, J., Ibid.

"In a newsletter mention. .." *Health Revelations,* by Dr. Robert Atkins, November 1998

CHAPTER 4

"... premature aging and disease conditions." Worlitschek, Michael, M.D. *Dacidification: A Basic Theory,* "Acids & Bases Require Equilibrium in the Organism," Germany (1995), referenced in Ion & Light Company, San Francisco, Calif.

"... particularly digestive, kidney, and immunity function." Ibid.

"... sugars do not have this effect." Bernstein, et al. "Depression of Lymphocyte Transformation Following Oral Glucose Ingestion," *American Journal of Clinical Nutrition,*1977; 30:613; Sanchez, et al. "Role of Sugars in Human Neutrophilic Phagocytosis," *American Journal of Clinical Nutrition,* 1973; 26:1180–1184.

"... gasoline on a smoldering fire." RossiFanelli, F., et al. *Journal of Parenteral and Enteral Nutrition,* 1991; 15:680, referenced in Quillin, Patrick, Quillin, Noreen, *Beating Cancer with Nutrition* (Tulsa, Okla.: Nutrition Times Press, Inc., 1994), p. 295.

"The pH Scale" References (partial): #64; Manufacturer's information, *New England Journal of Medicine,* 1985, 1351; Whang, Sang. *Reverse Aging,* 1990.

"... fruits actually acidify the blood." Katase, Tan. *Calcium Medicine* (Osaka, Japan: Ningen No Igaku Co., 1948).

"... acetic acid, carbonic acid, etc.)." Guyton, Aurther. *Textbook of Medical Physiology* (Philadelphia: W. B. Saunders Co., 1956), reference in Aihara, Herman. *Acid & Alkaline* (Oroville, Calif: GOMF Press, 1986).

"... sacrificing quality for quantity." Olarsch, I., Gerald, N. D., Stockton, Susan. "Why Are Kids Killing? The Nutrition-Mind Connection," *Townsend Letter for Doctors & Patients,* vol. 201, April 2000, Point Townsend, Wash., www.tldp-.com.

"... filtering organs (liver and kidneys)." Wood, Revecca. *The New Whole Foods Encyclopedia* (New York: Penguin/Arkana, 1999), p. xxii.

"... insomnia and other sleep disorders." Cherniske, Stephen. *Caffeine Blues* (New York: Warner Books, 1998).

"... health problems caused by overacidity." Ibid.

"... consumption paints a nastier picture; ..." Ibid.

CHAPTER 5

". . . might be from animal sources." Kradjian, Robert, M. *Save Yourself from Breast Cancer* (New York: Berkley Books, 1994), p. 104.

". . . of butter, margarine, and lard." Klapper, Michael. *Vegan Nutrition: Just What the Doctor Ordered,* Ahimsa Videotape, no. 12 (Malaga, N. J.: American Vegetarian Society, 1993).

"A 1992 Hawaiian study . . ." White, E., et al. "Maintenance of a Low-Fat Diet: Follow-Up of the Women's Health Trial," *Cancer Epidemiology, Biomarkers and Prevention,* 1992;1(4):315–322.

". . . and height, and breast cancer." Waard, F. De. "Breast Cancer Incidence and Nutritional Status with Particular Reference to Body Weight and Height," *Cancer Research,* 1975;35:p. 3351.

"A Historical Perspective" Historical references drawn from Kradjian, Robert, M., *Save Yourself from Breast Cancer* (New York: Berkley Books, 1994), p. 103.

". . . disease was reduced by 34%." Hindhede, M. "The Effect of Food Restriction During War on Mortality in Copenhagen," *Journal of the American Medical Association,* 1920;74(6):381–382.

". . . consistently ingested for many years." Kradjian, Robert, M. *Save Yourself from Breast Cancer,* p. 108.

". . . also offers broader health benefits." Quote source: www.healthscout.com, April 19, 2000, by Edward Edelson.

"The American Institute Research . . ." "Cancer Researchers Agree: New Colon Cancer Studies Send Wrong Message," April 2000, www.vegsource.com.

". . . egg, butter, and cheese consumption." Hirayama, T. "Epidemiology of Breast Cancer with Special Reference to the Role of Diet," *Journal of Preventive Medicine,* 1978;7:173–174.

". . . cancer present in meat eaters." Hepner, G. "Altered Bile Acid Metabolism in Vegetarians," *American Journal of Digestive Diseases,* 1975;20:935.

". . . however, still warrants additional research." Block, Keith, Gyllenhaal, Charlotte. *Nutrition: An Essential Tool in Cancer Therapy,* Report for OTA, U.S. Congress, 1990, p. 4.

". . . that increases their growth rate." Sanders T. A. B., Ellis, F. R., Dickerson, J. W. T. "Studies of VegansL the Fatty Acid Composition of Choline Phosphoglycerides, Erythrocytes, Adipose Tissue, Breast Milk and Some Indicators of Susceptibility to Ischemic Heart Disease in Vegans and Omnivore Controls," *American Journal of Clinical Nutrition,* 1978;31:805–813; Mead, J.R. "The Essential Fatty Acids: Past, Present and Future, *Prog Lipid Res,* 1981;20:1–6; Phinney, S. D., Odin, R. S., Johnson, S. B., Holman, R.T. "Reduced Arachdonate in Serum Phopholipids and Cholesteryl Esters Associated with Vegetarian Diets in Humans," *American Journal of Clinical Nutrition,* 1990;51:385–392.

". . . growth and longer tumor induction." Schmahl, D., Daisman, A., Habs, M., et al. "Experimental Investigations on the Influence upon the Chemical Carcinogenesis. Third Communication: Studies with 1,2-Dimethylhydrazine," *Z. Krebsforch* (abstract in English) 1976;86:89–94, referenced in Block, Keith, Gyllenhaal, Charlotte. *Nutrition: An Essential Tool in Cancer Therapy,* p. 13

"... the risk of endometrial cancer." Goodman, M., Wilkens, L., et al. "Association of Soy and Fiber Consumption with the Risk of Endometrial Cancer," *American Journal of Epidemiology,* 1997; 146(4):292–306.

"... author of *Hawaii Diet, ...*" *Shintani, Terry.* Hawaii Diet *(New York: Pocket Books, 1997), p. 73.*

"... reveals similar percentages of each, ..." McDougall, John. *The McDougall Plan* (Clinton, N.J.: New Win Publishing, 1983), Table 5.1, pp. 49–50.

"In a Harvard study ..." Cramer, D.W., et al. "Galactose Consumption and Metabolism in Relation to the Risk of Ovarian Cancer," *Lancet,* 1989; 2:66–71.

"... production of galactose from lactose." Physicians Committee for Responsible Medicine (PCRM), Washington, D.C., "What's Wrong With Dairy Products?"

"In a July 19, 1985 issue ..." Robbins, John. *Diet for a New America* (Walpole, N.H.: Still Point Publishing, 1987), pp. 268–270.

"... insulin-like growth factor (IGF)." Outwater, J. L., Nicolson, A., Bernard, N. "Dairy Products and Breast Cancer: The IFG-1, Estrogen, and bGH Hypothesis," *Medical Hypothesis,* 1997; 48:453–461.

"... linked to increased cancer risk." Cohen, P. "Serum Insulin-Like Growth Factor-I Levels and Prostate Cancer Risk—Interpretating the Evidence," *Journal of the National Cancer Institute,* 1998; 90:876–879.

"... products on a regular basis." Cadogan, J., Eastell, R., Jones, N., Barker, M. E. "Milk Intake and Bone Mineral Acquisition in Adolescent Girls: Randomised, Controlled Intervention Trial," *BMJ,* 1997; 315:1255–1269.

"... who had the lowest levels." Chan, J. M., Stampfer, M. J., Giovannucci, E., et al. "Plasma Insulin-Like Growth Factor-1 and Prostate Cancer Risk: A Prospective Study," *Science,* 1998; 279:563–565.

"... product consumption and prostate cancer." World Cancer Research Fund/American Institute for Cancer Research, *Food, Nutrition and the Prevention of Cancer: A Global Perspective* (Washington, D.C.: American Institute for Cancer Research, 1997), p. 461; Physicians Committee for Responsible Medicine (PCRM), "What's Wrong With Dairy Products?"

"... dairy products, eggs, and meat." Pusateri, D. J., Roth, W. T., Ross, J. K., Shultz, T. D. "Dietary and Hormonal Evaluation of Men at Different Risks for Prostate Cancer: Plasma and Fecal Hormone-Nutrient Interrelationships," *American Journal of Clinical Nutrition,* 1990; 51:371–377, referenced in Block, Keith, Gyllenhaal, Charlotte, *Nutrition: An Essential Tool in Cancer Therapy.*

"... the study began in 1982." Report taken from www.healthscout.com April 5, 2000, by Neil Sherman.

"... meats, dairy, and oil excess." MacDonald, P. "Effect of Obesity on Conversion of Plasma Androstenedione to Estrone in Postmenopausal Women With and Without Endometrial Cancer," *American Journal of Obstetician Gynecology,* 1978; 130:448.

"... of no milk at all." Block, Keith, Gyllenhaal, Charlotte. *Nutrition: An Essential Tool in Cancer Therapy.*

"Concluding a report ..." Phillips, R. "Role of Lifestyle and Dietary Habits in Risk of Cancer, " *Cancer Research,* 1975; 35:3513.

"Nutrition and Cancer study in 1989 ..." From Mead, Nathaniel. "Don't' Drink Your Milk!" *Natural Health,* July/August, 1994.

". . . to weakening of immune function." Cunningham, A. "Lymphomas and Animal Protein Consumption," *Lancet,* 1976; 2:1184.

". . . not as carnivores (meat consumers)." Collens, W. "Phylogenetic Aspects of the Cause of Human Atherosclerotic Disease," *Circulation,* 1965; (supp II) 31–32:II–7; Prosser, C. *Comparative Animal Physiology,* 2nd ed. (Philadelphia: W. B. Saunders, 1961), p. 116; Nasset, E. "Movements of the Small Intestine," P. Bard, *Medical Physiology,* 11th ed. (St. Lan's: C. V. Mosby, 1961), p. 116; Dietschy, J. "Regulation of Cholesterol Metabolism," (third of three parts), *New England Journal of Medicine,* 1970; 282:1241; *What's Wrong with Eating Meat?,* Ananda Marga Publications, 1977; Stewart, J. "Response of Dietary Vitamin B_{12} Deficiency to Psyciological Oral Doses of Cyanocobalamin," *Lancet,* 1970; 2:542.

". . . to cause blood sugar instability, . . ." Yam, D. *Medical Hypothesis,* 1992; 38:111.

". . . fatigue, mood swings, suppressed immunity, . . ." Berstein, J., et al. *American Journal of Clinical Nutrition,* 1977; 30:613; Sanchez, A., et al. *American Journal of Clinical Nutrition,* 1973; 26:180; McDougall, John. *The McDougall Plan;* Herbert, V. "Multivitamin Mineral Food Supplements Containing Vitamin B_{12} May Also Contain Dangerous Analogues of Vitamin B_{12}" letter, *New England Journal of Medicine,* 1982; 307:255; "Harmful B_{12} Breakdown Products in Multivitamins?" *Med World News* (Sept. 28, 1981):12.

". . . have an anti-B_{12} effect."

". . . such as this are rare, . . ." Murphy, M. "Vitamin B_{12} Deficiency Due to a Low-Cholesterol Diet in a Vegetarian," *Annals of Internal Medicine,* 1981; 94:57; Winawer, S. "Gastric and Hematological Abnormalities in a Vegan with Nutritional B_{12} Deficiency: Effects of Oral Vitamin B_{12}," *Gastroenterology,* 1967; 53:130; Immerman, A. "Vitamin B_{12} Status of a Vegetarian Diet—A Critical Review," *World Review of Nutritional Diet," 1981; 37:38; Stewart, J. "Response of Dietary Vitamin B_{12} Deficiency to Psyiological Oral Doses of Cyanocobalamin," Lancet, 1970; 2:542.*

Chapter 6

". . . physiological basis for the craving." Hunt, Douglas. *No More Cravings* New York: Warner Books, (1987), pp 22–23.

". . . feed behavior. One study . . ." Ibid. p. 23–24

". . . treatment. In another report . . ." Ibid.

". . . absent from the current diet." Ibid. p. 23–24.

". . . using kaolin or white clay . . ." *National Geographic,* "Nature's Rx," April 2000, p. 89.

". . . dreaded early-pregnancy morning sickness." Whang, Sang. *Reverse Aging* (Miami: JSP Publishing, 1990), p. 63.

". . . used dirt in their diet, . . ." Hunter, John, M. "Geophagy in Africa and in the United States: A Culture-Nutrition Hypothesis," "Geographical Review, April, 1973, pp. 170–195.

". . . physician and author, Douglas Hunt . . ." Hunt, Douglas. *No More Cravings,* p. 25.

". . . by some cultural folk medicines . . ." Kushi, M., Hannetta, Phillip. *Macrobiotics and Oriental Medicine* (New York: Japan Publications, Inc., 1991), p. 140.

". . . developing infant receives the following:" Mother's milk model referenced from Anna Marie Colbin, *Food and Healing* (New York: Ballentine Books, 1986).

". . . numerous books on Asian medicine, . . ." Books of Michio Kushi, Kushi Institute, Becket, Massachusetts.

"One theory . . ." Aihara, Herman. *Acid and Alkaline,* Table 10: The Calcium and Phosphorus Ratio (GOMF Publications, 1986), p. 43.

". . . unpasteurized milk, butter, yogurt, ghee . . ." Ghee is also known as clarified butter and is frequently used in East Indian Ayurvedic medicine.

"Recommendations . . ." Atlanta Center for Eating Disorders.

". . . and not the disease itself." Kradjian, Robert, M. *Save Yourself from Breast Cancer* (New York: Berkley Publishing Group, 1994), p. 62.

". . . the natural laws between them." Ohsawa, George. Seven Principles of the Order of the Universe, *The Book of Judgement.*

CHAPTER 7

". . . simple sugars, and fatty acids." Shurtleff, William, Aoyagi, Akiko. *The Book of Miso* (New York: Ballentine, 1976).

". . . humanity's health, longevity, and happiness." Kushi, Aveline, Jack, A. *The Complete Guide to Macrobiotic Cooking* (New York: Warner Books, 1985), pp. 11; 128–129.

". . . as 30 to 40 percent." Shurtleff, William, Aoyagi, Akiko. *The Book of Miso.*

". . . types of traditionally produced miso." Takahshio, Jusaku. Studies on Sources of Vitamin B_{12}, *Eiyo to Shokuryo,* 1955; 8(2):25–27.

". . . have been reproduced by spores." Leonard, Thom. "Fermentation: Why Cultured Foods Are a Smart Choice," *East West Journal,* Dec. 1984.

". . . bacteria, known as gut microflora." McDougall, John. "The Gut & Its Micro-Flora." *The McDougall Newsletter,* July/Aug. 1999.

". . . feces is composed of bacteria." Ibid.

". . . aerobic bacteria than meat eaters." *Journal of Nutrition,* 1975; 105:878, reference in McDougall, *The Gut and Its Micro-Flora.*

". . . three requirements are frequently overlooked:" Ibid.

". . . colonize within the human intestine." *American Jounral of Clinical Nutrition,* 1999:69:1035S.

". . . negative qualities of dairy products:" McDougall, John. "The Gut & Its Micro-Flora."

". . . all nonpasteurized forms of miso:" Shurtleff, William, Aoyagi, Akiko. *The Book of Miso.*

". . . no findings of any toxins." Ibid., pp. 34–35.

". . . our metabolic balance. Recent experiments . . ." Ibid., pp. 30–31.

". . . cooking meat at high temperatures." *J Diary Sci,* 1990; 73:2702.

". . . substances such as, *N*-nitrosamines." *Appl Microbiol,* 1975; 29:7.

". . . engulf and destroy tumor cells." *Bifidobacteria and Microflora,* 1994; 13:65.

"An Alabama study . . ." Baggott, J. E., Ha, T., Vaughn, W. H., Juliana, M.M., Hardin, J. M., Grubbs, C.J. "Effects of Miso and NaCl on DMBA-Induced Rat Mammary Tumors, *Nutr Cancer,* 1990; 14(2):103–109.

". . . medical school reported the following:" Santiago, L. A., Hiramatsu, M., Mori, A. *Japanese Soybean Paste Miso Scavenges Free Radicals and Inhibits Lipid Peroxidation, Dept. of Neurochemistry, Okayama University Medical School, Japan.*

". . . coverage in Japan's major newspapers." Shurtleff, William, Aoyagi, Akiko, *The Book of Miso,* pp. 36–37.

". . . easily destroyed by prolonged cooking." Ibid., p. 92.

". . . Aoyagi's *The Book of Miso.*" Ballantine Books, New York (1976).

CHAPTER 8

". . . basis for their reputed claims." Walters, Richard. *Options: The Alternative Cancer Therapy Book* (New York: Avery Publishing, 1993).

". . . even a waste of money." Yance, Donald R., Jr., Valentine, Arlene. *Herbal Medicine, Healing & Cancer* (Chicago: Keats Publishing, 1999), pp. 83–84.

". . . benefits while minimizing their toxicity." Simon, David. *Return to Wholeness* (New York: John Wiley & Sons, 1999), pp. 72–73.

". . . the wisdom of the herb." Simon, David. *Return to Wholeness,* p. 73.

". . . and bring it to market." Walters, Richard. *Options: The Alternative Cancer Therapy Book* (Garden City, N.Y.: Avery Publishing, 1993), p. 93.

". . . this pharmaceutical practice, Richard Walters . . ." Ibid.

". . . for most types of cancer." Broadhurst, C. Leigh. "How Do Plants Prevent Cancer?" *Herbs for Health,* Jan./Feb. 2000, p. 57.

". . . take place at three levels:" Yance, Donald R., Jr., Valentine, Arlene. *Herbal Medicine, Healing & Cancer,* pp. 110–111.

". . . nutrition author C. Leigh Broadhurst, . . ." Broadhurst, C. Leigh. "How Do Plants Help Prevent Cancer?" pp. 57–58.

". . . percent protection against this poison." Tierra, Michael. *The Way of Herbs* (New York: Pocket Books, 1990), p. 189.

". . . itself from hydrogen peroxide production." Werbach, L., et al. *Botanical Influences on Illness* (Tarzana, Calif.: 1994).

"Research has shown . . ." Hobbs, Christopher. *Herbal Adaptogens Fitting into the Modern Age,* 1996.

". . . reproduction of this "mutation error." Broadhurst, C. Leigh. "How Do Plants Help Prevent Cancer?," pp. 57–58.

". . . Yance, author and clinical herbalist, . . ." Yance, Donald R., Jr., Valentine, Arlene. *Herbal Medicine, Healing & Cancer,* p. 113.

". . . author, David Simon recommends . . ." Simon, David. *Return to Wholeness,* p. 82.

". . . dispel heaviness, congestion, and mucus." Ibid., pp. 77–78.

". . . balance with the great spirit." Thomas, Richard. *The Essiac Report* (Los Angeles: The Alternative Treatment Information Network, 1993).

". . . her meeting with Rene Caisse." Olsen, Cynthia, Chan, Jim. *Essiac: A Native Herbal Cancer Remedy* (Pagosa Springs, Colo.: Kali Press, 1996).

". . . cancer, I would use it." Thomas, Richard. *The Essiac Report.*

". . . more years with no reoccurrence." Olsen, Cynthia, Chan, Jim. *Essiac: A Native Herbal Cancer Remedy.*

". . . abnormal ones as "nature intended." Thomas, Richard. *The Essiac Report,* p. 107.

". . . Leroi and his wife, Rita, . . ." Moss, Ralph. *Herbs Against Cancer: History & Controversy* (Brooklyn, N.Y.: Equinox Press, Inc., 1998), p. 148.

". . . that specifically destroy tumor cells." Hajto, Tibor, Hostanka, K. "An Investigation of the Ability of *Viscum Album*-Activated Granulocytes to Regulate Natural Killer Cells *in Vivo,*" *Clin Trials J,* 1986; 23(6):345–358; and Heusser, Perer. *Immunological Results of Mistletoe Therapy, in Iscador: Compendium of Research Papers, 1986–1988* (Spring Valley, N.Y.: Mercury Press, 1991).

". . . in some cases cause remission." Walters, Richard. *Options; The Alternative Cancer Therapy Book,* p. 120.

". . . respond well to mistletoe therapy." Ibid., p. 122.

". . . essential mediators of immune response." Ibid., p. 126, from Hajto, Tibor, et al. "Increased Secretion of Tumor Cenrosis Factor a, Interluekin 1, and Interleukin 6 by Human Mononuclear Cells Exposed to B-Glactoside-Specific Lectin from Clinically Applied Mistletoe Extract," *Cancer Research,* 1990; 50:3322–3326.

". . . recommendation advises against self-administering." Leung A. Y., Foster, Y. *Encyclopedia of Common Natural Ingredients Used in Foods, Drugs and Cosmetics,* 2nd ed. (New York: John Wiley & Sons, 1996).

". . . natural properties include the following:" Lee, William, H., Friedrich, Joan, A. *Medicinal Benefits of Mushrooms* (New Canaan, Conn.: Keats Publishing, Good Health Guides 1997), p. 28.

". . . fungi polysaccharides are due to . . ." Ibid.

". . . carcinogenic unless neutralized through cooking." Shirota, Mike. "What You Should Know about Medicinal Mushrooms," *Explore!,* 1996; 7(2).

". . . referred to as beta 1,3-glucan, . . ." Ibid., pp. 30–31.

". . . Institute in Japan in 1969." Chihara, G., et al. "Fractionation and Purification of the Poly Saccharides with Marked Antitumor Activity, Especially Lentinan, from Lentinus Edodes (Berk.) Sin (an inedible mushroom)," *Cancer Research,* 30:2776–2781.

". . . benefits, and positive cardiovascular effects." Lee, William, H., Friedrich, Joan, A. *Medicinal Benefits of Mushrooms,* pp. 30–31.

". . . its ability to produce interferon." Freuhauf, Bonnard, Herberman. "The Effects of Lentinan on Production of Interleukin-1 by Human Monocytes," *Immunopharmacology,* 1982; 6:65–74.

". . . a part of combination therapy." Yance, Donald R., Jr., Valentine, Arlene. *Herbal Medicine, Healing & Cancer,* p. 156.

". . . in some cases preventing recurrence." Chang, Raymond, Y. *Role of Ganoderma Supplementation in Cancer Management,* Meridian Medical Group at the Institute of East-West Medicine and Department of Medicine, Cornell Medical College, 1996.

". . . syngeneic tumor systems in animals." Ibid.

". . . its supplemental use in cancer." Ibid.

". . . the final stages of cancer." Mizuno, T. *Antitumor Active Substances of Mushroom Fungi, Based Science and Latest Technology on Mushroom* (Tokyo: Nohson Bunka Sha, 1991), pp.121–135; and Mizuno, T. *Studies on Bioactive Substances and Medicinal Effects of Reishi, Ganoderma lucidum in Japan,* Shizuoka University.

". . . a wide variety of ways:" Lee, William, H., Friedrich, Joan, A. *Medicinal Benefits of Mushrooms,* p. 37.

". . . of up to six months." Hobbs, Christopher. *Herbal Adaptogens Fitting into the Modern Age.*

". . . recommend the following Reishi tea:" Lee, William, H., Friedrich, Joan, A. *Medicinal Benefits of Mushrooms,* p. 39.

". . . viral, fungal, and bacterial conditions." Yance, Donald R. Jr., Valentine, Arlene. *Herbal Medicine, Healing & Cancer,* p. 156.

". . . or liver function is impaired." Tsyukagoshi, S., et al. "Krestin (PSK)," *Cancer Treatment Review,* 1984; 11(2):131–155; reference in Yance, Donald R., Jr. Valentine, Arlene. *Herbal Medicine, Healing & Cancer,* p. 158.

". . . its healing potential becomes known." Takashi, M., Ahuang, C. "Maitake—Griffola Frondosa: Pharmacological Effects," *Food Reviews International,* 1995; 11(1):135–149, and Gray, S.F. "Grifola Frondose," *Medicinal Fungi Monographs,* p. 110, courtesy Maitake Products, Inc., Paramus, N.J.

". . . and small quantities of minerals." Ibid.

". . . provided increased immune protection by . . ." Hishida, I., Nanba, H. Kuroda, H. "Antitumor Activity Inhibited by Orally Administered Extract from Fruit Body of *Grifola frondosa* (Maitake)," *Chem Pharm Bulletin,* 1987; 5:1819–1827.

". . . the body's self-healing power." Nanba, H. "The Healing Properties of Hen of the Woods," *Healthy & Natural Journal,* 1995; 2(1):92–93.

". . . mushrooms discussed in this section." Chart model reference: Yance, Donald R., Jr., Valentine, Arlene. *Herbal Medicine, Healing & Cancer,* p. 159.

CHAPTER 9

". . . optimum dose for different nutrients." Challem, Jack. "The Past, Present and Future of Vitamins," *The Nutrition Reporter,* 1997.

". . . schizophrenics with vitamins C and B$_3$." Ibid.

". . . free radical theory of aging, . . ." Ibid.

". . . afford expensive preparations and formulas." Kushi, Michio. *The Seminars of Michio Kushi,* compiled by Jim Ledbetter (Boston: East West Publications, 1973).

". . . falling into the following categories . . ." Statistics obtained from Simone, Charles B., *Cancer & Nutrition* (Garden City, N.Y.: Avery Publishing Group), Chapter 6.

". . . the B group (vitamin B$_6$, . . ." Pao, E., Mickle, S. "Problem Nutrients in the United States," *Food Technology,* September 1981; and Nationwide Food Consumption Survey, *U.S. Dept. Agriculture* (Md.: Beltsville, Science & Education Admin., 1980).

". . . thiamine, folate, riboflavin, niacin) . . ." Dietary intake source data, United States, 1976–1980; and Kirsch, A., Bidlack, W. R. "Nutrition and the Elderly: Vitamin Status and Efficacy of Supplementation," *Nutrition,* 3:305–314.

". . . vitamin C, . . ." Schorah, C. J. "Inappropriate Vitamin C Reserves: Their Frequency and Significance in an Urban Population," *The Importance of Vitamins to Health,* Ed. T. G. Taylor (Lancaster, England: MTP Press, 1978), pp. 61–72.

". . . and vitamin D." Gary, P. J. Goodwin, J. S., Hunt, W. C. Hooper, E. M., Leonard, A. G. "Nutritional Status in a Healthy Elderly Population: Dietary and Supplemental Intakes," *American Journal of Clinical Nutrition,* 36:319–331.

". . . malnutrition can impair immune function." Bristrian, Bruce, et al. "Prevalence of Malnutrition in General Medical Patients," *JAMA,* April 12, 1976; 235(15); Lemoine, et al. "Vitamin B$_1$, B$_2$, B$_6$ and Status in Hospital Patients," *American Journal of Clinical Nutrition,* October 17, 1965; Driezen, S. "Nutrition and the Immune Response—Review," *International Journal of Vitamin Nutrition,* Res. 49, 1979; Beisel, et al. "Single-Nutrient Effects on Immunologic Functions," *JAMA,* Jan. 2, 1981; Pollack, S. V. "Nutritional Factors Affecting Wound Healing," *Journal of Dermatology Surgical Oncology,* 1979;5:8.

". . . percent lower than in nonsmokers." Pelletier, O. "Vitamin C and Cigarette Smokers—Second Conference on Vitamin C; *Ann NY Acad Sci,* 258:156–166; Hornig, D. H., Glatthaar, B. E. "Vitamin C and Smoking: Increased Requirement of Smokers," *Int J Vit Nutr Res Suppl,* 27:139–155; Menkes, M. S., Constock, G. W., Vuilleumier, J. P., Helsing, K. J. Rider, A. A., Brookmeyer, R. "Vitamin C Is Lower in Smokers," *NEJM,* 1986; 315:1250–1254.

". . . low levels in heavy smokers." Chow, C. K., Thacker, R. R., Changchit, C., Bridges, R. B., Rehm, S. R. Humble, J., Turbeck, J. "Lower Levels of Vitamin C and Carotenes in Plasma of Cigarette Smokers," *J Am Coll Nutr,* 5:305–312; Witter, F. R., Blake, D. A., Baumgardner, R., Mellitis, E. D., Niebyl, J. R., "Folate, Carotene and Smoking," *Am J Obstet Gynecol,* 144:857; Gerster, H. "Beta-Carotene and Smoking," *J Nutr Growth Cancer,* 1982; 4:45–49; Pacht, E. R., Kaseki, H., Mohammed, J. R., Cornwell, D. G., Davis, W. B. "Deficiency of Vitamin E in the Alveolar Fluid of Cigarette Smokers: Influence on Alveolar Marcrophage Cytotoxicity," *J Clin Invest,* 1986; 77:789–796; Serfontein, W. J., Ubbink, J. B., Devilliers, L. S., Becker, P. J. "Depressed Plasma Pyridoxal-5-Phasphate Levels in Tobacco-Smoking Men," *Atherosclerosis,* 59:341–346.

". . . are estimated to be alcoholic." Sheils, M. "Portrait of America," *Newsweek* (Special Report), Jan. 17, 1983.

". . . vitamin B$_{12}$, magnesium, and zinc." Pao, E., Mickle, S. "Problem Nutrients in the United States," *Food Technology,* September 1981; Leevy, C. M., Baker, H. "Vitamins and Alcoholism," *American Journal of Clinical Nutrition,* 1968; 21:11; Leiber, C. S. *Alcohol and Malnutrition in the Pathogenesis of Liver Disease and*

Nutrition, Veterans Administration Hospital and Dept. of Medicine, Mt. Sinai School of Medicine of the City University of New York, Bronx, N. Y., Sept. 1975); Lumeng, L., Li, T. K. "Vitamin B_6 Metabolism in Chronic Alcohol Abuse," *Journal of Clinical Investigation,* 1974; 53; Leevy, C. M., Baker, H., Ten Hove, W., Frank, O., Cherrick, G. R. "B Complex Vitamins in Liver Disease of the Alcoholic," *American Journal Clinical of Nutrition,* 1965; 16:4; Halsted, C. H., Heise, C. "Ethanol and Vitamin Metabolism," *Pharmac Ther,* 1987; 34:453–464; Aoki, K., Ito, Y., Sasake, R., Ohtani, M., Hamajima, N., Asano, A. "Smoking, Alcohol Drinking and Serum Carotenoids Levels," *Japan Journal of Cancer Research Gann,* 1987; 78:1049–1056; Fazio, V., Flint, D. M., Wahlqvist, M. L. "Acute Effects of Alcohol on Plasma Ascorbic Acid in Healthy Subjects," *Ameican Journal of Clinical Nutrition,* 1981; 34:2394–2396.

". . . C, folic acid, and beta-carotene." Roe, D. A. *Drug-Induced Nutritional Deficiencies* 2nd ed. Westport, Conn.: AVI Publishing Co., Inc., 1987); Brin, M. "Drugs and Environmental Chemicals in Relation to Vitamin Needs," in *Nutrition and Drug Interrelations,* eds. J. N. Hathcock and J. Coon (New York: Academic Press, 1987), vol. 87, pp. 813–821; Driskell, J. A., Geders, J. M., Urban, M. C. "Vitamin B_6 Status of Young Men, Women and Women Using Oral Contraceptives," *J Lab Clin Med,* 1976; 87:813–821; Prasad, A. S., Lei, K. Y., Oberleas, D., Moghissi, K. S., Stryker, J. C. "Effect of Oral Contraceptive Agents on Nutrients: II. Vitamins," *American Journal of Clinical Nutrition,* 1975; 28:385–391.

". . . those sensitive to other yeasts." Mangels, Reed. "Vitamin B_{12} in the Vegan Diet," *Simply Vegan: Quick Vegetarian Meals,* Wasserman, Debra, Mangels, Reed.

". . . other immune cells against tumors." Goldfarb, R. H., Herberman, R. B. "Natural Killer Cell Reactivity: Regulatory Interactions Among Phorbol Ester, Interferon, Cholera Toxin and Retinoic Acid," *J Immunol,* 1981; 126; 2129; Dennert, G. et al. "Retionic Acid Stimulation of Killer-T Cell Induction," *Euro J of Immuno,* 1978; 8:23; Dennert G., et al. "Retinoic Acid Stimulation of the Induction of Mouse Killer T-Cell in Allogeneic and Syngeneic Systems," *J Nat Cancer Instit,* 1979; 62:89.

". . . risks of developing colon cancer." *New England Journal of Medicine,* 1994; 331:141–147.

". . . from smoking and smog exposure." La Vecchia, C., et al. "Dietary Vitamin A and the Risk of Invasive Cervical Cancer," *International Journal of Cervical Cancer,* 1984; 34:3,319–322; Menkes, M. S., et al., "Serum Beta-Carotene, Vitamins A and Selenium and the Risk of Lung Cancer," *New England Journal of Medicine,* 1986; 315:1250.

". . . to fight cancer and infection, . . ." "The Effect of Vitamin E on Immune Responses," *Nutrition Reviews,* 1987; 45(1):27.

". . . of chemotherapy agents against tumors . . ." Prasad, K. N., et al. "Vitamin E Increases the Growth Inhibitory and Differentiating Effects of Tumor Therapeutic Agents on Neuroblastoma and Glioma Cells in Culture," *Proceedings of the Society for Experimental Biology and Medicine,* 1980; 164(2):158–163.

". . . protect against radiation treatment-toxicity." Myers, C. E., et al. "Effect of Tocopherol and Selenium on Defenses against Reactive Oxygen Species and Their Effect on Radiation Sensitivity," *Ann of the NY Acad Sci,* 1981; 393:429–425.

". . . seeds, pistachios, walnuts, and spinach." Bliznakov, Emile, Hunt, Gerald. *The Miracle Nutrient Coenzyme Q10* (New York: Bantam Publishing, 1987).

". . . after exposure to a carcinogen." Shamsuddin, A. M. "Inositol Hexaphosphate Inhibits Large Intestinal Cancer in F344 Rats 5 Months after Induction by Azoxymethane," *Carcinogenesis,* 1989; 10(3):635–626.

". . . taken up by malignant cells." Shamsuddin, A. M. "Inositol Phospates Have Novel Anticancer Function," *Journal of Nutrition,* 1995; 125:725S–732S.

". . . ability to destroy cancer cells." Panush, R. S., Delafuente, J. C. "Vitamins and Immunocompetence: Group B Vitamins—World Review," *Nutrition Digest,* 1985; 45:97–132; Posner, B. M., et al. "Nutrition in Neoplastic Disease," *Advances in Modern Human Nutrition and Dietetics,* 1980; 29:139–169.

". . . vitamin B_6 inhibit tumor growth." Ibid.

". . . development of chemically-induced tumors." Basu, T. K. "Significance of Vitamins in Cancer," *Oncology,* 1976; 33:183.

". . . the efficacy of cancer treatment." Diamond, J., Cowden, Lee W., Goldburg Burton. *Alternative Medicine Definitive Guide to Cancer (Future Medicine Publishing, 1997), p. 785.*

". . . for a healthy immune system." Cameron, E. T., et al. "Ascorbic Acid and Cancer: A Review," *Cancer Research,* 1979; 39:663–681.

". . . large amounts of vitamin C." Yonemoto, R. H. "Vitamin C and Immunological Response in Normal Controls and Cancer Patients," *Medico Dialoga,* 1979; 5:23–30.

". . . large doses of vitamin C, . . ." Park, C. H. Vitamin C in Leukemia and Preleukemia Cell Growth," *Nutrition, Growth and Cancer,* eds. Tryflates and Prassad (New York: Alan R. Liss, 1988), pp. 321–330.

". . . D has shown antitumor qualities." Good, R. A., et al. "Nutrition, Immunity and Cancer—A Review," *Clinical Bulletin,* 1979; 9:3–12, 63–75.

". . . suicide" (apoptosis) in cancer cells." Boik, J. "Conducting Research on Natural Agents: Vitamin D Metabolites," *Cancer and Natural Medicine* (Princeton, Minn.: Oregon Medical Press, 1995), p. 181.

". . . could offer prostate cancer protection." Martin, Wayne. "Anti-Cancer Effect of Vitamin D," *Townsend Newsletter for Doctors and Patients,* October, 1996, p. 111.

". . . enhancing its cancer-fighting potential, . . ." Rotruck, J. T., et al. "Selenium: Biochemical Role as a Component of Glutahione Peroxidase," *Science,* 1973, 588–590, referenced in *Alternative Medicine Definitive Guide to Cancer,* Diamond J., Cowden, Lee W., Goldburg, Burton.

". . . often deficient in cancer patients." Schrauzer, G. N. "Selenium for the Cancer Patient," *Adjuvant Nutrition in Cancer Treatment Symposium,* Tampa, Florida, Sept. 25, 1995 Schrauzer is based at the Biological Trace Element Research Institute in San Diego, California.

". . . whose tumors regressed following ovariectomy." Ip, C. "Prophylaxis of Mammary Neoplasaia by Selenium Supplementation in the Initiation and Promotion Phases of Carcinogenesis," *Cancer Research,* 1981; 41:4386–4393.

". . . offers protection against colon cancer." Alattery, M. L., Sorenon, A. W., Ford, M. H. "Dietary Calcium Intake as a Mitgating Factor in Colon Cancer," *Am J Epidm,* 1988; 128(3):504–514.

". . . synthesis of RNA and DNA, . . ." Blondell, J. M. "The Anticarcinogenic Effect of Magnesium," *Medical Hypothesis,* 1980; 6:8, 863–871.

". . . and repair of all tissues." Standel, V. W. "Dietary Iodine and the Risk of Breast, Endometrial and Ovarian Cancer," *The Lancet,* 1976; 1:7965, 890–891.

". . . and for enhanced immune function." Prudden, J. "Use of Cartilage in Cancer Treatment," Lecture at the 1995 Adjuvant Nutrition for Cancer Treatment Symposium, Tampa, Florida, (Sept. 30, 1995.) Cited in *Alternative Medicine Definitive Guide to Cancer,* Diamond, J., Cowden, Lee W., Goldburg, Burton, p. 756.

". . . acids can inhibit breast cancer." Wynder, E. I., et al. "Diet and Breast Cancer in Causation and Therapy, Cancer, *1986; 58:8 suppl., 1804–1831.*

". . . in animals receiving corn oil." Fritsche, K. L., Johnston, P. V. "Effect of Dietary Alpha-Linolenic Acid on Growth, Metastasis, Fatty Acid Profile, and Prostaglandin Production of Two Murine Mammary Adenocarcinomas," *Journal of Nutrition,* 1990; 120, 1601–1609. Cited in *Alternative Medicine Definitive Guide to Cancer,* Diamond, J., Cowden, Lee W., Goldburg, Burton, p. 769.

". . . survival times in laboratory animals." Kidd, P. "Germanium-132: Homeostatic Normalizer and Immunostimulant: A Review of its Preventive and Therapeutic Efficacy," *Internat Clin Nutr Rev,* 1987; 7:1, 11–20.

". . . researcher Keiichi Morishita, M.D., suggests . . ." Morishita, Keiichi. *Overcoming Cancer: The Natural Medicine Diet Therapy* (Los Angeles: Living Naturally Learning Center, 1998), translated from Shogan Sakusen (1995) Gan Wa Korede Naoseru, Korede Fusegeru (1980) by Sinichi Kishi, Los Angeles.

". . . and spread of cancer cells." Referenced from Gaynor, Mitchell L., M.D., Hickey, Jerry, R.Ph., *Dr. Gaynor's Cancer Prevention Program,* New York; Kensington Books, 2000, pg. 291.

". . . I and II breast cancer." *The Doctor's Prescription for Health Living,* vol. 4, no. 10, pg. 12.

". . . stem from high-dose supplements." *Vitamin and Nutritional Supplements,* "Medical Essay," Supplement to *Mayo Clinic Health Lettter,* June 1997.

"Here are some miscellaneous facts . . ." Cited in *Position of the American Dietetic Association: Vitamin and Mineral Supplementation,* Janet R. Hunt, October 1995.

". . . iron and other trace elements." Food and Nutrition Board. *Recommended Dietary Allowances,* 10th ed. (Washington, D.C.: National Academy Press, 1989).

". . . result in irreversible neuroligic damage." Ibid.

". . . high-density lipoprotein cholesterol levels." Ibid.

". . . effect of coumadin anticoagulant drugs." Bendich, A., Machlin, L. J. "Safety of Oral Intake of Vitamin E," *American Journal of Clinical Nutrition,* 1988; 48:612–619.

". . . bone problems, and liver damage." HealthNotes.com (1998).

". . . with cranial neural crest defects." Rothman, K. J., Morre, L. L., Singer, M. R., Nguyen, U. D. T., Mannino, S., Milunsky, A. "Teratogenicity of High Vitamin A Intake," *New England Journal of Medicine,* 1995; 333:1369–1373.

". . . deaths in the United States." U.S. Preventive Services Task Force. "Routine Iron Supplementation during Pregnancy; Policy Statement and Review Article," *JAMA,* 1993; 270:2846–2848.

". . . carcinomas, is still highly debatable." Moss, Ralph. *Questioning Chemotherapy* (Brooklyn, N.Y.: Erquinox Press, 1995), pp.163–164.

"Most of the following suggestions . . ." Referenced from HealthNotes, Inc., *www.healthnotes.com,* 1125 SE Madison, Suite 209, Portland, Oregon, 92714.

". . . and vomiting caused by chemotherapy." de Blasio F., et al. "N-Acetyl Cysteine (NAC) in Preventing Nausea and Vomiting Induced by Chemotherapy in Patients Suffering from Inoperable No Small Cell Lung Cancer (NSCLC)," *Chest,* 1996; 110(4 Suppl):103S.

". . . according to double-bind research, . . ." Wadleigh, R. G., Redman, R. S., Graham, M. L., et al. "Vitamin E in the Treatment of Chemotherapy-Induced Mucositis," *American Journal of Medicine,* 1992; 92:481–484.

". . . increase the effectiveness of chemotherapy." Nakagawa, M., Hamaguchi, T., Ueda, H., et al. "Potentiation by Vitamin A of the Action of Anticancer Agents against Nurine Tumors," *Japan Journal of Cancer Research,* 1985; 76:887–894; Prasad, K. N., Edwards-Prasad, J., Ramanujam, S., et al. "Vitamin E Increases the Growth Inhibitory and Differentiating Effects of Tumor Therapeutic Agents in Neuroblastoma and Glioma Cells in Culture," *Proc Soc Ex Biol Med,* 1980; 164: 158–163; Taper, H. S., de Gerlache, J., et al. "Non-Toxic Potentiation of Cancer Chemotherapy by Combined C and K3 Vitamin Pre-Treatment," *International Journal of Cancer,* 1987; 40:575–579.

". . . Livingston in the journal *Oncology*." Labriola D., Livingston, R., M.D., Possible interactions between dietary antioxidants and chemotherapy. *Oncology* 1999; 13:1003-11.

". . . in his, *Antioxidants Against Cancer.*" Moss, Ralph W., Ph.D., *Antioxidants Against Cancer,* New York; Equinox Press, 2000, pg. 20–21.

". . . increased free radical damage to fats." Ladner, C., et al. Effect of etoposide (VP16-213) on lipid peroxidation and antioxidant status in a high-dose radiochemotherapy regimen. *Cancer Chemotherapy Pharmacology*, 1989; 25(3):210-2.

". . . (alpha-tocopherol) levels by 20 percent . . ." Clemens MR, et al. Plasma vitamin E and beta-carotene concentrations during radiochemotherapy preceding bone marrow transplantation. *American Journal of Clinical Nutrition*, 1990 Feb; 51(2):216-9.

". . . recommendations of 90 to 120 milligrams." Folkers, K., Wolanjuk, A. "Research on Coenzyme Q10 in Clinical Medicine and in Immunomodulation," *Drugs Exptl Clin Res,* 1985; 11:539–545.

". . . to give enough heart protection . . ." Fujita, K., Shinpo, K., Yamada, K., et al. "Reduction of Adriamycin Toxicity by Ascorbate in Mice and Guinea Pigs," *Cancer Research,* 1982; 42:309–316.

". . . from damage when taking adriamycin." Ogura, R., Humon, Y., Young, R. "Adriamycin Amelioration of Toxicity by Alpha-Tocopherol," *Cancer Treat Rep,* 1976; 60:961–962.

". . . to 1600 IU per day." Wood, L. A. "Possible Prevention of Adriamycin-Induced Alopecia by Tocopherol," *New England Journal of Medicine,* 1985; 312:1060 (letter).

". . . leads to depletion of magnesium." Buckley, J. E., Clark, V. L., Meyer, T. J., Pearlman, N. W. "Hypomagnesemia after Cisplatin Combination Chemotherapy," *Arch Intern Med,* 1984; 144:2347–2348.

". . . administered intravenously by a physician." Cascinus, S., Cordella, L., Del ferro, E., et al. "Neuroprotective Effect of Reduced Glutathione on Cioplatin Based

Chemotherapy in Advanced Gastric Cancer: A Randomized Double-Bind Placebo-Controlled Trial, *J Clin Oncol,* 1995; 13:26–32; Smythe, J. F., Bowman, A., Perren, T., et al. "Glutathione Reduces the Toxicity and Improves Quality of Life of Women Diagnosed with Ovarian Cancer Treated with Cisplatin: Results of a Double-Bind, Randomized Trial," *Ann Oncol,* 1997; 8:569–573.

". . . B₆ can eliminate this pain." Vukelja, S. J., Lombardo, F., James W. D., Weiss, R. B. "Pyroxidine [sic] for the Palmar-Plantar Erythrodysesthesia Syndrome," *Ann Intern Med,* 1989; 111:688–689 (letter); Molina, R., Gabian, C., Slavik, M., Dahlberg, S. "Reversal of Palmar-Plantar Erythrodysesthesia (PPE) by B₆ Without Loss of Response in Colon Cancer Patients Receiving 200/mg/m2/Day Continuous 5FU, *Proc Am Soc Clin Oncol,* 1987; 6:90 (abstract).

". . . is a sample supplement recommendation . . ." Referenced from Gaynor, Mitchell L., M.D., Hickey, Jerry, R. Ph.D., *Dr. Gaynor's Cancer Prevention Program,* New York: Kensington Books, 2000, pg. 195.

". . . *Herbal Medicine, Healing & Cancer,* . . ." Yance, Donald R., Jr., Valentine, Arlene. *Herbal Medicine, Healing & Cancer* (Lincolnwood, Ill.: Keats Publishing, 1999), pp. 120–159.

CHAPTER 10

"In Will Durant's historical books, . . ." Durant, Will. *Our Oriental Heritage,* (1954); *The Life of Greece,* (1939); and *Caesar and Christ,* (1957) (New York: Simon & Schuster).

"Natural breakfast cereals . . ." If the familiar fast breakfast cereals are desired, it is best to use them on a transition diet with the addition of diluted (water) soy milk and a small amount of fruit. Although there might be emotional comfort in this familiar kind of breakfast, it is not an energizing or whole breakfast.

". . . vegetables may trigger arthritic symptoms . . ." Childers, Norman Franklin. *Arthritis: Childer's Diet to Stop It!* Somerville, N.J. Somerset Press, 1986).

"Vegetarian burgers" Free of persevatives, coloring, MSG, and artificial flavorings.

"Nori . . ." Nori is frequently used to wrap around rice in sushi preparations.

"Kombu . . ." Kombu is generally used in soup and bean stocks for its rich mineral content. I often refer to it as *oriental bay leaf.*

"Dulse . . ." A popular Eastern Canadian sea vegetable, dulse is often used as a dried flaked condiment.

"Wakame . . ." Wakame is generally used in soups and resembles cooked spinach.

"Organic Seeds/Nuts . . ." Seeds and nuts should be minimally processed, free of sugar, sugar substitutes, preservatives, and hydrogenated oils. Added sea salt can add enhance flavor, prolong shelf life, and aid digestion. Organic quality is essential since pesticide residues are held within fatty acids.

"Fermented Foods/Pickles . . ." Pickles should be made with naturally dried sea salt and eaten in very small quantities (or avoided for salt-sensitive or restricted individuals) with a meal to aid digestion. Only a small amount (several slivers) is necessary.

CHAPTER 11

" Methods of Cooking . . ." Reference: Wood, Rebecca. *Be Nourished; The Complete Guide and Cookbook Celebrating Whole Foods,* 1995, Naturally Grand Cooking School, PO Box 40408, Grand Junction, Colo. 81504.

". . . range or in the microwave?" Ibid.

". . . to macrobiotic teacher Michio Kushi, . . ." Kushi, Michio. The Seminars of Michio Kushi, Seminar Reports, 1971–1973, East West Foundation, Boston, Mass.

"According to the *Lancet, . . ." Lancet,* December 9, 1989.

". . . researcher/author John Ott suggests . . ." Ott, John. *Light, Radiation & You ; How to Stay Healthy* (Devin-Adair Pub., 1985).

". . . *Journal of the American Dietetic Association . . ." Journal of the American Dietetic Association, May 1989.*

"Another study . . ." *Lipids,* 1988; 23:367–369.

". . . books, offers the following comments . . ." Quoted from *Ask Dr. Weil @ www.about.com* April 18, 1997.

". . . with a slightly salty seasoning." Matesz, Rachel Albert, Matesz Don. *The Nourishment for Life Cookbook* (Seattle, Wash.: Nourishment for Life Press, 1994).

" Cookbook author . . ." Kushi, Aveline. *Aveline Kushi's Complete Guide to Macrobiotic Cooking* (New York: Warner Books, 1985).

". . . more PAHs than leaner cuts." Lefferts, Lisa. "Great Grilling," *Nutrition in Action Newsletter,* CSIP, Classic Series Archives.

". . . National Laboratory in Livermore, California." Schardt, David, Corcoran, Leila. *Beat the Heat,* Safe Cooking, www.about.com.

". . . convenient referencing, the following chart . . ." Chart inspired by Baum, Lenore, *Lenore's Natural Cuisine* (Farmington Hills, Mich.: Culinary Publications, 1999).

". . . scallions and sometimes, brine pickles." Original reference: Matesz Rachel Albert , Matesz, Don. *The Nourishment for Life Cookbook* (Seattle, Wash.: Nourishment for Life Press, 1994).

". . . can bind steroids and carcinogens." Sparandeo, James J. "Foods and Tumor Growth Inhibition," Chapter 4, "Immune System Enhancement Diet," Comprehensive Nutritional News, Easton, Pa., 1991.

". . . to be discharged by elimination." Matesz, Rachel Albert, Matesz Don. *The Nourishment for Life Cookbook.*

". . . lower incidence of breast cancer." Cohen, Thompson Teas. *Seaweed Blocks the Mammary Tumor Promoting Effects of High Fat Diets,* International Breast Cancer Research Conference, Denver, Colorado, March 1983, Abstract 53, Wilmington, Del.: Stuart Pharmecueticals, 1983.

". . . against other forms of cancer." Yamamoto, et al. "Antitumor Activity of Edible Marine Algae: Effect of Crude Fucoidan Freactions Prepared from Edible Brown Seaweeds Against L-12100 Leukemia, *Hydrobiologia,* 1984; 116/117:145–148.

". . . lung cancer in laboratory animals." Furusawa, et al. "Anticancer Activity of a Natural Product viva Natural, Extracted from Undaria Pinnantifida on Intraperitoneally Implanted Lewis Lung Carcinoma," *Oncology,* 1985; 42:364–369.

"... because they selectively bind strontium." Tanaka, Y. "Studies on Inhibition of Intestinal Absorption of Radioactive Strontium," *Ca Med Assoc J,* 1986, 99:169.

"... some cases, complete tumor regression." Teas, Jan, et al. "Dietary Seaweed and Mammary Carcinogenesis in Rats," *Cancer Research,* 1984, 44:2758.

"... *Salt & the Human Condition, ...*" Tisdale, Sallie. *Lot's Wife—Salt & the Human Condition (New York: Henry Holt & Co., 1988).*

"... "free flowing" in humid conditions." Table salt reference: *Salt—Walking the Briny Line* (Boston: Talking Food Company, 1976).

"... "When it rains, it pours" ..." Slogan © Morton International, Inc., Morton Salt Company, Chicago, Illinois.

"... Langre offered the following observation ..." Interview with D. Jacques De Langre, *The Newsletter of Advanced Natural Therapies* (1992).

CHAPTER 12

"... Zealand cookbook author Cheryl Beere, ..." Beere, Cheryl, Reynolds, Patrick. *The Atomic Café Cookbook* (Auckland, New Zealand: Goodwit Publishing, 1995).

"... authors Mary Estella and Lenore Baum." Estella, Mary. *Natural Foods Cookbook* (New York: Japan Publications, 1988); Baum, Lenore. *Lenore's Natural Cuisine* (Farmington Hills, Mich.: Culinary Publications, 1999).

"... and cookbook author Christina Pirello's ..." Pirello, Christina. *Cooking the Whole Foods Way* (New York: HP Books, 1997).

"... award-winning author Rebecca Wood, ..." Wood, Rebecca. *The Splendid Grain* (New York: William Morrow & Co., 1997), p. 158.

"... this one from Lenore Baum ..." Baum, Lenore. *Lenore's Natural Cuisine.*

"Author Aveline Kushi ..." This recipe appears in *Aveline Kushi's Complete Guide to Marcobiotic Cooking* (New York: Warner Books, 1985), with Alex Jack.

"... author and writer Cheryl Beere." Beer, Cheryl, Reynolds, Patrick. *The Atomic Café Cookbook.*

"Creamy Cauliflower Soup" Thanks to Anna MacKenzie, courtesy of *Kushi Summer Conference,* 1997, Poultney, Vermont.

"Roasted Root Vegetables" Thanks to Arisha Wemhoff for this recipe.

"Peach Mousse" Thanks to cook and author Melanie Waxman for this delicious treat.

"Almond Drop Cookie" Thanks to chef and master baker Robert Pezdirt of Omaha, Nebraska.

"... soup, inspired by Jody Main, ..." Spiller, G., Hubbard, R. *Nutrition Secrets of the Ancients* (Rocklin, Calif.: Prima Publishing, 1996), p. 56, by Jody Main.

"Apple Glaze" Thanks to Christina Pirello, *Cooking the Whole Foods Way,* p. 491.

"Halibut with Lemon & Capers" A variation from an original Christina Pirello recipe.

AFTERWORD

"... West Foundation in Oriental Medicine ..." This is now known as the Kushi Institute and headquartered in Becket, MA.

INDEX

A

N-acetyl cysteine (NAC), 194
Acid/alkaline balance, 59-84
    alkaline water, 79-80
    antacids, 72
    caffeine, 74-78
        coffee, decaffeinated, 75
        methylxanthines, 76
    and cancer cell growth, 83-84
    carbohydrate digestion, 68-69
    carbonic acid, 63, 71
    as cause of cravings, 112
    concept, 59-60
    confusion about, 69-70
        titration, 69-70
    controls, four, 62-63
    demystifying, 66-68
    electrolytes, 74
    excess acidity, effects of, 81-84
    extracellular fluids, 63-64
    fatigue, 81
    homeostasis, 60
    Hunza's of northern Pakistan, 79
    indigestion, 72
    ionizing water, 79-80
    kidney stones, 82
    lactic acid, 62
    minerals, loss of, 71-73
        N-P-K fertilizer, 73-74
        osteoporosis, 73
    Peyer's patches, 81
    pH scale, 61-62, 64
    potency, 64-65
    stress, effects of, 78-79
    sugar and acid production, 70-71
    terrain medicine, 65
    Umeboshi plum, 72, 77
Adaptogens, 154-155

Adriamycin, 196
Aerobic/anaerobic bacteria, 141
Agaritin, 165
Aihara, Herman and Cornelia, 312
Akizuki, Dr. Shinichiro, 144
Alcohol, 11
Alcohol consumers, supplements for, 183
Alka-Seltzer®, 77
Alkaline/acid balance, 59-84 (*see also*
        Acid/alkaline balance)
Alkaline water, 79-80
Allergy response as cause of cravings,
        117-119
Alternative health movement, growth of,
        3-4
Alternatives to familiar foods, 219
American Herbal Products Association, 163
American Institute, 91
American Medical Association (AMA), 148
Amino acids, 39
Ammonia, excess of from high-protein
        diets, 40-41
Animal fats, 11
Animal protein categories, 215-216
American Cancer Society, xxi, 34, 91
Antacids, 72
Anthroposophy, 161
Antibiotics, 164
Antioxidants, 43-58
    and cancer, 58
    for cancer protection, 185-188, 195
    vs. free radicals, 43-45
    phytochemicals, 44-53
        burdock, 53
        cancer preventive research, 50-52
        phenolic group, 46,48
        sources, 47
        supplements, 56-58
    sources, 45-46

Antioxidants (*cont'd.*)
vegetables, 44-46
"veggie-phobia," prescription for, 55-56
Antioxidants against Cancer, 195
Aoyagi, Akiko, 146
Apoptosis, 189
Arame, 252
Astragalus, 198
Atkins, Dr. Robert, 80
Atropine, 148

B

Baking, 236
Balance, 4
Beans, categories of, 214
Benzopyrene, 90
Bernard, Dr. Neal, xviii
Beta 1,3-glucan 167
Beta-carotene, 44-45, 185-186 (*see also*
Antioxidants)
Beta-lactoglobulin, 95
Beverages, categories of, 218-219
Bile acids, 12
Blanching, 235
Blood quality, strengthening, xxiii-xxiv
Blood sugar, 25-29
imbalance as cause of cravings, 112-113
regulating, xxiv
Boiling, 235
The Book of Miso, 146
Bovine growth hormone (BGH), 89
Bovine leukemia, 88-89
Breakfast, 240-246
menus and recipes, 263-273
Breast cancer, dairy-eating patterns and, 95
British Journal of Cancer, 37
Broadhurst, C. Leigh, 153
Broiling, 236
Burdock, 53
Burkitt, Dr. Dennis, 21

C

Caffeine, 74, 78
Caisse, Rene, 158-160
Calcium, 189
deficiencies, 105
Campbell, Prof. I. Colin, 9
Cancer:
and carbohydrates, 31-32
detection vs. prevention, 7-8

Cancer: (*cont'd.*)
and diet, 8-10 (*see also* Eating habits)
and fats, 37-38
Cancer Institute: *see also* National
Cancer Institute
Cannibalism, 107
Capsules, supplement, 177-178 (*see also*
Supplement)
Caragheenan, 250
Carbohydrate digestion, 68-69
Carbohydrates, 13-32
as fuel for body, 13-14
grains, whole, 14-32
avoidance, reasons for, 18-19
fiber, 21-24 (*see also* Fiber)
glycemic index, 15, 27-29
phytates, 22-23
products, popular, 20-21
reasons for eating, five, 17-18
what they are, 16
sugars, 13-32
and cancer, 31-32
insulin, 27-29, 31-32
simple, 23-26
Carbonic acid, 63, 71
Carcinogens, xxii
CCK PZ, 111
Cell mutations, prevention of by medicinal
herbs, 155-156
Cereal, 208
Chelation, 251
Chemotherapy toxicity, minimizing, 193-200
antioxidants, 185-188, 195
herbal support, 198-200
questioning effectiveness of, 193
recommendations, 194-196
supplement protocol, 196-198
Chewing, 135, 222
China Project (CP), 9-10, 33-34
Chitin, 164-165
Chylomicrons, 36
Cisplatin, 196
"Cloud Fungus," 171
Coenzyme Q10, 186, 194-195
Coffee, 74-78
decaffeinated, 75
Colon, protecting, 12
Comfort foods, 116-117, 132
dangers in, xix
Compulsive overeating, 114-116
Cooking for health benefits, 227-261 (*see
also* Food preparation)
cookware, 260

Cooking for health benefits (*cont'd.*)
  methods, 231-237
Cookware, 260
CoQ10, 186, 194-195
Cramer, Dr. Daniel, 93
Cravings for what body needs, 105-121
  cannibalism, 107
  categories, 8, 107
  causes, 108-121
    acid/alkaline balance, 112
    allergy response, 117-119
    blood sugar, 112-113
    elimination/detoxification, 119-120
    emotional, 114-116
    expansion/contraction, 120-121
    genetics, 116-117
    nutritional, 108-111
  endocannibalism, 107
  for fat, six ways to defeat, 129-132
  geophagia, 106
  how to handle, 121
  pica, 106
  for salt, 105
  substitutions, 123-125
  sugar, ten strategies to eliminate, 126-128

D

Dairy foods, 11, 85-101 (*see also* Meat and
    dairy foods)
  categories of, 216
Dandelion, 153
Death cap mushroom, 153
DeCosse, Dr. Jerome, 12
Deficiencies for vegetarians, 98
DeLangre, Jacques, 256
Deoxycholic acid, 90
Detection of cancer, 7-8
Detoxification:
  ability, strengthening, xxiv
  as cause of cravings, 119-120
  by medicinal herbs, 152-154
Dietary change, xix
Digitalis, 148
Dinner menus and recipes, 287-301
Dulse, 252
Durant, Will, 206

E

Eating habits, cancer prevention and, 1-12
  alternative health movement, growth
    of, 3-4

Eating habits, cancer prevention and
    (*cont'd.*)
  cancer: detection vs. prevention, 7-8
  colon, protecting, 12
  and diet, 8-10
    China Project (CP), 9-10
    free radicals, 8
    heterocyclic amines, 11-12
    phytoestrogens, 10
    studies, confirming, 11-12
  metastasis, 8
  pleasure foods, 6-7
  shifts, seven major, 1-3
  staple foods, 4-6
  supportive foods, 6
  vegetables, three categories of, 6
Elderly, supplements for, 182
Electrical cooking, 232
Electrolytes, 74
Eleuthero, 198
Elimination/detoxification as cause of
    cravings, 119-120
Emotional causes of cravings, 114-116
Endocannibalism, 107
Environmental causes of cancer, 8
Essiac, 158-160
Estradiol, 37
Estrogens, 10, 37, 95
Etoposide, 150
Excipients, 187
Exercise to manage acid-producing stress,
    78-79
Expansion/contraction as cause of crav-
    ings, 120-121
Extracellular fluid, 63-64

F

Familial factor, 117
Fat cravings, six ways to defeat, 128-132
Fatigue as sign of excess acidity, 81
Fats, 32-38
  and cancer risks, 37-38
  chylomicrons, 36
  as comfort foods, 132
  fatty acids, 34-35
  fish oils, 35
  monounsaturated, 35
  and oxygen, 35-37
  rouleaux formation, 36
  saturated, 34
  sticky blood cell syndrome, 36
Felton, James, 237
Fermented foods, 217

Fiber, 21-24
  phytates, 22-23
  roughage, 24
Fish oils, 35
Flax, 52
Fleming, Sir Alexander, 164
Flurouracil, 196
Food inhalation, 135
Food plan for natural cancer-fighting,
    201-225
  alternatives, 219
  animal protein, 215-216
  assessing dietary plan, 202-205
  beans, 214
  beverages, 218-219
  change, making, two theories about,
      224-225
  chewing, art of, 222
  dairy, 216
  fermented foods, 217
  fruits, 216-217
  grains, whole, 206-209, 211-212
    categories, 211-212
    cereal, 208
    history, 206-209
  individualized needs, 201-202
  organic oils, 218
  pickles, 217
  Prevention/Therapeutic Plan, 206,
      221-224
  sea vegetables, 214-215
  seeds/nuts, organic, 215
  sweeteners, natural, 217
  Therapeutic Plan, 206, 221-224
  Transition Plan, 205, 220-221
  vegetables, 212-214
  water, 209-211
Food preparation and cooking for health,
    227-261
  breakfast, 240-246
  cooking methods, 231-237
    electrical, 232
    gas, 231-232
    microwave, 232, 233
    wood, 231
  cooking styles, 232-237
    baking, 236
    blanching, 235
    boiling, 235
    broiling, 236
    grilling, 237
    kombu, use of, 234-235
    marinating, 236
    pot cooking, 234

Food preparation and cooking for health
    (cont'd.)
    pressing, 236
    pressure cooking, 234
    raw, 235
    sauté, 235
    soups, 234-235
    steaming, 234
  gas, avoiding, 258-261 (see also Salt)
  grains, 246-248 (see also Grains)
  ingredient amounts, 248-249
  salt, rethinking, 252-258
  sea vegetables, 249-252 (see also Sea
      vegetables)
  shopping hints, 229
  substitutions, 249
  tastes, five savory, 238-240
    food categories, 239
  variety, 230-231
Food quality, cancer prevention and, 1-12
    (see also Eating habits)
Foods That Fight Pain, xviii
Fred Hutchinson Cancer Research
    Center, 50
Free radicals, xvi, 8
  and aging theory, 180-182
  and antioxidants, 43-58 (see also
      Antioxidants)
Friedrich, Joan A., 171
Fruit:
  alkaline-forming, 67
  categories of, 216-217
  not staple food, 6
Fu Zhen therapy, 148-149
Fundamentals of Therapy, 162
Fun, Casimir, 179-180

G

Galactose, 93-94
Gas cooking, 231-232
Gas factor, avoiding, 258-261
Genetics as cause of cravings, 116-117
Gentian, 157
Geophagia, 106
Germanium, 169, 190-191
Ginseng, 198
Glossary for recipe products, 302-305
Glucone, 13
Glutathione S-transferase (GST), 52
Glycemic index, 15, 27-29
Glycemic Research Institute, 27
Glycogen, 14, 29-30

Gobo, 53
Grains, 14-32, 98-100, 206-209, 211-212, 246-248
  avoidance, reasons for, 18-19
  categories, 211-212
  cereal, 208
  chewing thoroughly, 99
  cooking times, 246
  fiber, 21-24 (*see also* Fiber)
  glycemic index, 15, 27-29
  history, 206-209
  phytates, 22-23
  products, popular, 20-21
  reasons for eating, 5, 17-18
  and vegetable combinations, 247-248
  what they are, 16
Green tea as nutrient supplement, 191
Grilling, 237

H

Harman, Dr. Denham, 180
HCAs, 11-12, 237
HDPs, 164, 165
Health strategies, four, xxiii-xxiv
Herbs, medicinal, 147-176
  as basis for modern drugs, 198
  and cancer prevention, 151-158
    adaptogens, 154-155
    antioxidant protection, 157
    calming, 157-158
    cell mutations, preventing, 155-156
    detoxification, 152-154
    digestion and elimination, 156-157
    immune response, 154-155
    inflamed tissues, soothing, 156
    liver cleansing, 153-154
    mucositis, 156
    nervines, 157-158
    sedative, 157-158
    supportive lifestyle and diet critical, 151-152
  and drug companies, 150
  Essiac, 158-160
  etoposide, 150
  Fu Zhen therapy, 148-149
  Hoxsey s formula, 160-161
  Iscador, 161-163
  mistletoe, 161-163
  mushrooms, 163-176 (*see also* Mushrooms)
  standardizing, 149-151

Herbs, medicinal (*cont'd.*)
  taxol, 150
  vinca alkaloids, 150
Heredity in predisposition to cravings, 116-117
Heterocyclic amines (HCAs), 11-12, 237
High protein diets, supplements for, 183
Hiziki, 251-252
Hobbs, Christopher, 170
Hoffer, Dr. Abram, 180
Homeostasis, 60, 104-105
Hopkins, Frederick, 178-180
Host defenses potentiators (HDPs), 164, 165
Hoxsey, Harry, 160-161
Hyperinsulinism, 112
Hunza s of northern Pakistan, 79
Hypoglycemia, 113

I

Immunity, strengthening, xxiv
Inositol (IP6), 186-188
Insulin, 27-29, 31-32
Insulin-like growth factor (IGF), 94
Interferon, 168
Intracellular fluid, 66
Inulin, 53
Iodine, 190, 254
Ionizing water, 79-80
Iscador, 161-163

J

Journal of American Medical Association, 94
Journal of Nutrition, 141
The Jungle, 88
"Junk-dessert schizophrenia," 122-123
Junshi, Dr. Chen, 9

K

Kelp, 234-235, 250, 251
Kidney stones, 82
Klenner, Dr. Frederick R., 180
Knize, Mark, 237
Koji, 141
Kombu, 234-235, 250, 251
Kristal, Dr. Alan, 50
Kushi, Aveline, 236, 312
Kushi, Michio, 110, 181, 232, 312

L

Labriola, Dan, 195
Lactic acid, 62
Lambe, William, 87
Lee, William H., 171
Lentinan, 167-168, 172
Leroi, Dr. Rita, 162
Leucovorin, 194
Lind, James, 179
Liquids, need for, 209-211
Liver cleansing by medicinal herbs,
    153-154
Livingston, Robert, 195
*Lot's Wife —Salt and the Human
    Condition*, 253
Lunch menus and recipes, 274-286
Lung cancer, dairy-eating patterns and, 95

M

Macrobiotics, 311-312
Magnesium, 189-190
Maitake mushrooms, 172-176
    anti-HIV activity, 175-176
    D-fraction, 172, 174-175, 176
    "dancing mushroom," 172, 173
    health benefits, 175
    history, 173
    and immunity, 174
    tastiest of mushrooms, 176
Marinating, 236
Meat:
    not staple food, 6
Meat and dairy foods, 85-101
    body design and function, 95-97
    dairy food consumption, 92-95
        beta-lactoglobulin, 95
        and breast cancer, 95
        insulin-like growth factor (IGF), 94
        and ovarian cancer, 93-94
        and prostate cancer, 94
    history, 87-88
    meat cravings, reducing with oil, 98
    meat-eating and cancer research,
        89-92
        benzopyrene, 90
        deoxycholic acid, 90
        in endometrial cancer, 90
    quality of meat, 88-89
        bovine growth hormone (BGH), 89
        bovine leukemia, 88-89

Meat and dairy foods (*cont'd.*)
    statistics, 85-87
    vegetarian option, 97-100
        deficiencies, 98
        grains, 99-100
        sodium, need for, 97
Medication users, supplements for, 184
The Metabolism of Tumors, 83-84
Metastasis, 8
Methotrexsate, 194
Methylxanthines, 76
Microflora, 140-141
Micronutrients, 184
Microwave:
    cooking, 232
    warnings, 233
Milk, 11, 92-93
Milk thistle, 153
Miller, Dr. Edgar K., 45
Mindell, Earle, 187
Minerals, loss of, 71-73
Miso soup, 137-146
    aerobic/anaerobic bacteria, 141
    amino acids, 139
    cancer fighting role, 144-145
    for digestion and assimilation, 141-144
    heavy metals, bonding to, 144
    molds, 140-141
    salt content, 143
    using, 145-146
    vegetable quality protein, 139
Mistletoe, 161-163
Molds, 140-141
    use of to fight infections, 163-176 (*see
        also* Mushrooms)
Monounsaturated fats, 35
Morishita, Dr. Keiichi, 191
Moss, Ralph, 193, 195
Mucositis, 156, 194
Mushrooms, 163-176
    agaritin, 165
    antibiotics, 164
    chitin, 164-165
    chlorophyll, absence of, 166
    host defenses potentiators (HDPs), 164,
        165
    Maitake, 172-176 (*see also* Maitake)
    penicillin, 164
    probiotic, 164
    PSK, 171-172 (*see also* PSK)
    Reishi, 168-171 (*see also* Reishi)
    Shiitake, 166-168 (*see also* Shiitake)
Mycelium, 168

N

NAC (*N*-acetyl cysteine), 194
Nature, 191
N-P-K fertilizer, 73-74
National Academy of Sciences, xxi, 149
National Cancer Institute, xxi, 8, 11-12, 24, 50, 83-84, 190, 237
National Department of Health and Human Services, xxi
National Research Council, 41
Natural killer (NK) cells, xvi
Nervines, 157-158
The New England Journal of Medicine, 91
The New York Times, 87
Nishime, 235
Non-Hodgkin's lymphoma, dairy-eating patterns and, 95
Nori, 250
Notes on the Causation of Cancer, 87
Nursing women, supplements for, 183
Nutrition, role of in fighting cancer, xvi-xix
  medical schools, lack of training in, xvii-xviii
  preventive power, xvii
  redemptive powers, xvii
Nutritional cravings, 108-111 (*see also* Cravings)
Nuts, organic, categories of, 215

O

Oats, 208
Oil-sautéing, 235, 249
Omega-3 fatty acids, 190
Oral contraceptive users, supplements for, 184
Organic oils, 218
Organocholorine chemicals, 88
Osteoporosis, 73
Ovarian cancer, dairy-eating patterns and, 93-94
Overeating:
  compulsive, 114-116
  reasons for, six, 133-135
Oxygen, fatty diet and, 35-37

P

Pagophagia, 110
PAHs (polycyclic aromatic hydrocarbons), 237

Pauling, Dr. Linus, 180
Peyer s patches, 81
pH scale, 61-62, 64
Phenolic group of phytochemicals, 46, 48, 50-52
Phytates, 22-23
Phytochemicals/nutrients, xxii, 44-53 (*see also* Antioxidants)
Phytoestrogens, 10
Pica, 106
Pickles, 217
Pills supplement, 177-178 (*see also* Supplement)
Pirquet, C.E., 117
Pleasure foods, 6-7
Polycyclic aromatic hydrocarbons (PAHs), 237
Pot cooking, 234
Potassium, 256
Potions supplement, 177-178 (*see also* Supplement)
Pregnant women, supplements for, 183
Pressing salad, 236
Pressure cooking, 234
Prevention/Therapeutic Plan, 206, 221-224
  Swing Percentage, 221
Prolactin, 41-42
Prostaglandins, 111
Prostate, 10
  cancer, dairy-eating patterns and, 94
Proteins, 38-42
  amino acids, 39
  ammonia, excess of, 40-41
  critical to life, 39
  myths about, 38-39
  poisoning from, 40-42
PSK mushrooms, 171-172
  "Cloud Fungus," 171
  documented results as advantage, 172
  health benefits, 175
  and immunity, 174
  and lentinan, 172
  number one selling anticancer agent in world, 171
  "Turkey Tail," 171
Psychological stresses, acid-forming effects of, 78-79

Q

Questioning Chemotherapy, 193
Quinones, 186

R

Raw foods, 235
Recipe product glossary, 302-305
Regan, Dr. Timothy, 36
Reishi mushrooms, 168-171
   benefits, 170
   germanium, 169
   health benefits, 175
   in highest class of tonics, 168-169
   and immunity, 174
   mycelium, 168
   recipe, 170-171
   triterpenoids, 169, 170
Resource guide, 325-334
Restaurant tips, 306-309
Roughage, 24
Rouleaux formation, 36
Russell, Rolo, 87

S

Salitos, 258
Salt, rethinking, 252-258
   controversy, 252-253
   how much is too much, 257
   need for, 253-254
   sea salt vs. table salt, 255
   sodium and potassium, 256
   table salt, danger in, 254
   Umeboshi salt plums, 256-258
Salt cravings, 105
Saturated fats, 34-35
Sauté, 235
Schrauzer, Gerhard, 189
Scientific American, 87
Scurvy, 179
Sea salt vs. table salt, 255
Sea vegetables, 249-252
   arame, 252
   and cancer prevention, 251
   categories of, 214-215
   dulse, 252
   hiziki, 251-252
   kombu, 250, 251
   nori, 250
   wakame, 251
Sedative herbs, 157-158
Seeds/nuts, organic, categories of, 215
Selenium, 189
Sex hormones, 10

Shamsuddin, Dr. A.M., 188
Shiitake mushrooms, 166-168
   vs. cholesterol, 167
   health benefits, 175
   and immunity, 174
   interferon, 168
   lentinan, 167-168, 172
Shintani, Dr. Terry, 92
Shoyu, 137-146 (*see also* Miso)
Shurtleff, William, 146
Shute, Dr. Evan, 180
Simon, David, 149,156
Sinclair, Upton, 88
Smokers, supplements for, 183
Smoking, xix
Snowden, Dr. John, 94
Snyderwine, Elizabeth, 237
Soup that heals, 137-146 (*see also* Miso)
Soups, 234-235
Soy sauce, 137
Soybeans, 52, 137-146 (*see also* Miso)
Standardizing, 149-151
Staple foods, 4-6
Steaming, 234
Steel-cut oats, 245
Steiner, Rudolph, 161
Sticky blood cell syndrome, 36
Stir fry, 235
Strategies for eliminating sugar, fat, and
      overeating, 103-135
   chewing, 135
   craving for what body needs, 105-121
      (*see also* Cravings)
   fat, six strategies to defeat, 129-132
   food inhalation, 135
   homeostasis, 104-105
   "junk-dessert schizophrenia," 122-123
   overeating, six reasons for, 133-135
   sugar cravings, ten strategies to elimi-
      nate, 126-128
   will power, role of, 103-104
Stress, acid-forming effects of, 78-79
Substitutions for familiar foods, 219
Sugar cravings, ten strategies to elimi-
      nate, 126-128
Sugars, 13-32 (*see also* Carbohydrates)
   and acid production, 70-71
   diseases from excess, 30-31
   glycemic index, 15, 27-29
   glycogen, 29-30
   simple, 23-26
   what happens in body, 29

Supplements for health support, 56-58, 177-200
  cancer-protection supplement plan, 185-193
    antioxidants, 185-188
    nutrients, 188-191
  capsules, pills and potions, 177-178
  caution, 191-193
  chemotherapy toxicity, minimizing, 193-200 (*see also* Chemotherapy)
    antioxidants, 185-188, 195
    supplement protocol, 196-198
  dependence on, avoiding, 181
  free radical theory of aging, 180-182
  medical acceptance, 177-178
  micronutrients, 184
  natural vs. artificial, 187
    excipients, 187
  vitamins, 178-182
    balanced diet debate, 181
  who can benefit from, 182-185
Supportive foods, 6
Sweeteners, natural, categories of, 217
Sweets cravings, 112-113
Szent-Gyorgyi, Dr. Albert, 180

T

Tamari, 137-146 (*see also* Miso)
Tastes, five savory, 238-240
  food categories, 239
Taxol, 150
Taylor, Dr. Lawrence, 186
Terrain medicine, 65
Testosterone, 10
Therapeutic Plan, 206, 221-224
Tisdale, Sallie, 253
Titration, 69-70
Toniolo, Paulo, 37-38
Toxicity discharge, whole grain and, 18
Transition Plan, 205, 220-221
Traveling tips, 306-309
"Turkey Tail," 171

U

Ubiquinone, 186
Ullah, Dr. A., 188
Umeboshi plum, 72, 77, 256-258
Urokinase, 191

V

Variety as natural spice, 230-231
Vegetables:
  categories of, 212-214
  and grain combinations, 247-248
  raw vs. cooked, 56
  recommendations, 57
  as source of phytochemicals, 44-46
  supplements, 56-58
  three categories of, 6
  "veggie-phobia," five-step prescription for, 53-56
Vegetarian diets, 37-38
  acid-forming, 69
  deficiencies, 98
  as option, 97-100
  pitfalls, 3, 100
  sodium, need for, 97
  supplements for, 185
Vinca alkaloid drugs, 150
Visek, Willard J., 40-41
Vitamins, 178-182, 184
  A, 194
  B complex, 188
  B_2, 195
  B_6, 196
  balanced diet debate, 181
  C, 188-189, 194, 195
  caution, 191-193
  D, 189
  E, 186, 194
  excesses, dangers in, 191-193
  micronutrients, 184

W

Wakame, 251
Warburg, Dr. Otto, 83-84
Water, 209-211
"Water-fry" cooking, 249
Wegman, Dr. Ita, 161-162
Weight gain, 27-29
Weight loss regimes, supplements for, 183
Weil, Dr. Andrew, 233
Will power, role of, 103-104
Williams, Roger, 180-181
Wolever, Dr. Tomas, 27-28
Wood, Rebecca, 231, 279
Wood cooking, 231
World Cancer Research Fund, xxi
World Health Organization (WHO), 22-23

Y

Yance, Donald R., 155
Yeasts, 140-141
Yogurt, 142

Z

Zinc, 190